T0227238

Pelvic Floor Disorders

Editor

DARREN M. BRENNER

GASTROENTEROLOGY CLINICS OF NORTH AMERICA

www.gastro.theclinics.com

Consulting Editor
ALAN L. BUCHMAN

March 2022 • Volume 51 • Number 1

ELSEVIER

1600 John F. Kennedy Boulevard • Suite 1800 • Philadelphia, Pennsylvania, 19103-2899
http://www.theclinics.com

GASTROENTEROLOGY CLINICS OF NORTH AMERICA Volume 51, Number 1
March 2022 ISSN 0889-8553, ISBN-13: 978-0-323-81343-3

Editor: Kerry Holland
Developmental Editor: Hannah Almira Lopez

© **2022 Elsevier Inc. All rights reserved.**

This periodical and the individual contributions contained in it are protected under copyright by Elsevier, and the following terms and conditions apply to their use:

Photocopying

Single photocopies of single articles may be made for personal use as allowed by national copyright laws. Permission of the Publisher and payment of a fee is required for all other photocopying, including multiple or systematic copying, copying for advertising or promotional purposes, resale, and all forms of document delivery. Special rates are available for educational institutions that wish to make photocopies for non-profit educational classroom use. For information on how to seek permission visit www.elsevier.com/permissions or call: (+44) 1865 843830 (UK)/ (+1) 215 239 3804 (USA).

Derivative Works

Subscribers may reproduce tables of contents or prepare lists of articles including abstracts for internal circulation within their institutions. Permission of the Publisher is required for resale or distribution outside the institution. Permission of the Publisher is required for all other derivative works, including compilations and translations (please consult www.elsevier.com/permissions).

Electronic Storage or Usage

Permission of the Publisher is required to store or use electronically any material contained in this periodical, including any article or part of an article (please consult www.elsevier.com/permissions). Except as outlined above, no part of this publication may be reproduced, stored in a retrieval system or transmitted in any form or by any means, electronic, mechanical, photocopying, recording or otherwise, without prior written permission of the Publisher.

Notice

No responsibility is assumed by the Publisher for any injury and/or damage to persons or property as a matter of products liability, negligence or otherwise, or from any use or operation of any methods, products, instructions or ideas contained in the material herein. Because of rapid advances in the medical sciences, in particular, independent verification of diagnoses and drug dosages should be made. Although all advertising material is expected to conform to ethical (medical) standards, inclusion in this publication does not constitute a guarantee or endorsement of the quality or value of such product or of the claims made of it by its manufacturer.

Gastroenterology Clinics of North America (ISSN 0889-8553) is published quarterly by Elsevier Inc., 360 Park Avenue South, New York, NY 10010-1710. Months of issue are March, June, September, and December. Business and Editorial Offices: 1600 John F. Kennedy Blvd., Suite 1800, Philadelphia, PA 19103-2899. Customer Service Office: 6277 Sea Harbor Drive, Orlando, FL 32887-4800. Periodicals postage paid at New York, NY and additional mailing offices. Subscription prices are $368.00 per year (US individuals), $100.00 per year (US students), $973.00 per year (US institutions), $395.00 per year (Canadian individuals), $100.00 per year (Canadian students), $1002.00 per year (Canadian institutions), $468.00 per year (international individuals), $220.00 per year (international students), and $1002.00 per year (international institutions). Foreign air speed delivery is included in all *Clinics* subscription prices. All prices are subject to change without notice. **POSTMASTER**: Send address changes to *Gastroenterology Clinics of North America*, Elsevier Health Sciences Division, Subscription Customer Service, 3251 Riverport Lane, Maryland Heights, MO 63043. **Telephone: 1-800-654-2452 (U.S. and Canada); 314-447-8871 (outside U.S. and Canada). Fax: 314-447-8029. E-mail: journalscustomerservice-usa@elsevier.com (for print support); journalsonlinesupport-usa@elsevier.com (for online support).**

Reprints. For copies of 100 or more, of articles in this publication, please contact the Commercial Reprints Department, Elsevier Inc., 360 Part Avenue South, New York, New York 10010-1710. Tel. 212-633-3874, Fax: 212-633-3820, E-mail: reprints@elsevier.com.

Gastroenterology Clinics of North America is also published in Italian by Il Pensiero Scientifico Editore, Rome, Italy; and in Portuguese by Interlivros Edicoes Ltda., Rua Commandante Coelho 1085, 21250 Cordovil, Rio de Janeiro, Brazil.

Gastroenterology Clinics of North America is covered in *MEDLINE/PubMed (Index Medicus), Excerpta Medica, Current Contents/Clinical Medicine, Science Citation Index, ISI/BIOMED,* and *BIOSIS.*

Contributors

CONSULTING EDITOR

ALAN L. BUCHMAN, MD, MSPH, FACP, FACN, FACG, AGAF
Professor of Clinical Surgery (Gastroenterology), Medical Director, Intestinal Rehabilitation and Transplant Center, University of Illinois Chicago/UI Health, Chicago, Illinois, USA

EDITOR

DARREN M. BRENNER, MD, FACG, AGAF, RFF
Associate Professor of Medicine and Surgery, Irene D. Pritzker Foundation Research Scholar, Director, Northwestern Neurogastromotility and Interdisciplinary Bowel Dysfunction Programs, Director, Motts Tonelli GI Physiology Laboratory, Northwestern University Feinberg School of Medicine, Department of Medicine, Division of Gastroenterology/Hepatology, Northwestern University, Chicago, Illinois, USA

AUTHORS

MARY A. ATIA, MD
Consultant, Arizona Digestive Health

ADIL E. BHARUCHA, MBBS, MD
Professor of Medicine, Division of Gastroenterology and Hepatology, Mayo Clinic, Rochester, Minnesota, USA

DARREN M. BRENNER, MD, FACG, AGAF, RFF
Associate Professor of Medicine and Surgery, Irene D. Pritzker Foundation Research Scholar, Director, Northwestern Neurogastromotility and Interdisciplinary Bowel Dysfunction Programs, Director, Motts Tonelli GI Physiology Laboratory, Northwestern University Feinberg School of Medicine, Department of Medicine, Division of Gastroenterology/Hepatology, Northwestern University, Chicago, Illinois, USA

BROOKS D. CASH, MD, AGAF, FACG, FACP, FASGE
Dan and Lillie Sterling Professor of Medicine, Division of Gastroenterology, Hepatology and Nutrition, The University of Texas Health Science Center at Houston, Houston, Texas, USA

WILLIAM D. CHEY, MD
Professor of Medicine, Division of Gastroenterology and Hepatology, Department of Internal Medicine, Michigan Medicine Health System, Ann Arbor, Michigan, USA

SARAH COLLINS, MD
Associate Professor, Department of Obstetrics and Gynecology, Division of Female Pelvic Medicine and Reconstructive Surgery, Northwestern University Feinberg School of Medicine, Chicago, Illinois, USA

ENRIQUE COSS-ADAME, MD
Department of Gastroenterology, Instituto Nacional de Ciencias Médicas y Nutrición "Salvador Zubirán", México City, México

BETHANY DOERFLER, MS, RDN
Senior Clinical Research Dietitian, Division of Gastroenterology and Hepatology, Northwestern University Feinberg School of Medicine, Chicago, Illinois, USA

TANMAY GAGLANI, MD
Department of Internal Medicine, The University of Texas Health Science Center at Houston, Houston, Texas, USA

SEIFELDIN HAKIM, MD
Division of Gastroenterology, Hepatology and Nutrition, The University of Texas Health Science Center at Houston, Houston, Texas, USA

LUCINDA A. HARRIS, MS, MD
Associate Professor of Medicine, Division of Gastroenterology and Hepatology, Alix School of Medicine, Mayo Clinic, Scottsdale, Arizona, USA

ANAM HEREKAR, MD
Division of Gastroenterology/Hepatology, Medical College of Georgia, Augusta University, Augusta, Georgia, USA

ELIZABETH F. HOOVER, DO
Resident Physician, Department of Obstetrics and Gynecology, University of Virginia, Charlottesville, Virginia, USA

SUAKA KAGBO-KUE, MD
Fellow, Division of Gastroenterology and Hepatology, Mayo Clinic, Scottsdale, Arizona, USA

TENNEKOON KARUNARATNE, MD, PhD
Division of Gastroenterology/Hepatology, Medical College of Georgia, Augusta University, Augusta, Georgia, USA

CHRISTINA LEWICKY-GAUPP, MD
Associate Professor, Department of Obstetrics and Gynecology, Division of Female Pelvic Medicine and Reconstructive Surgery, Northwestern University Feinberg School of Medicine, Chicago, Illinois, USA

JOY J. LIU, MD
Fellow, Department of Medicine, Division of Gastroenterology/Hepatology, Northwestern University, Chicago, Illinois, USA

TISHA N. LUNSFORD, MD
Assistant Professor of Medicine, Division of Gastroenterology and Hepatology, Alix School of Medicine, Mayo Clinic, Scottsdale, Arizona, USA

STACY MENEES, MD, MS
Associate Professor of Medicine, Division of Gastroenterology, Michigan Medicine Health System, Veterans Affairs Ann Arbor Healthcare System, Ann Arbor, Michigan, USA

STACEY A. MISSMER, ScD
Professor, Department of Obstetrics, Gynecology, and Reproductive Biology, College of Human Medicine, Michigan State University, Grand Rapids, Michigan, USA; Adjunct

Professor, Department of Epidemiology, Harvard T.H. Chan School of Public Health, Boston, Massachusetts, USA

RAVINDER K. MITTAL, MD
Professor of Medicine, Department of Medicine/Gastroenterology, University of California, San Diego, La Jolla, California, USA

SARAH QUINTON, PsyD
Director, Q Wellness

SATISH S.C. RAO, MD, PhD
Division of Gastroenterology/Hepatology, Medical College of Georgia, Augusta University, Augusta, Georgia, USA

GREGORY S. SAYUK, MD, MPH
Professor of Medicine and Psychiatry, Division of Gastroenterology, Department of Psychiatry, Washington University School of Medicine, St. Louis Veterans Affairs Medical Center, St Louis, Missouri, USA

AMOL SHARMA, MD, MS, FACG
Associate Professor of Medicine, Division of Gastroenterology/Hepatology, Medical College of Georgia, Augusta University, Augusta, Georgia, USA

SUKHBIR S. SINGH, MD, FRCSC
Professor, Department of Obstetrics and Gynecology, The Ottawa Hospital, University of Ottawa, Women's Health Center, Ottawa, Ontario, Canada

ELISA R. TROWBRIDGE, MD, FACOG
Associate Professor, Department of Obstetrics and Gynecology/Urology, University of Virginia, Division Director, Female Pelvic Medicine and Reconstructive Surgery, Charlottesville, Virginia, USA

FRANK F. TU, MD, MPH
Clinical Professor, Department of Obstetrics and Gynecology, NorthShore University HealthSystem, Pritzker School of Medicine at the University of Chicago, Evanston, Illinois, USA

LORI J. TUTTLE, PT, PhD
Professor of Physical Therapy, Department of Medicine/Gastroenterology, University of California, San Diego, Doctor of Physical Therapy Program, San Diego State University, San Diego, California, USA

YUN YAN, MD, PhD
Division of Gastroenterology/Hepatology, Medical College of Georgia, Augusta University, Augusta, Georgia, USA

Contents

> Anatomy of pelvic floor muscles has long been controversial. Novel imaging modalities, such as three-dimensional transperineal ultrasound imaging, MRI, and diffusion tensor imaging, have revealed unique myoarchitecture of the external anal sphincter and puborectalis muscle. High-resolution anal manometry, high-definition anal manometry, and functional luminal imaging probe are important new tools to assess anal sphincter and puborectalis muscle function. Increased understanding of the structure and function of anal sphincter complex/pelvic floor muscle has improved the ability to diagnose patients with pelvic floor disorders. New therapeutic modalities to treat anal/fecal incontinence and other pelvic floor disorders will emerge in the near future.

> Disorders of defecation, including constipation and fecal incontinence, are very common. The digital rectal examination (DRE) is a key component in the early evaluation of patients with these complaints. Confident performance of a DRE requires dedicated training for the clinician and hands-on experience with the technique. DRE can yield a diagnostic accuracy comparable to specialized physiologic tests, including anorectal manometry. This review will describe in detail the steps required to perform a thorough DRE evaluation, as well as the proper interpretation of observations. Thereafter, the current evidence-based findings supporting the value of DRE in defecatory disorders will be summarized.

> This article reviews the indications, techniques, interpretation, strengths, and weaknesses of tests (anal manometry, anal surface electromyography, rectal balloon expulsion test, barium and MRI defecography, assessment of rectal compliance and sensation, and colonic transit) that are used diagnose defecatory disorders in constipated patients. The

selection of tests and the sequence in which they are performed should be individualized to and interpreted in the context of the clinical features. Because anorectal functions are affected by age, results should be interpreted with reference to age- and sex-matched normal values for the same technique.

Constipated patients are frequently referred to gastroenterologists for symptoms refractory to lifestyle modifications and laxatives. Dyssynergic defecation, the dyscoordination of rectoanal, abdominal, and pelvic floor muscles to facilitate defecation, is a major cause of refractory primary constipation. Understanding of the diagnosis, evaluation, and management of dyssynergic defecation and other evacuation disorders will allow providers to effectively manage these patients. This review focuses on the definition, pathophysiology, evaluation, and treatment of dyssynergic defecation and other evacuation disorders. Emerging treatments for these disorders include home biofeedback therapy for dyssynergic defecation and translumbosacral neuromodulation therapy for levator ani syndrome.

Fecal incontinence (FI) is defined as the involuntary loss or passage of solid or liquid stool in patients. FI is a common and debilitating condition in men and women. The incidence increases with age and also often goes unreported to health care providers. It is crucial that providers ask at-risk patients about possible symptoms. Evaluation and management is tailored to specific symptoms and characteristics of the incontinence. If conservative methods fail to improve symptoms, then other surgical options are considered, such as sacral nerve stimulation and anal sphincter augmentation. This review provides an update on current and future therapies.

Spinal cord injury and neurogenic bowel dysfunction (NBD) are life-changing events for affected patients. The clinical manifestations of NBD vary depending on the level and severity of the spinal cord lesion. Managing patients with NBD can be complicated by comorbidities, such as immobility, bladder dysfunction, progressive neurologic decline, psychological factors, loss of independence, and social withdrawal, and ideally involves a multimodal, multidisciplinary approach. Evaluation and management should be individualized, depending on the residual neurologic capabilities of the patient and their predominant gastrointestinal symptoms, and commonly involves lifestyle modifications, physical therapy, laxative medications, and surgical interventions.

Opioid-related constipation encompasses constipation directly caused by opioid use (opioid-induced constipation [OIC]) as well as pre-existing constipation worsened by opioid use (opioid-exacerbated constipation [OEC]). Over-the-counter laxatives should be used as first-line agents for both OIC and OEC, given their efficacy, low cost, and high safety profiles. Symptoms of OIC and responses to therapy can be assessed with the Bowel Function Index. Individuals with OIC refractory to laxatives may be responsive to peripherally acting μ-opioid receptor antagonists. Although data supporting the superiority of one prescription agent over another is lacking, all have proven effective for the treatment of OIC.

Painful and bothersome anorectal syndromes can be a diagnostic and therapeutic challenge for clinicians because structural and functional abnormalities may often coexist and require a multidisciplinary approach to management. Although it is often difficult to attribute all of a patient's anorectal symptoms to a singular disorder with definitive intervention and cure, improving quality of life, treating coexistent conditions such as functional constipation and/or defecation disorders, addressing psychological comorbidities if present, and confirming there is no evidence of inflammatory or malignant conditions are top priorities.

This article discusses the role of psychological and nutritional factors in gastrointestinal pelvic floor disorders such as dyssynergic defecation and explores the use of multidisciplinary strategies to enhance treatment.

This review focuses on the diagnosis, evaluation, and treatment of urinary incontinence (UI). UI is a common diagnosis that is encountered among women in their lifetime. Stress, urge (overactive bladder), and overflow are the most commonly encountered types of incontinence, but anatomic and neurologic causes are important to rule out. There are many treatment options available for the management of UI, and most patients will benefit from conservative strategies including weight loss, timed voiding, fluid intake reduction, pelvic floor strengthening exercises, and medications. For those who do not achieve adequate improvement with conservative measures, surgical intervention can provide good symptom relief.

Pelvic organ prolapse (POP) is defined as the descent of one or more of the anterior and posterior vaginal walls, uterus (cervix), or apex of the vagina (vaginal vault or cuff scar after hysterectomy). Although POP can be asymptomatic, if the bulge extends beyond the opening of the vagina, it can have a significant impact on a woman's quality of life. Findings include vaginal bulging toward or through the vaginal introitus that the patient may feel, palpate, or see with a mirror. If a woman is bothered by her prolapse, she should be offered both nonsurgical and surgical treatments.

Endometriosis, affecting 5-10% of reproductive-age women, is a common contributor to dysmenorrhea and chronic pelvic pain. Diagnosis requires laparoscopic tissue biopsy, but careful pelvic examination, and/or imaging with either ultrasound or MRI, may identify patients who should receive empiric first-line therapy. The presence of dyschezia, particularly with cyclical exacerbation, should raise suspicion for bowel or rectovaginal septum involvement, and a greater need for surgical management. Treatment of dysmenorrhea includes hormonal suppression of the menstrual cycle, and/or analgesics; more severe cases with strong pain and disability may require earlier surgical intervention to excise disease while preserving fertility desires.

GASTROENTEROLOGY
CLINICS OF NORTH AMERICA

SERIES OF RELATED INTEREST

Gastrointestinal Endoscopy Clinics of North America
(Available at: https://www.giendo.theclinics.com)
Clinics in Liver Disease
(Available at: https://www.liver.theclinics.com)

THE CLINICS ARE AVAILABLE ONLINE!
Access your subscription at:
www.theclinics.com

Foreword

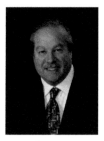

Alan L. Buchman, MD, MSPH
Consulting Editor

The pelvic floor includes essentially all ligaments, muscles, and nerves that are connected to and interact with the pelvic floor organs, rectum, bladder, uterus, and vagina. When the support of these organs weakens, the organs themselves are affected. Both men and women may experience problems in this realm.

Dr Brenner has assembled a group of talented clinicians who are experts in the assessment and treatment of pelvic and rectal pain and various anorectal disorders, urinary and/or fecal incontinence, leakage, and straining. Although seemingly benign, these disruptive symptoms have a significant effect on quality of life.

This group of authors provides a functional basis for the understanding of these pelvic disorders, their identification through functional diagnostic techniques, and potential treatment strategies that cover nutrition, medical, surgical, and behavioral/psychological approaches.

Indeed, this issue of *Gastroenterology Clinics of North America* should be viewed as a primer to educate clinicians in the nuances of these frequently overlooked disorders, just as Dr Brenner has described.

Alan L. Buchman, MD, MSPH
Intestinal Rehabilitation and Transplant Center
Department of Surgery/UI Health
University of Illinois at Chicago
840 South Wood Street
Suite 402 (MC958)
Chicago, IL 60612, USA

E-mail address:
a.buchman@hotmail.com

Gastroenterol Clin N Am 51 (2022) xiii
https://doi.org/10.1016/j.gtc.2021.12.002
0889-8553/22/© 2021 Published by Elsevier Inc.

gastro.theclinics.com

Preface

The Pelvic Floor: Complex Interplay Between Gastrointestinal and Urogenital Structures and Function

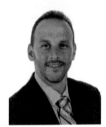

Darren M. Brenner, MD, FACG, AGAF, RFF
Editor

Pelvic floor disorders are common and defined as a group of conditions affecting the neurologic and muscular structures of the pelvis. While many gastroenterologists consider this synonymous with constipation and/or fecal incontinence, the reality is that these disorders cover a spectrum inclusive of but not limited to the bowel, bladder, uterus, and vagina. That said, individuals seeking care from gastroenterologists will predominately present with chief complaints of constipation and/or fecal incontinence, and in most circumstances, when initial therapies focused on modifying stool frequency and texture have failed, more advanced diagnostic and therapeutic assessments occur at academic institutions.

Given the anatomy and physiology of the pelvic floor, there is significant overlap between gastrointestinal conditions and disorders of the urogential/urogynecologic systems. These include urinary incontinence, pelvic organ prolapse, and chronic pelvic pain syndromes. Unfortunately, gastroenterologists receive little to no formal didactic or hands-on training focused on pathophysiology, diagnostic, and treatment strategies for these maladies. Consequently, these conditions may remain undiagnosed and unaddressed, limiting the therapeutic impact of gastrointestinal intervention.

Accordingly, the initiative of this issue of *Gastroenterology Clinics of North America* is to serve as a primer highlighting the underlying pathophysiology, diagnosis, and treatment of gastrointestinal as well as nongastrointestinal pelvic floor disorders across a spectrum of subspecialties. From the gastrointestinal perspective, this issue provides an in-depth, up-to-date, evidence-based overview of the anatomy and physiology of the pelvic floor, highlights key features of an appropriate digital rectal

Gastroenterol Clin N Am 51 (2022) xv–xvi
https://doi.org/10.1016/j.gtc.2021.12.001
0889-8553/22/© 2021 Published by Elsevier Inc.

gastro.theclinics.com

examination, and focuses on current assessments and treatments for multiple gastro-intestinal pelvic floor illnesses, including functional defecation disorders, fecal incontinence, neurogenic and opioid-related bowel dysfunction, rectal pain, and common perianal complaints. We also highlight the importance of dietary interventions and the impact that psychiatric conditions and trauma has on these issues, focusing on the role of behavioral therapy for these conditions. While the predominant focus remains on gastrointestinal illnesses, articles on urinary incontinence, pelvic organ prolapse, and endometriosis have been provided by expert urogynecologists from across the country. A better understanding of the associations between gastrointestinal and urogenital illnesses should improve patient outcomes.

Darren M. Brenner, MD, FACG, AGAF, RFF
Northwestern University—
Feinberg School of Medicine
676 North Saint Clair Avenue
Suite 1400
Chicago, IL 60611, USA

E-mail address:
darren-brenner@northwestern.edu

Anorectal Anatomy and Function

Ravinder K. Mittal, MD[a],*, Lori J. Tuttle, PT, PhD[b,c]

KEYWORDS

- External anal sphincter • Morphology • Pelvic floor • Anal incontinence
- Fecal continence

KEY POINTS

- Novel imaging techniques, such as 3D ultrasound and diffusion tensor MRI, have revealed the unique myoarchitecture of the external anal sphincter and puborectalis muscle, which is relevant from the point of view of understanding their precise function and preventing obstetric/surgical damage to these muscles.
- Studies show that the external anal sphincter and puborectalis muscle operate at the short sarcomere length, which has important implications for designing novel surgical approaches to treat anal incontinence.
- High-resolution manometry, high-definition manometry, and functional luminal imaging probe are important new modalities to assess the strength of the anal sphincter. However, 3D ultrasound imaging and diffusion tensor imaging can assess the integrity of anal sphincter muscles with much greater certainty than the traditional imaging modalities.

INTRODUCTION

Fecal incontinence (FI) is defined as the recurrent uncontrolled passage of fecal material for at least 3 months or more. Anal incontinence, however, includes difficulty in controlling passage of fecal material and gas. A recent study[1] investigated FI symptoms using a mobile app "MyGiHealth" and found that 14% (one in seven) of the people reported FI symptoms in the past, and 33% in the past 7 days. FI is age-related and more prevalent among individuals with inflammatory bowel disease, celiac disease, irritable bowel syndrome, and diabetes. The cause of FI is multifactorial; stool consistency, rectal reservoir function, and anal sphincter function play important roles.[2,3] However, consensus is that the anal sphincter function is the most important player in the development of FI symptoms.[4,5] Recent studies that used a novel functional

[a] Department of Medicine/Gastroenterology, University of California, San Diego, ACTRI, 9500 Gilman Drive, MC 0061, La Jolla, CA 92093-0990, USA; [b] Department of Medicine/Gastroenterology, University of California, San Diego, USA; [c] San Diego State University, San Diego, CA, USA
* Corresponding author.
E-mail address: rmittal@ucsd.edu

Gastroenterol Clin N Am 51 (2022) 1–23
https://doi.org/10.1016/j.gtc.2021.10.001
0889-8553/22/© 2021 Elsevier Inc. All rights reserved.

gastro.theclinics.com

luminal imaging probe (FLIP) to assess anal sphincter function found that in most subjects referred to the tertiary care centers, anal canal distensibility is higher in patients with FI as compared with control subjects.[6,7] Even though the prevalence of FI is reported to be the same in men and women, severe FI symptoms are more often observed in women as compared with men. One of the reasons for this is most likely related to the susceptibility of women to the anal sphincter and pelvic floor muscles during vaginal childbirth. Some 20% to 35% of women develop damage to the external anal sphincter (EAS) and puborectalis muscle (PRM) during vaginal childbirth.[8,9] A review of literature reveals that 80% of patients in the clinical trials for the treatment of FI are women.[10–12] Why there is a delay of two to three decades or more between the timing of obstetric trauma (childbearing years of 20s and 30s) and development of symptoms later in life is not known. The previously mentioned observations suggest that the anal sphincter or anal closure mechanism is the major continence mechanism. However, FI symptoms can clearly occur in women who have never given vaginal birth, albeit infrequently, reminding care providers that factors other than the anal sphincter complex muscles must be relevant to the genesis of FI. Advances in imaging (ultrasound [US] and MRI), and function measurement tools have improved our understanding of the anal sphincter complex. The focus of this review is to provide the reader with up-to-date information on the anal sphincter complex and pelvic floor anatomy and function. Three distinct anatomic structures, the internal anal sphincter (IAS), EAS, and PRM, the last one being a part of the pelvic floor or levator ani muscle, contribute to the anal closure/sphincter mechanism.

INTERNAL ANAL SPHINCTER

The circular muscle layer of the rectum extends caudally into the anal canal to become the IAS (**Fig. 1**). The circular muscles in the sphincter region are thicker than those of the rectum with discrete septa in between the muscle bundles.[13,14] The longitudinal

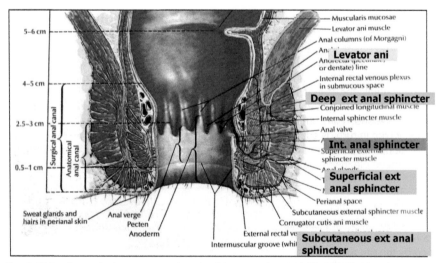

Fig. 1. This schematic shows external anal sphincter to be made up of subcutaneous, superficial, and deep parts. The deep external anal sphincter is actually the puborectalis muscle. (*Modified from* Netter F. Atlas of Human Anatomy. In: Kelly P, ed. 3rd edition ed. Teteboro, New Jersey: Icon Learning system 2003:Plates 361 & 364; with permission)

muscles of the rectum extend into the anal canal and end up as thin septa that penetrate into the circular muscle layer of IAS, PRM, EAS, and perianal fat.[15] The longitudinal muscle of the anal canal is also known as the conjoined tendon (muscle) because the skeletal muscles of the pelvic floor may also contribute to its formation. However, the longitudinal muscle of the rectum is the major contributor to the longitudinal muscles of anal canal. The intersphincteric plane between the longitudinal muscle and EAS is important to surgeons; it is used to separate the anal canal from EAS and adjacent structures during abdominoperineal resection for rectal cancer. The function of the longitudinal muscle in anal sphincter function and dysfunction is not known.[14] The IAS is a major contributor to the resting or baseline anal sphincter/closure pressure, contributing greater than 50% to 70% of resting pressure as measured using manometry. The IAS tone is myogenic in origin, a unique property of the IAS smooth muscle cells, as compared with the adjacent muscle of the rectum. Isolated muscle strips of the IAS in a muscle-bath, devoid of endocrine and neural influences, can maintain tonic contraction.[16] Studies show that the source of calcium, crucial for muscle contraction, is extracellular in the phasic (eg, rectal muscle) but intracellular in the tonic muscle of the IAS.[17] There is a difference in the intracellular messenger RhoA/ROCK pathway in the phasic (rectal) versus tonic (IAS) muscles.[18] The critical intracellular step in contraction of the smooth muscle is phosphorylation of the myosin light chain through a kinase (MLCK). The MLCK is dephosphorylated by myosin light chain phosphatase (MLCP), which results in muscle relaxation. The critical difference between phasic and tonic muscle is that the RhoA/ROCK machinery is more active in a tonic muscle, such as the IAS. The activation of RhoA/ROCK by intracellular calcium (also known as calcium sensitization) leads to inhibition of MLCP resulting in sustained elevation of phosphorylated MLC, which induces sustained tonic contraction. The known extracellular signals that activate RhoA/ROCK are the products of renin-angiotensin system (angiotensin II) and arachidonic acid pathway (thromboxane A_2 and prostaglandin $F_{2\alpha}$).[19] Platelet activating factor, a product of inflammation, is a major cause of low LES tone[17] and could be relevant for the IAS tone. There is also evidence that the interstitial cells of Cajal, present in the IAS and other smooth muscle sphincters, play a significant role in the genesis of IAS tone.[20]

Neural Control of Internal Anal Sphincter

The autonomic nerves, sympathetic (spinal nerves) and parasympathetic (pelvic nerves), supply the IAS.[21,22] Sympathetic fibers originate from the lower thoracic ganglia to form the superior hypogastric plexus. Parasympathetic fibers originate from the second, third, and fourth sacral nerves and form the inferior hypogastric plexus, which in turn gives rise to superior, middle, and inferior rectal nerves that ultimately supply the rectum and anal canal. These nerves are thought to synapse with the myenteric plexus of rectum. Sympathetic nerves mediate IAS contraction through the stimulation of α-adrenergic receptors,[23] and relaxation through β_1, β_2, and β_3 adrenergic receptors.[24,25] Studies show predominance of low-affinity β_3 receptors in the IAS. Stimulation of parasympathetic or pelvic nerves causes relaxation of the IAS through nitric oxide–containing neurons located in the myenteric plexus of the rectum.[16,26] There are no myenteric neurons in the IAS itself; however, it is richly innervated by the processes of myenteric inhibitory neurons located in the rectum. Besides nitric oxide, vasoactive intestinal peptide, carbon monoxide, and ATP are inhibitory neurotransmitters that likely play limited roles in the IAS relaxation.[27] Degeneration of myenteric neurons results in impaired IAS relaxation, a hallmark of the Hirschsprung disease.

EXTERNAL ANAL SPHINCTER

The anatomy of EAS has been a subject of significant debate for long time. Santorini (1769)[28] described the EAS to be composed of three separate muscles bundles: (1) subcutaneous, (2) superficial, and (3) deep. In many schematics published in the literature, including the one by Netter (see **Fig. 1**), the EAS is also made of three components. A close inspection of these schematics, however, reveals that the PRM is missing from these drawings. It is possible that even though not labeled as such, the PRM is part of the levator ani muscle complex. Shafik[29] described that the EAS consisted of three loops, with PRM located cranial to them. The subcutaneous portion of the EAS sits caudal to the IAS and the superficial portion surrounds the distal IAS. Several investigators have argued that only the subcutaneous and superficial muscle bundles constitute the EAS. Histologic study by Fritsch and coworkers[30] and MRI study of Hussain and coworkers[31] found that the EAS is composed of only the subcutaneous and superficial portions. Based on three-dimensional (3D) US imaging, we found that the deep part of the EAS is likely to be the PRM because it is shaped like a "U." It does not surround the anal canal in circumferential fashion.[32]

Another intriguing aspect of the EAS anatomy, based on published literature, is that it is attached to the perineal body at the ventral end.[33,34] The perineal body is a midline fibrotendinous structure to which, besides EAS, several other muscles of perineum (ie, superficial and deep transverse perinea, and bulbospongiosus) are also attached. These perineal muscles along with the EAS are referred to as the superficial muscles of the perineum. Recent studies show that the perineal body is not the site of insertion of superficial muscles of the perineum; instead, it is the site of crossing of the superficial muscles of the perineum.[35,36] The EAS muscles from the right and left side cross over to the other side in the midline structure of perineal body to continue as transverse perinea and bulbospongiosus muscles (**Fig. 2**).[35] The superficial transverse perinea muscle may not have definitive attachment to the bone; fibers seem to merge into septa of ischiorectal fat. However, the two bulbospongiosus muscles are attached to the pubic rami close to the symphysis pubis. Posterior to the anal canal, the EAS continues as anococcygeal raphe. Micro computed tomography imaging and histologic study show that the muscle fibers of the EAS, from right and left side, decussate at the posterior end of anal canal and then continue as anococcygeal raphe, which is attached to the tip of coccyx (anococcygeal raphe) (**Figs. 3** and **4**). Contrary to published literature, it may be that the EAS is not a donut-shaped ring of circular muscles fibers; instead, it has a unique myoarchitecture with crossing of muscle fibers in the midline at the ventral and dorsal ends of the anal canal with attachments to the pubic rami at the ventral end and coccyx at the dorsal end. In that regard, the EAS is no different from other skeletal muscles in the body that originate from a bone (fixed end) and are inserted into a bone (mobile end). In the case of EAS, its origin is from the pubic rami (fixed end) and insertion is into the coccyx (mobile end). Dynamic MRI studies show that the coccyx moves 8 to 10 mm in the ventral and cranial direction with the contraction of EAS and pelvic floor muscles.[37] Magnetic resonance diffusion tensor imaging (MR-DTI) is a novel technique to determine the myoarchitecture at a mesoscale level (in between histology or microscopic and macroscopic)[38,39] and the EAS is visualized by MR-DTI.[35] Future studies are needed to determine if MR-DTI is a better imaging technique to assess the anatomic integrity of the EAS than the current gold standard US imaging.

The unique morphology of the EAS has many implications for clinicians. Endoanal US imaging is the current gold standard to assess damage to the EAS muscle. It assumes an annular morphology of the EAS, which is not the case, and hence US

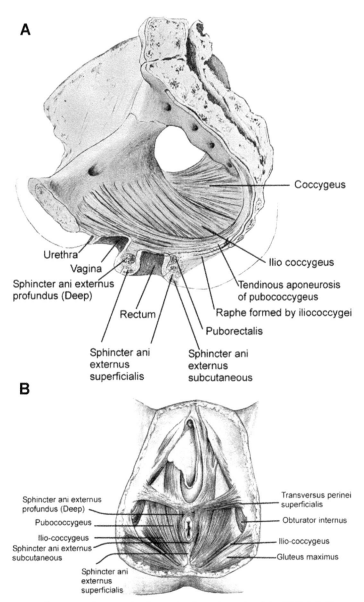

A

Coccygeus

Urethra
Vagina
Sphincter ani externus
profundus (Deep)

Ilio coccygeus

Tendinous aponeurosis
of pubococcygeus

Rectum

Raphe formed by iliococcygei

Puborectalis

Sphincter ani
externus
superficialis

Sphincter ani
externus
subcutaneous

B

Sphincter ani externus
profundus (Deep)
Pubococcygeus
Ilio-coccygeus
Sphincter ani externus
subcutaneous

Transversus perinei
superficialis

Obturator internus

Ilio-coccygeus

Gluteus maximus

Sphincter ani
externus
superficialis

Fig. 2. (*A*) Pelvic floor muscles seen in the sagittal section of pelvis. (*B*) Pelvic floor muscles as seen from the perineal surface. (*Adapted from* Raizada V, Mittal RK. Pelvic floor anatomy and applied physiology. Gastroenterol Clin North Am. 2008;37(3):493-vii. https://doi.org/10.1016/j.gtc.2008.06.003; with permission)

imaging cannot provide complete information on the structural integrity of EAS in patients with FI. Lateral episiotomy that sections through the bulbospongiosus and transverse perinea muscle is not a sphincter-sparing operation. Sphincteroplasty for the surgical repair of EAS muscle restores a circular shape to the EAS. However, if it is not an annular muscle to begin with, sphincteroplasty cannot be an effective

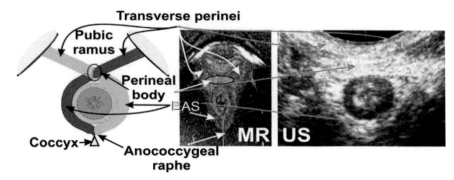

Transverse Perinea are the part of External Anal Sphincter Muscle

Fig. 3. Morphology of external anal sphincter: a "purse string," not a donut structure. (*From* Mittal RK, Bhargava V, Sheean G, Ledgerwood M, Sinha S. Purse-string morphology of external anal sphincter revealed by novel imaging techniques. Am J Physiol Gastrointest Liver Physiol. 2014;306(6):G505-G514. https://doi.org/10.1152/ajpgi.00338.2013; with permission)

surgical procedure to restore EAS function. Long-term studies indeed show that the sphincteroplasty is not an effective operation for the treatment of FI.[40]

Neural Control of External Anal Sphincter

The muscle fibers of EAS are composed of fast and slow twitch types, which allow it to maintain sustained tonic contraction at rest and allow it to contract rapidly with voluntary squeeze. Motor neurons in Onuf nucleus (located in the sacral spinal cord) innervate EAS muscle through the inferior rectal branches of right and left pudendal nerves.

PUBORECTALIS AND DEEP PELVIC FLOOR MUSCLES (LEVATOR ANI)

According to Sappey (1869), "the levator-ani is one of those muscles that has been studied the most, and at the same time about which we know the least."[33,41] Sappey also mentioned that the "The doctrine of continuity of fibers between two or more muscles of independent actions has been applied to the levator-ani at various scientific epochs, and this ancient error, renewed without ceasing, has singularly contributed

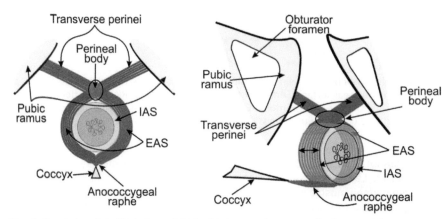

Fig. 4. Frontal and sagittal view of EAS with its attachment to the bony pelvis.

to complicate its study." It is interesting that even in 2021, the nomenclature of various pelvic floor muscles, precise anatomy, neural innervation, and functions of the levator ani/pelvic diaphragm are still being debated. Holl (1897)[42] suggested that some of the pubococcygeus muscle fibers, instead of inserting into the coccyx, loop around the rectum, and to these fibers he gave the name "puborectalis" or "sphincter recti." Prior depictions of the pelvic floor only show pubococcygeus, iliococcygeus, and ischiococcygeus as deep pelvic floor or levator ani muscles (see **Fig. 2**). Whether puborectalis and pubococcygeus are two separate muscles is not clear but clearly the puborectalis is located caudal to the iliococcygeus muscle. In the obstetrics/gynecology and urogynecology literature many authors use the term pubovisceral muscle,[43] for what is referred to as puborectalis by others. Irrespective of the previously mentioned controversies, puborectalis is a U-shaped muscle with ventral attachment to the two pubic rami. Dorsally, muscles from the two sides loop around the anorectum and possibly attach to the coccyx. From a functional point of view, puborectalis has unique function; it is responsible for the formation of the "anorectal angle," best seen on a midsagittal image of the pelvis during barium or MR defecography (**Fig. 5**). With contraction and relaxation of the PRM, the anorectal angle becomes more acute and obtuse, respectively. During defecation, the anorectal angle becomes obtuse and in patients with FI, with damage to the PRM the anorectal angle stays obtuse and does not change significantly with squeeze.

3D-US imaging of the pelvic floor provides better understanding of the morphology and function of PRM. The entire U-shaped PRM is visualized exquisitely by 3D-US imaging (**Fig. 6**); it forms the inferior margin of pelvic floor hiatus through which the urethra and anal canal emerge from the pelvis to the exterior in males, and in females, the urethra, vagina, and anal canal. Contraction of PRM reduces the size of pelvic floor hiatus and it also lifts the anal canal ventrally, thus compressing three orifices (ie, anal

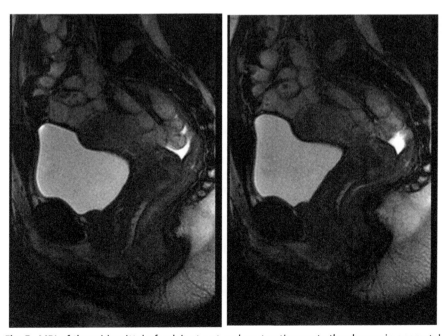

Fig. 5. MRI of the midsagittal of pelvis at rest and contraction: note the change in anorectal angle with contraction.

Pelvic Floor Hiatus at Rest & Squeeze

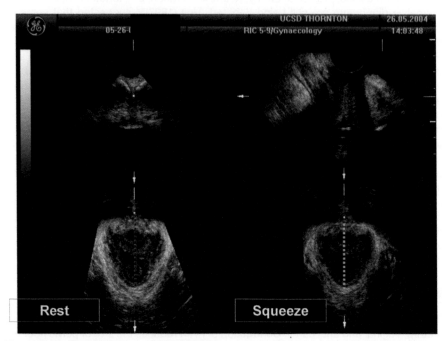

Fig. 6. Pelvic floor hiatus imaged by 3D-ultrasound transducer. Note the U-shaped puborectalis muscle at rest and during contraction. Note reduction in the dimensions of hiatus with contraction. Dorsoventral dimension of the hiatus becomes smaller during contraction resulting in compression of all the structures against the back of symphysis pubis.

canal, vagina, and urethra) against each other and in turn against the back of pubic symphysis. This results in dorsoventral closure of the vagina. Existence of a vaginal high-pressure zone related to the pelvic floor muscle is well known. Characteristics of the vaginal high-pressure zone have been described in detail in recent years using many different types of pressure measurement techniques, such as infusion manometry (side hole and sleeve sensor technique),[44,45] 3D-US imaging,[46] high-definition manometry (**Fig. 7**),[47] and most recently by FLIP (**Fig. 8**).[48] These studies prove that the vaginal high-pressure zone is related to PRM contraction, which has important clinical implications in that the PRM function may be easily assessed by recording vaginal pressure. Traditional measurements of the anorectal angle to assess PRM function require imaging studies, such as MRI and barium defecography, and are somewhat subjective. However, vaginal pressure measurement is a simple technique that can provide objective and quantitative assessment of PRM function. One can use 3D manometry and FLIP to record the vaginal high-pressure zone accurately. In patients with FI, not only anal pressures, but vaginal pressures are lower as compared with control subjects suggesting that the PRM function is impaired in significant numbers of patients with FI (**Fig. 9**).[49] Recent studies have identified weakness of the vaginal high-pressure zone using FLIP.[50,51] The PRM contraction, in addition to increasing anal and vaginal pressure, also increases urethral pressure.[52] Thus, it is highly likely that the PRM is also important in the urethral continence mechanism; further studies are needed to validate the previously mentioned hypothesis.

High-Definition Vaginal Canal Manometry

Rest   Squeeze

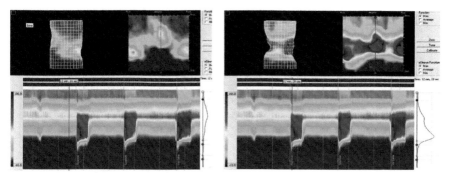

Fig. 7. High-definition manometry of vaginal anal high-pressure zone. (*Top*) Cylindrical and two-dimensional surface plot of pressure profile at rest and with voluntary squeeze. (*Bottom*) Vaginal pressure profile as seen with high-resolution manometry (at rest and voluntary contraction). (*From* Raizada V, Bhargava V, Jung SA, et al. Dynamic assessment of the vaginal high-pressure zone using high-definition manometry, 3-dimensional ultrasound, and magnetic resonance imaging of the pelvic floor muscles. Am J Obstet Gynecol. 2010;203(2):172.e1-172.e1728. https://doi.org/10.1016/j.ajog.2010.02.028; with permission)

Neural Innervation of the Puborectalis Muscle

Branches from the sacral nerve roots, S2, S3, and S4 innervate the pelvic floor muscles. The three deep pelvic floor muscles, pubococcygeus, iliococcygeus, and ischiococcygeus (also known as coccygeus) are innervated by branches from S2, S3, and S4 that enter these muscles from their abdominal surface. However, the EAS and other superficial muscles of the perineum are innervated by pudendal nerve branches. There is considerable controversy whether pudendal nerves innervate the PRMs. An electrophysiologic study by Percy and colleagues[53] found that electrical stimulation of the pudendal nerve did not activate PRM. It is possible that in their study the electrodes were not precisely located in the puborectalis portion of the levator ani muscle. The authors of this review believe that the PRM is the middle layer of pelvic floor musculature,[45] and similar to EAS, PRM is innervated by the pudendal nerve (from the perineal/inferior surface of pelvic floor muscle). Conversely, deep pelvic floor muscles (pubococcygeus, iliococcygeus, and coccygeus) are innervated by direct branches of the sacral nerve roots S3 and S4 from the superior (abdominal) surface of the pelvic floor. The clinical significance of this is that pudendal nerve damage may cause dysfunction of the puborectalis and EAS (both constrictor muscles), which in turn may cause FI.

Relationship Between Anatomy and Function of the Levator Ani

The name levator ani implies an elevator of anus. Pelvic floor muscles have two important functions: physical support or actual floor to the pelvic viscera; and constrictor function to the anal canal, urethra, and vagina. These two functions may be distinct and related to different components of the pelvic floor musculature. The pubococcygeus, iliococcygeus, and ischiococcygeus likely provide the physical support or act as "floor" for the pelvic/abdominal organs. However, PRM provides the constrictor

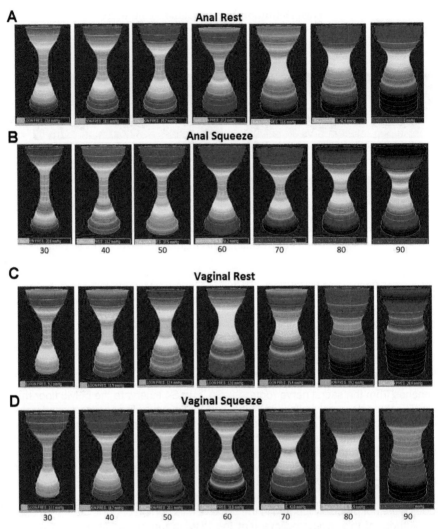

Fig. 8. (A–D) Anal and vaginal high-pressure zone visualized with FLIP at various balloon volumes of the FLIP bag. Note the hourglass shape of the anal and vaginal high-pressure zone.(*From* Tuttle LJ, Zifan A, Sun C, Swartz J, Roalkvam S, Mittal RK. Measuring length-tension function of the anal sphincters and puborectalis muscle using the functional luminal imaging probe. Am J Physiol Gastrointest Liver Physiol. 2018;315(5):G781-G787. https://doi.org/10.1152/ajpgi.00414.2017; with permission)

function for anal canal, vagina, and urethra. The urethra and anal canal have two constrictors or sphincters of their own. In the case of the anal canal these are the IAS (smooth muscle) and EAS (skeletal muscle), and in the case of the urethra they are the smooth muscle sphincter located at the bladder neck (internal urethral sphincter, also known as lissosphincter) and rhabdosphincter (external urethral sphincter). The PRM is the third constrictor or sphincter of the anal canal and urethra. The vagina, however, has only one constrictor mechanism, which is caused by the puborectalis portion of pelvic floor muscles. The PRM is relevant to multiple subspecialties: gastroenterology, colorectal surgery, urology, urogynecology, radiology, and neurology.

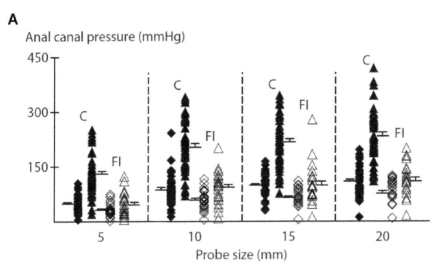

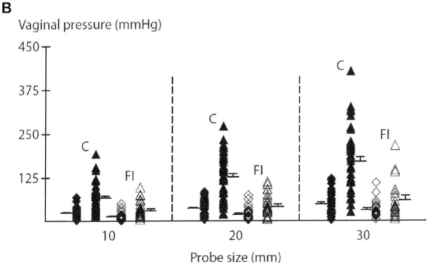

Fig. 9. Anal (*A*) and vaginal pressure (*B*) at rest (*diamonds*) and voluntary squeeze (*triangles*) in control subjects (*filled symbols*) and patients with FI (*open symbols*). Note an increase in pressure with probe size increase and with squeeze. Pressures are significantly lower in patients compared with control subjects at rest and squeeze. C, control subjects. (*From* Kim YS, Weinstein M, Raizada V, et al. Anatomical disruption and length-tension dysfunction of anal sphincter complex muscles in women with fecal incontinence. Dis Colon Rectum. 2013;56(11):1282-1289. https://doi.org/10.1097/DCR.0b013e3182a18e87; with permission)

LENGTH-TENSION FUNCTION OF THE EXTERNAL ANAL SPHINCTER AND PUBORECTALIS MUSCLES

The basic unit of all muscles is the sarcomere, which is made of actin and myosin filaments. The sarcomere length is a major determinant of the force that any muscle generates during its maximal contraction. The length-tension relationship, best known as Starling curve in the context of myocardium, is well described.[54] It is a bell-shape curve, that is, muscle tension increases with increase in muscle length to a certain length and then it decreases. The degree of overlap between actin and myosin filaments determines the force generated by the sarcomere.[55] At optimal length there is maximum overlap between the actin and myosin filaments. The length at which a muscle/sarcomere operates in vivo (operational length) and the length at which it generates maximal tension (optimal length) are different. Myocardium under physiologic conditions operates at a short sarcomere length and when stretched it increases the force of contraction. Different muscles in the body operate at different operational lengths. Studies show that like myocardium, the EAS and PRM also operate at a short sarcomere length.[56–58] Studies of the rabbit EAS reveal that the optimal sarcomere length of EAS is approximately 20% larger than its operational length. In humans, the EAS and PRM when stretched (eg, by placing probes of increasing diameters in the anal and vaginal canals) generate greater tension.[57,58] Hence, the anal and vaginal pressures increase with an increase in the diameter of the manometry probe used to record pressure. Like normal healthy subjects, in patients with FI who have damaged EAS and PRM, these muscles operate at the suboptimal length even though the slope of the length-tension curve is steeper in normal subjects compared with patients with damaged muscle.[49] The clinical significance of knowing the length-tension relationship is that it may be possible to change/adjust the sarcomere length to gain muscle function. Plication of the EAS muscle in rabbits led to an increase in the sarcomere length and increase in anal closure pressure that were sustained for 6 months (the duration of the study) (**Fig. 10**).[59] Whether plication of the EAS and PRM can improve anal closure function and FI in humans requires study.

ASSESSING THE ANATOMY OF ANAL CLOSURE MECHANISMS

The current gold standard to assess anatomic integrity of the anal closure mechanism is endoanal US. The endoanal US probe is approximately 15 mm in diameter, and it is placed in the lumen of the anal canal. The previously mentioned methodology has been in use since the early 1990s. Using mechanical US transducers, one can image the entire length of the anal canal and using computer software can display the anal canal anatomy in 3D; many studies have proven the previously mentioned modality as reliable.[60–62] However, the limitations of endoluminal US technique are: (1) the US probe is large in size (15 mm) and may not be tolerated well by subjects; (2) anal distention caused by US probe causes artifactual thinning of the muscles; (3) the caudal-most portion of EAS, located below the IAS, is not well visualized; (4) perineal body, an important part of the EAS, is not seen; and (5) anal canal descends caudally more in the ventral than in dorsal direction, and hence one has to be careful in the interpretation of axial US images in the dorsal part of anal canal. US images show that in most patients, damage to the IAS and EAS is located between 11- and 2-o'clock positions of anal canal (12 o'clock being the ventral midline location), the location of the perineal body. The latter is an extremely important location, the site of crossing of muscle fibers from the two sides of EAS. Transperineal, also known as translabial, 3D-US imaging is an important technique to visualize muscles of the anal sphincter complex.[60,61,63,64] In this technique, the US transducer is placed on the perineum and one can capture a US volume of pixels that is visualized off-line using computer software. The transperineal/translabial US technique is patient friendly because it does not require insertion of a US probe into the anal canal and US imaging quality is excellent. One can see the caudal parts of the anal canal, EAS, and perineal body well in these US images (**Fig. 11**). For imaging of the anal canal, the US

EAS Plication to Treat Anal Incontinence

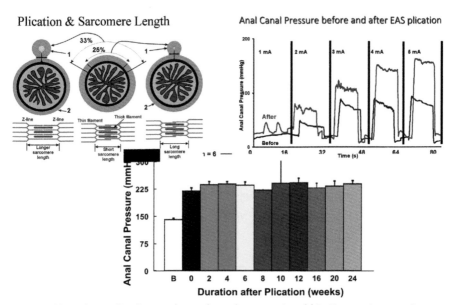

Fig. 10. Effect of EAS plication on the anal canal pressure in rabbit. Note an increase in pressure following plication length of 20% of the EAS circumference. Also note that the increase in anal canal pressure following plication is sustained for 24 weeks. (*From* Mittal RK, Sheean G, Padda BS, Rajasekaran MR. Length tension function of puborectalis muscle: implications for the treatment of fecal incontinence and pelvic floor disorders. J Neurogastroenterol Motil. 2014;20(4):539-546. https://doi.org/10.5056/jnm14033; with permission)

transducer is directed in the dorsal direction. However, to visualize the pelvic floor hiatus and PRM the US transducer is directed toward the head end of the subject. Using the previously mentioned technique, one can capture the images of anal canal and pelvic floor hiatus in real time during contraction and therefore study dynamic changes in the pelvic floor hiatus during anal sphincter squeeze and Valsalva maneuver. Another US imaging technique that can provide useful information on the integrity of anal sphincter muscle is high-frequency US imaging[65]; it allows one to visualize individual muscle fascicles inside the body of the EAS (**Figs. 12** and **13**). A recent study demonstrated crossing of muscle fascicles of EAS in the perineal body in normal subjects, and damage to the myoarchitecture of EAS using high-frequency US imaging.[66]

MRI of the pelvic floor and anal sphincter muscles has been successfully performed by several investigators.[35,36,39,67,68] The coils to capture MRIs are usually placed on the abdomen of subjects; however, endoanal and endovaginal coils (probes) have also been used to capture pelvic floor, IAS, and EAS images. One can visualize the EAS much better in MRI than US images. However, the IAS is better visualized in the US images. MR defecography is a dynamic study to assess the defecatory process and stool evacuation. It is used to identify pelvic floor dyssynergia, rectocele, and other anatomic abnormalities that may occur during the defecation process. MRI during defecography is usually performed in the supine position; however, open MRI magnets to perform defecography in the seated position are available at a few centers. MR-DTI to study the myoarchitecture of anal sphincter and pelvic floor

Multiple Slice View- Distal Anal Canal

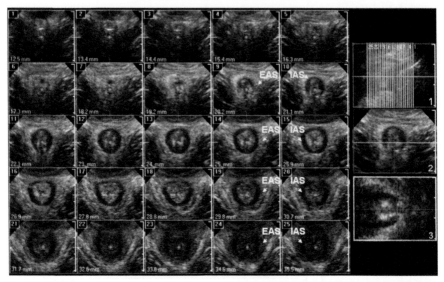

Fig. 11. US images of the anal sphincter muscles obtained with transperineal 3D-US transducer. Axial slices 1 mm apart from caudal (1) to cranial (25) end of the anal canal. Dark (*black*) ringlike structure is IAS. EAS is located outside the IAS.

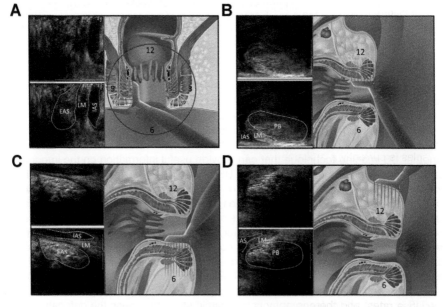

Fig. 12. (*A–D*) High-frequency US images of the anal canal with the hockey stick–shaped US transducer placed at different locations inside and outside the anal canal. EAS, external anal sphincter; IAS, internal anal; sphincter; LM, longitudinal muscle. (*From* Ledgerwood-Lee M, Zifan A, Kunkel D, Sah R, Mittal R.K. High-frequency ultrasound imaging of the anal sphincter muscles in normal subjects and patients with fecal incontinence. Neurogastroenterol Motil. 2019 Apr; 31(4): e13537.)

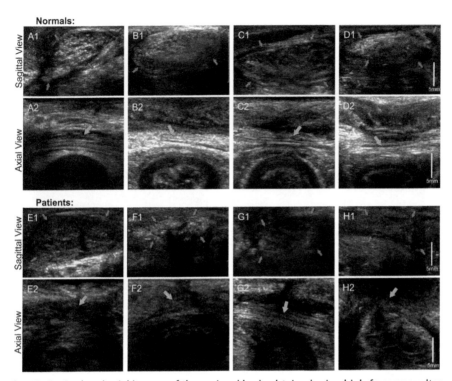

Fig. 13. Sagittal and axial images of the perineal body obtained using high-frequency ultrasound transducer. *Top two rows* are from four different normal subjects and *bottom two rows* are from four different patients with FI. Note individual muscle fascicles in the perineal body in normal subjects and loss of muscle fascicles in patients with FI. *Orange arrows* show the outline of the perineal body. *Blue arrows* show the muscle fascicles inside the perineal body. (*From* Ledgerwood-Lee M, Zifan A, Kunkel D, Sah R, Mittal R.K. High-frequency ultrasound imaging of the anal sphincter muscles in normal subjects and patients with fecal incontinence. Neurogastroenterol Motil. 2019 Apr; 31(4): e13537.)

muscles is currently a research tool. It provides information on the myoarchitecture. We have successfully visualized crossing of muscle fibers of the EAS in the perineal body (**Fig. 14**).[35,36]

Functional Assessment of the Anal Closure Mechanism

Schuster balloon, infusion manometry, and solid-state sensors to assess the function of the anal closure mechanism have been replaced by high-resolution manometry, and high-resolution manometry is currently considered the gold standard of clinical anorectal testing.[69] There are many advantages of high-resolution manometry over the old pressure measurement techniques; the sensors have high fidelity (faster response rates) and there is no concern with regards to the relative movement between pressure transducers and anal canal structures during various maneuvers used in anorectal motility testing. Furthermore, the display (color topography) is reader friendly. High-definition anorectal manometry is another system[70] that provides information on the asymmetry of anal sphincter pressure profile (**Fig. 15**).[71–73] The high-definition anorectal manometry probe is larger than the high-resolution anorectal

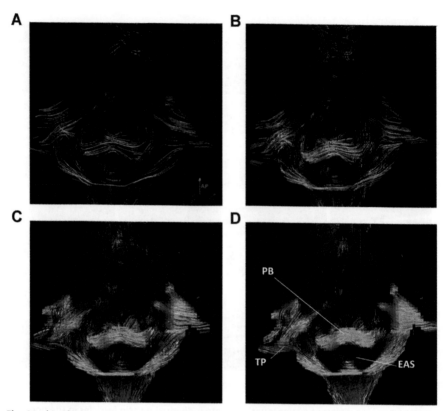

Fig. 14. (*A–D*) Magnetic resonance diffusion tensor image of the external anal sphincter and other muscles of perineum. EAS, external anal sphincter; TP, transverse perinea; PB, perineal body. (*From* Zifan, A., Reisert, M., Sinha, S. et al. Connectivity of the Superficial Muscles of the Human Perineum: A Diffusion Tensor Imaging-Based Global Tractography Study. Sci Rep 8, 17867 (2018). https://doi.org/10.1038/s41598-018-36099-4; with permission)

manometry probe (10 mm vs 4.5 mm). The anal canal pressure recorded by high-definition anorectal manometry is higher than high-resolution anorectal manometry because of the length-tension principle described previously. One of the promises of high-definition anorectal manometry was that it may be able to detect locations of damage in the EAS and IAS has not borne out in studies. FLIP is the "latest kid on the block" to assess the anal closure functions. It provides information on the anal canal distensibility as a measure of the strength of anal closure mechanism.[6,7] The anal canal distensibility is greater in patients with FI as compared with control subjects. One study reported high sensitivity and specificity to diagnose FI based on the anal canal distensibility at rest; squeeze values were not necessarily better than rest values in discriminating normal subjects from patients. Distending the anal canal with FLIP brings back the length-tension principle of anal sphincter muscle in the equation (**Figs. 16–18**).[48,50,51] Vaginal manometry has also been used to assess the PRM function in normal control subjects and patients with FI.[49–51] The vaginal high-pressure zone shows significant circumferential asymmetry, because the force responsible for the genesis of vaginal high-pressure zone is directed in the dorsoventral direction (ie, lift of the anal canal by PRM contraction in the ventral direction). The

High Definition Manometery-Anal Canal Pressure

Rest   Squeeze

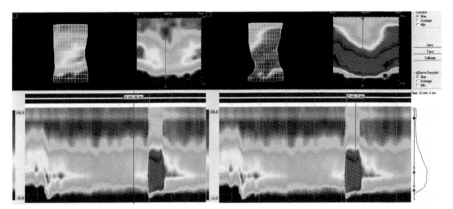

Fig. 15. High-definition manometry of the anal high-pressure zone. (*Top*) Cylindrical and two-dimensional surface plot of pressure profile at rest and with voluntary squeeze. (*Bottom*) Pressure profile of the anal canal seen with high-resolution manometry at rest and contraction.

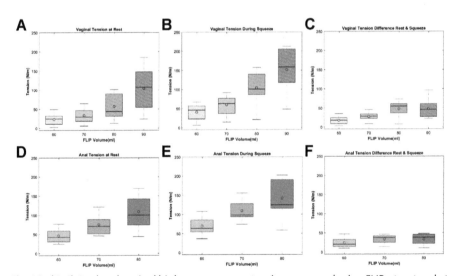

Fig. 16. (*A–F*) Anal and vaginal high-pressure zone tension measured using FLIP, at rest and at maximal voluntary contraction. Note the increase in the tension with increase in the FLIP bag volume, which represents the length-tension property of the anal sphincter and puborectalis muscle. (*From* Kim YS, Weinstein M, Raizada V, et al. Anatomical disruption and length-tension dysfunction of anal sphincter complex muscles in women with fecal incontinence. Dis Colon Rectum. 2013;56(11):1282-1289. https://doi.org/10.1097/DCR.0b013e3182a18e87; with permission)

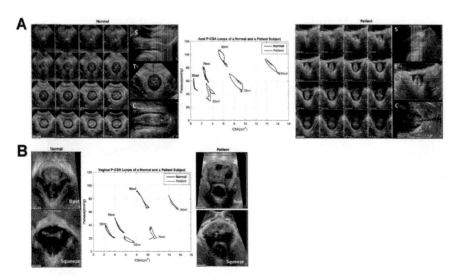

Fig. 17. Anal (*A*) and vaginal (*B*) length-tension loops in normal subjects (*black*) and patients with FI (*red*) at different bag volumes of the FLIP. Note the shift of loops to the right and upward with increase in FLIP bag volumes. In patients the loops are shifted to the right. P-CSA, pressure-cross sectional area. (*From* Tuttle LJ, Zifan A, Sun C, Swartz J, Roalkvam S, Mittal RK. Measuring length-tension function of the anal sphincters and puborectalis muscle using the functional luminal imaging probe. Am J Physiol Gastrointest Liver Physiol. 2018;315(5):G781-G787. https://doi.org/10.1152/ajpgi.00414.2017; with permission).

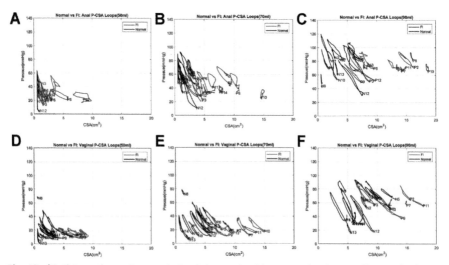

Fig. 18. (*A–F*) Length-tension analysis of the anal sphincter and puborectalis muscle shown in the form of loops. These data are obtained from the FLIP. Each loop represents a contraction cycle and shows changes in muscle tension as a function of the length of muscle over time. Loops move to the right and upward with the increase in FLIP bag volume. In the patients, loop is shifted to the right as compared with normal subjects. P-CSA, pressure-cross sectional area. (*From* Tuttle LJ, Zifan A, Sun C, Swartz J, Roalkvam S, Mittal RK. Measuring length-tension function of the anal sphincters and puborectalis muscle using the functional luminal imaging probe. Am J Physiol Gastrointest Liver Physiol. 2018;315(5):G781-G787. https://doi.org/10.1152/ajpgi.00414.2017; with permission).

vaginal pressures are higher in the dorsoventral as compared with lateral direction. The ventral or anterior pressure are highest in the vaginal high-pressure zone.

SUMMARY

Muscles in general are straightforward in their function; they only shorten and lengthen with contraction and relaxation, respectively. It is the architecture, or the arrangement of the muscle fascicles inside the body of the muscle that determines the physical function of muscle in vivo. Flexion and extension at the elbow are achieved by simple arrangement of muscle fibers organized in a linear direction from the origin (shoulder) to the insertion (elbow). However, muscle fibers of EAS, placed in the configuration of figure-of-eight, can cause circumferential closure of the anal canal. Future studies need to focus on the architecture of muscle fibers of pelvic floor muscles to better understand their function.

Pelvic floor disorders are many and are generally lumped together. However, they are broadly classified into disorders of pelvic floor support (prolapse, descending perineal syndrome) and constrictor function (urinary and FI). Furthermore, these disorders may be further divided into dysfunctions of pelvic floor contraction (FI and urinary incontinence) and relaxation (constipation and urinary retention). As a clearer picture of the anatomy and function of pelvic floor muscles emerges, it is likely that different components of the pelvic floor muscles will be implicated in different pelvic floor disorders. With such a functional classification, it may be possible to identify specific targets and more effective therapeutic strategies to treat various pelvic floor disorders. A better understanding of the correct anatomy of anal sphincter and pelvic floor muscles is crucial for the understanding of precise function. Most importantly, prevention of damage or surgical restoration of the sphincter and other pelvic floor muscles' function requires understanding of their correct anatomy.

CLINICS CARE POINTS

- Correct understanding of the muscle architecture is essential in defining the function of muscle, preventing damage and restoring function of the muscle. Anatomy of the anal sphincter and pelvic floor muscles has been an area of controversy.
- Novel imaging technique has revealed unique myoarchitecture of the pelvic floor and anal sphincter muscles.
- High resolution anal manometry, 3D high definition anal manometry and functional luminal imaging probe are important new tools to measure anal sphincter function.
- Length-tension principle, well described for the cardiac muscle is also applicable to the anal sphincter muscle and using this principle, it may be possible to devise novel strategies to treat anal/fecal incontinence.

DISCLOSURE

Authors have no conflict of interest.

Drs L.J. Tuttle and R.K. Mittal are supported by NIH Grant 1R01HD088688.

REFERENCES

1. Menees SB, Almario CV, Spiegel BMR, et al. Prevalence of and factors associated with fecal incontinence: results from a population-based survey. Gastroenterology 2018;154:1672–1681 e3.

2. Rao SS, Bharucha AE, Chiarioni G, et al. Functional anorectal disorders. Gastro-enterology 2016. https://doi.org/10.1053/j.gastro.2016.02.009.

3. Bharucha AE, Rao SS. An update on anorectal disorders for gastroenterologists. Gastroenterology 2014;146:37–45 e2.

4. Read NW, Haynes WG, Bartolo DC, et al. Use of anorectal manometry during rectal infusion of saline to investigate sphincter function in incontinent patients. Gastroenterology 1983;85:105–13.

5. Bharucha AE, Fletcher JG, Harper CM, et al. Relationship between symptoms and disordered continence mechanisms in women with idiopathic faecal inconti-nence. Gut 2005;54:546–55.

6. Gourcerol G, Granier S, Bridoux V, et al. Do endoflip assessments of anal sphincter distensibility provide more information on patients with fecal inconti-nence than high-resolution anal manometry? Neurogastroenterol Motil 2016;28: 399–409.

7. Sorensen G, Liao D, Lundby L, et al. Distensibility of the anal canal in patients with idiopathic fecal incontinence: a study with the functional lumen imaging probe. Neurogastroenterol Motil 2014;26:255–63.

8. DeLancey JO, Kearney R, Chou Q, et al. The appearance of levator ani muscle abnormalities in magnetic resonance images after vaginal delivery. Obstet Gyne-col 2003;101:46–53.

9. Sultan AH, Kamm MA, Hudson CN, et al. Anal-sphincter disruption during vaginal delivery. N Engl J Med 1993;329:1905–11.

10. Graf W, Mellgren A, Matzel KE, et al. Efficacy of dextranomer in stabilised hyal-uronic acid for treatment of faecal incontinence: a randomised, sham-controlled trial. Lancet 2011;377:997–1003.

11. Hull T, Giese C, Wexner SD, et al. Long-term durability of sacral nerve stimulation therapy for chronic fecal incontinence. Dis Colon Rectum 2013;56:234–45.

12. Heymen S, Scarlett Y, Jones K, et al. Randomized controlled trial shows biofeed-back to be superior to pelvic floor exercises for fecal incontinence. Dis Colon Rectum 2009;52:1730–7.

13. Kumar L, Emmanuel A. Internal anal sphincter: clinical perspective. Surgeon 2017;15:211–26.

14. Al-Ali S, Blyth P, Beatty S, et al. Correlation between gross anatomical topog-raphy, sectional sheet plastination, microscopic anatomy and endoanal sonogra-phy of the anal sphincter complex in human males. J Anat 2009;215:212–20.

15. Netter F. Atlas of human anatomy. In: Kelly P, editor. 3rd edition. Teteboro (NJ): Icon Learning system; 2003. p. 361–4.

16. Rattan S. The internal anal sphincter: regulation of smooth muscle tone and relax-ation. Neurogastroenterol Motil 2005;17(Suppl 1):50–9.

17. Harnett KM, Rieder F, Behar J, et al. Viewpoints on acid-induced inflammatory mediators in esophageal mucosa. J Neurogastroenterol Motil 2010;16:374–88.

18. Rattan S. Ca2+/calmodulin/MLCK pathway initiates, and RhoA/ROCK maintains, the internal anal sphincter smooth muscle tone. Am J Physiol Gastrointest Liver Physiol 2017;312:G63–6.

19. Rattan S, Singh J, Kumar S, et al. Nature of extracellular signal that triggers RhoA/ROCK activation for the basal internal anal sphincter tone in humans. Am J Phys-iol Gastrointest Liver Physiol 2015;308:G924–33.

20. Cobine CA, Hannah EE, Zhu MH, et al. ANO1 in intramuscular interstitial cells of Cajal plays a key role in the generation of slow waves and tone in the internal anal sphincter. J Physiol 2017;595:2021–41.

21. Bharucha AE. Pelvic floor: anatomy and function. Neurogastroenterol Motil 2006; 18:507–19.

22. Raizada V, Mittal RK. Pelvic floor anatomy and applied physiology. Gastroenterol Clin North Am 2008;37:493–509, vii.

23. Yamato S, Rattan S. Role of alpha adrenoceptors in opossum internal anal sphincter. J Clin Invest 1990;86:424–9.

24. Rathi S, Kazerounian S, Banwait K, et al. Functional and molecular characterization of beta-adrenoceptors in the internal anal sphincter. J Pharmacol Exp Ther 2003;305:615–24.

25. Li F, De Godoy M, Rattan S. Role of adenylate and guanylate cyclases in beta1-, beta2-, and beta3-adrenoceptor-mediated relaxation of internal anal sphincter smooth muscle. J Pharmacol Exp Ther 2004;308:1111–20.

26. Rattan S, Shah R. Influence of sacral nerves on the internal anal sphincter of the opossum. Am J Physiol 1987;253:G345–50.

27. Rattan S, Thatikunta P. Role of nitric oxide in sympathetic neurotransmission in opossum internal anal sphincter. Gastroenterology 1993;105:827–36.

28. Santorini J. Septemdecim tabulae, 1715.

29. Shafik A. A new concept of the anatomy of the anal sphincter mechanism and the physiology of defecation. The external anal sphincter: a triple-loop system. Invest Urol 1975;12:412–9.

30. Fritsch H, Brenner E, Lienemann A, et al. Anal sphincter complex: reinterpreted morphology and its clinical relevance. Dis Colon Rectum 2002;45:188–94.

31. Hussain SM, Stoker J, Lameris JS. Anal sphincter complex: endoanal MR imaging of normal anatomy. Radiology 1995;197:671–7.

32. Liu J, Guaderrama N, Nager CW, et al. Functional correlates of anal canal anatomy: puborectalis muscle and anal canal pressure. Am J Gastroenterol 2006; 101:1092–7.

33. Thompson P. The myology of the pelvic floor. Newton: McCorquoddale; 1899.

34. Hsu Y, Fenner DE, Weadock WJ, et al. Magnetic resonance imaging and 3-dimensional analysis of external anal sphincter anatomy. Obstet Gynecol 2005; 106:1259–65.

35. Mittal RK, Bhargava V, Sheean G, et al. Purse-string morphology of external anal sphincter revealed by novel imaging techniques. Am J Physiol Gastrointest Liver Physiol 2014;306:G505–14.

36. Zifan A, Reisert M, Sinha S, et al. Connectivity of the superficial muscles of the human perineum: a diffusion tensor imaging-based global tractography study. Sci Rep 2018;8:17867.

37. Bo K, Lilleas F, Talseth T, et al. Dynamic MRI of the pelvic floor muscles in an upright sitting position. Neurourol Urodyn 2001;20:167–74.

38. Zijta FM, Froeling M, Nederveen AJ, et al. Diffusion tensor imaging and fiber tractography for the visualization of the female pelvic floor. Clin Anat 2013;26:110–4.

39. Zijta FM, Froeling M, van der Paardt MP, et al. Feasibility of diffusion tensor imaging (DTI) with fibre tractography of the normal female pelvic floor. Eur Radiol 2011;21:1243–9.

40. Halverson AL, Hull TL. Long-term outcome of overlapping anal sphincter repair. Dis Colon Rectum 2002;45:345–8.

41. Sappey P. Traite d. (2nd ed). Anatomie Descriptive; 1739.

42. Holl M. Handbuch des Anatomie. Jena: Fischer; 1897.

43. Lawson JO. Pelvic anatomy. I. Pelvic floor muscles. Ann R Coll Surg Engl 1974; 54:244–52.

44. Guaderrama NM, Nager CW, Liu J, et al. The vaginal pressure profile. Neurourol Urodyn 2005;24:243–7.

45. Guaderrama NM, Liu J, Nager CW, et al. Evidence for the innervation of pelvic floor muscles by the pudendal nerve. Obstet Gynecol 2005;106:774–81.

46. Jung SA, Pretorius DH, Padda BS, et al. Vaginal high-pressure zone assessed by dynamic 3-dimensional ultrasound images of the pelvic floor. Am J Obstet Gynecol 2007;197:52.e1-7.

47. Raizada V, Bhargava V, Jung SA, et al. Dynamic assessment of the vaginal high-pressure zone using high-definition manometry, 3-dimensional ultrasound, and magnetic resonance imaging of the pelvic floor muscles. Am J Obstet Gynecol 2010;203:172 e1–8.

48. Tuttle L, Ali Z, Schwartz J, et al. Measuring Length-Tension Function of the Anal Sphincters and Puborectalis Muscle Using Functional Luminal Imaging Probe. Am J Physiol Gastrointest Liver Physiol 2018;315(5):G781–7.

49. Kim YS, Weinstein M, Raizada V, et al. Anatomical disruption and length-tension dysfunction of anal sphincter complex muscles in women with fecal incontinence. Dis Colon Rectum 2013;56:1282–9.

50. Tuttle LJ, Zifan A, Sun C, et al. Measuring length-tension function of the anal sphincters and puborectalis muscle using the functional luminal imaging probe. Am J Physiol Gastrointest Liver Physiol 2018;315:G781–7.

51. Zifan A, Mittal RK, Kunkel DC, et al. Loop analysis of the anal sphincter complex in fecal incontinent patients using functional luminal imaging probe. Am J Physiol Gastrointest Liver Physiol 2020;318:G66–76.

52. Rajasekaran MR, Sohn D, Salehi M, et al. Role of puborectalis muscle in the genesis of urethral pressure. J Urol 2012;188:1382–8.

53. Percy JP, Neill ME, Swash M, et al. Electrophysiological study of motor nerve supply of pelvic floor. Lancet 1981;1:16–7.

54. Gordon AM, Huxley AF, Julian FJ. The variation in isometric tension with sarcomere length in vertebrate muscle fibres. J Physiol 1966;184:170–92.

55. Huxley AF, Simmons RM. Proposed mechanism of force generation in striated muscle. Nature 1971;233:533–8.

56. Rajasekaran MR, Jiang Y, Bhargava V, et al. Length-tension relationship of the external anal sphincter muscle: implications for the anal canal function. Am J Physiol Gastrointest Liver Physiol 2008;295:G367–73.

57. Mittal RK, Sheean G, Padda BS, et al. The external anal sphincter operates at short sarcomere length in humans. Neurogastroenterol Motil 2011;23:643.e8.

58. Mittal RK, Sheean G, Padda BS, et al. Length tension function of puborectalis muscle: implications for the treatment of fecal incontinence and pelvic floor disorders. J Neurogastroenterol Motil 2014;20:539–46.

59. Rajasekaran MR, Jiang Y, Bhargava V, et al. Sustained improvement in the anal sphincter function following surgical plication of rabbit external anal sphincter muscle. Dis Colon Rectum 2011;54:1373–80.

60. Martinez Franco E, Ros C, Santoro GA, et al. Transperineal anal sphincter complex evaluation after obstetric anal sphincter injuries: with or without tomographic ultrasound imaging technique? Eur J Obstet Gynecol Reprod Biol 2021;257:70–5.

61. Subramaniam N, Dietz HP. What is a significant defect of the anal sphincter on translabial ultrasound? Ultrasound Obstet Gynecol 2020;55:411–5.

62. Murad-Regadas SM, da SFGO, Regadas FS, et al. Usefulness of anorectal and endovaginal 3D ultrasound in the evaluation of sphincter and pubovisceral

muscle defects using a new scoring system in women with fecal incontinence af-ter vaginal delivery. Int J Colorectal Dis 2017;32:499–507.

63. Dietz HP. Pelvic floor trauma in childbirth. Aust N Z J Obstet Gynaecol 2013;53: 220–30.

64. Weinstein MM, Pretorius DH, Jung SA, et al. Transperineal three-dimensional ul-trasound imaging for detection of anatomic defects in the anal sphincter complex muscles. Clin Gastroenterol Hepatol 2009;7:205–11.

65. Timor-Tritsch IE, Monteagudo A, Porges RF, et al. The use of a 15-7-MHz 'small parts' linear transducer to evaluate the anal sphincter in female patients. Ultra-sound Obstet Gynecol 2005;25:206–9.

66. Ledgerwood-Lee M, Zifan A, Kunkel DC, et al. High-frequency ultrasound imag-ing of the anal sphincter muscles in normal subjects and patients with fecal in-continence. Neurogastroenterol Motil 2019;31:e13537.

67. Goh V, Tam E, Taylor NJ, et al. Diffusion tensor imaging of the anal canal at 3 tesla: feasibility and reproducibility of anisotropy measures. J Magn Reson Imaging 2012;35:820–6.

68. Zijta FM, Lakeman MM, Froeling M, et al. Evaluation of the female pelvic floor in pelvic organ prolapse using 3.0-Tesla diffusion tensor imaging and fibre tractog-raphy. Eur Radiol 2012;22:2806–13.

69. Lee TH, Bharucha AE. How to perform and interpret a high-resolution anorectal manometry test. J Neurogastroenterol Motil 2016;22:46–59.

70. Chakraborty S, Feuerhak KJ, Zinsmeister AR, et al. Reproducibility of high-definition (3D) manometry and its agreement with high-resolution (2D) manometry in women with fecal incontinence. Neurogastroenterol Motil 2017;29. 10.1111/nmo.12950.

71. Raizada V, Bhargava V, Karsten A, et al. Functional morphology of anal sphincter complex unveiled by high definition anal manometry and three dimensional ultra-sound imaging. Neurogastroenterol Motil 2011;23:1013–9.e460.

72. Coss-Adame E, Rao SS, Valestin J, et al. Accuracy and reproducibility of high-definition anorectal manometry and pressure topography analyses in healthy subjects. Clin Gastroenterol Hepatol 2015;13:1143–11450.e1.

73. Cheeney G, Remes-Troche JM, Attaluri A, et al. Investigation of anal motor char-acteristics of the sensorimotor response (SMR) using 3-D anorectal pressure topography. Am J Physiol Gastrointest Liver Physiol 2011;300:G236–40.

The Digital Rectal Examination

Appropriate Techniques for the Evaluation of Constipation and Fecal Incontinence

Gregory S. Sayuk, MD, MPH

KEYWORDS

- Digital rectal examination • Physical examination • Anal sphincter
- Fecal incontinence • Constipation • Defecation • Dyssynergic defecation
- Functional defecation disorder

KEY POINTS

- The performance of a digital rectal examination (DRE) provides valuable information regarding anal sphincter tone, anatomic issues with the anorectum, and the physiology of the defecatory mechanism in health and in the symptomatic individual.
- There are several obstacles that have led to the underutilization of DRE in practice, including inadequate training, lack of physician comfort and confidence in performing the examination, concerns about patient comfort, and some conflicting literature regarding the value of DRE.
- DRE is particularly useful in evaluating patients with complaints relating to constipation (ie, functional defecation disorders) and fecal incontinence.
- A DRE protocol requires training and practice, but it can easily be mastered and lead to meaningful reductions in reliance on additional testing to make a diagnosis in patients with defecatory issues.
- Experienced practitioners can achieve a diagnostic accuracy comparable to that of a formal anorectal manometry and balloon expulsion protocol, particularly in patients with pelvic floor dyssynergia.

INTRODUCTION

The digital rectal examination (DRE) is an essential component of the complete physical examination of the gastrointestinal (GI) tract. DRE can provide valuable diagnostic information to the practitioner in certain clinical scenarios, including GI bleeding and particularly with disorders of defecation, such as constipation and fecal incontinence

Division of Gastroenterology, Washington University School of Medicine, 915 North Grand Boulevard, St. Louis, MO 63106, USA; Department of Psychiatry, Washington University School of Medicine, 915 North Grand Boulevard, St. Louis, MO 63106, USA; St. Louis Veterans Affairs Medical Center, St. Louis, MO, USA
E-mail address: gsayuk@wustl.edu

Gastroenterol Clin N Am 51 (2022) 25–37
https://doi.org/10.1016/j.gtc.2021.10.003
0889-8553/22/Published by Elsevier Inc.
gastro.theclinics.com

(FI). The performance of this straightforward evaluation yields a wealth of information beyond an assessment of anal sphincter tone and the contents of the rectal vault. A perianal inspection and DRE hold the potential to make diagnoses of anal and rectal malignancies, structural abnormalities such as hemorrhoids, fissures or fistulas, infections including condyloma acuminata ("anal warts") or perianal abscesses, detect the presence of blood, and even provide diagnostic clues regarding neuromuscular conditions. Yet, the value of this test is dependent on the training and experience of the clinician. For a variety of reasons, even gastroenterology providers often neglect to perform a DRE when clinically indicated. Unfortunately, deferral of a DRE in some cases may result in unnecessary, additional diagnostic testing and health care utilization, and even more importantly, delays in diagnosis, continued symptoms, and misguided therapeutic trials. This review will discuss the considerations and proper steps in the performance of the DRE, with a particular focus on patient complaints of constipation or FI, and it will summarize the data supporting the value of this examination in patients presenting with these defecatory disorders.

OBSTACLES TO PERFORMING DRE
Insufficient DRE Training in Medical Education

One major obstacle to the confident performance of a competent DRE is a lack of instruction and supervision in the performance of this examination while in training. A survey of Australian fourth-year medical students indicated that the vast majority regarded the DRE to be an essential skill for medical practitioners, and one that should be mastered before graduation.[1] Yet, the median number of rectal examinations conducted while in training by the students was 2, with nearly 1 in 5 students reporting that they had never performed a DRE. Hence only one-half of the students felt confident that they could perform a reasonable DRE. Another study of nearly 400 Irish medical students in their final year of training across 5 medical schools revealed that one-fourth of the medical students had no experience in performing a DRE, with an additional 20% indicating only having completed the maneuver on practice mannequins.[2] Of the 56% of the respondents who endorsed some experience with DRE, one-third of these students reported a lack of confidence in their ability to perform and interpret this examination. A survey of US physicians found that 93% reported DRE training in medical school, yet over one-fourth of these same individuals indicated that experience was "very little," or "not at all" sufficient.[3] Collectively, these data portray clear deficiencies in the adequacy of medical school training in DRE.

Lack of Physician Comfort and Confidence in Performing DRE

Inefficiencies and inexperience in training may result in many practitioners feeling uncomfortable with the performance of DREs. In the previously noted survey of US physicians, several other reasons for not performing DRE evaluations were cited, including concern for the modesty of the patient (43.8%), the perceived invasiveness of the evaluation (39.6%), and a deferral of the examination during the clinic visit due to a planned future colonoscopy (35.6%).[3] This indicates that DRE often is either not performed, or at a minimum is underutilized in the evaluation of patients with defecatory disorders.[4] Interestingly, junior physicians more often cited these concerns as reasons to defer the performance of a rectal examination.[4] However, the hesitancy on behalf of practitioners to perform DRE is not matched by patient refusal of the examination. The physician survey indicated that fewer than 10% of patients decline DRE when recommended, and that this patient deferral correlates with physician specialty (gastroenterologists < primary care) and physician experience (senior < junior).[4] In fact, patients are willing to undergo DRE, and when it is not performed were indicated, patients notice: a survey administered in the waiting room of a primary care clinic to over 400 patients found that 91% of patients "would have allowed" a rectal examination to be performed, and 56% thought DRE "should have been done by a reasonable health care provider", yet DRE was actually completed on only 16% of these respondents.[5]

Deferral of DRE to Future Testing

An oft-cited rationale for foregoing DRE evaluation in the office is the plan for additional imaging, manometric, and/or colonoscopic assessment of the patient's defecatory issue. There are, however, several shortcomings to this approach. Although anorectal manometry, defecography, and colonoscopy are all reasonable studies for the evaluation of FI and functional defecation disorders, and might indeed provide similar information as a DRE, some patients may ultimately cancel or not follow-through on recommendations for these tests leading to missed, or at a minimum, unnecessary delays in diagnosis.[6] Furthermore, the protocols of some of these studies include the use of a bowel preparation or enema, which might result in the loss of potentially valuable information and clinical clues—the content and texture of stool in the rectal vault, for example. Lastly, a rectal examination during colonoscopy is often performed in parallel with the administration of sedation. This may not only affect sphincter tone but also compromise the patient's ability to participate in the functional components (bear down and squeeze maneuvers) of the DRE.

Publications Calling into Question the Clinical Value of DRE

The DRE has been disparaged in the literature as an "unpleasant, invasive," and "useless examination," representing "flimsy thinking and bad medicine" on behalf of the provider.[7] However, this limited view in part comes from the perspective of general practitioners, with an interest in examination of the prostate and colon cancer screening (where admittedly the value of DRE is somewhat uncertain), rather than the more sophisticated pursuit of the DRE with functional maneuvers to evaluate disorders of defecation. It is generally agreed upon that performance of fecal occult blood testing on a DRE specimen is of little value given the higher potential for false-positive results.[8] It has also been suggested that symptom scales are necessary for the clinical assessment of defecation disorders, particularly FI, as the DRE is neither sufficient for evaluating the severity of defects in continence mechanisms, nor accurate in predicting response to therapy.[9]

In pediatric populations, the 2014 North American Society for Pediatric Gastroenterology, Hepatology, and Nutrition (NASPGHAN) and the European Society for Pediatric Gastroenterology, Hepatology, and Nutrition (ESGHAN) evidence-based recommendations for the evaluation and treatment of functional constipation concluded that "evidence does not support the use of digital rectal examination to diagnose functional constipation"[10] based on a single study assessing the ability of DRE to discriminate between radiographically constipated and nonconstipated children. In this study, DRE demonstrated a sensitivity of 77%, and a specificity of only 35%, yielding a likelihood ratio of 1.2 (95% confidence interval [CI], 1.0 to 1.4).[11] However experts have argued that this pediatric population did not reflect the broader pediatric GI population, that the DRE methodology used did not apply the more sophisticated application of this examination, and that the assessment of DRE application did not consider the detection of other conditions in the differential diagnosis.[6]

Underutilization of the DRE

As a result of these challenges and obstacles to the performance of DRE, it should come with little surprise that this examination is often neglected by practitioners, even at top academic institutions. A survey of nearly 200 medical students and over 400 clinicians (including 128 adult gastroenterology faculty or fellows) across 4 United States medical schools found that these clinicians self-reported having performed only a median of 10 DRE examinations in the prior year, with much higher utilization of this technique reported by more experienced and specialized physicians.[3] Indeed, over 500 annual DREs were reported by 10 gastroenterologists, and GI physicians in this cohort performed 10 times the number of DRE evaluations compared with their internist counterparts. Physicians who have graduated within the past 4 years reported performing an average of 29 DREs per year, whereas those who have been in practice for more than 20 years indicated that they performed 4 times this number.[3] These data strongly suggest that the DRE may represent a "dying art," particularly among general practices, again underscoring the importance of adequate training and supervision in the performance of this examination as an early, formative experience for medical trainees.

PERFORMING A PROPER DRE

> *"By far your greatest aide will be the finger. The majority of diseases which affect the rectum can be made out by the educated finger."*
> Joseph M. Mathews, M.D., A Treatise on Diseases of the Rectum, Anus, and Sigmoid Flexure, 1897[12]

The benefits of a properly performed rectal examination in the evaluation of defecatory disorders, including constipation and FI, have been appreciated for many decades. The aforementioned data regarding DRE training, and our anecdotal experience with GI trainees suggest it is worthwhile to review, in detail, the steps necessary to perform an appropriate DRE.

Anatomic Considerations

Pertinent anatomy evaluated during a DRE includes the terminal segment of large bowel, or rectum, which is positioned along the sacrum and estimated to be approximately 12 to 15 cm in length, the anal sphincters, which are 3 to 4 cm in length and composed of voluntary, external skeletal sphincter muscle and internal, involuntary smooth muscle (the latter responsible for the majority of the resting anal sphincter tone), and the levator ani muscle group composed of the pubococcygeus, iliococcygeus, and puborectalis muscles.[13] A very elegant study by Joguet and colleagues describes the pelvic anatomy relevant to DRE based on a cadaveric study, and moreover describes average measurements of the index finger in an adult male and female cohort, noting their fingers to be of sufficient length to palpate all of the anatomic landmarks of interest.[14] The anatomy and physiology essential to pelvic floor function is described in full detail in the Ravinder K. Mittal and Lori J. Tuttle ' article, "Anorectal Anatomy and Function," in this issue.

Contraindications

It has been suggested that the only absolute contraindication to the performance of a DRE is that the practitioner "has lost all of his or her fingers"![15] Relative contraindications of note, however, include patients who are acutely ill or immunosuppressed (particularly with neutropenia), the latter due to potential for development of perianal abscesses or sepsis due to bacterial seeding.[16] Other considerations wherein the risk-benefit of DRE must be assessed include patients who have recently undergone anorectal surgery, have experienced rectal trauma, have known anal or distal rectal strictures, stenoses, or ulcerations, or have evidence of thrombocytopenia or other coagulopathies. Patients reporting severe anal pain upon initiation of the rectal examination may be better served by an examination under anesthesia to identify the source of symptoms.

A Stepwise Approach to DRE

Preparing for the DRE

The first step in performing a DRE is the preparation of the patient for the examination. This includes a discussion of the indication for the evaluation and a description of the steps involved in the process. It is important to acknowledge that there may be some minor discomfort or a sense of urgency.[6] It is also helpful to reassure the patient that the majority tolerate the procedure very well, while also encouraging the patient to be forthcoming if the examination becomes exceedingly uncomfortable. A nearby bathroom is advisable, and we ask patients whether they feel the need to use the facilities before proceeding.

Next in the periprocedure planning is the gathering of necessary supplies including examination gloves, water-soluble lubrication, viscous lidocaine or lidocaine jelly (if a painful condition such as hemorrhoids or an anal fissure is anticipated), accessory lighting for adequate visualization, facial tissues, cotton swabs, a patient gown, and sheets for patient draping. It is suggested that all the examination rooms routinely used for DRE be routinely stocked with these supplies. It is also important to have a room with an appropriate examination table and a curtain for privacy. We perform all DRE evaluations in the presence of a nurse chaperone.

Patient positioning for DRE

Patients should change into an examination gown without removing their undergarments. Left lateral decubitus positioning is recommended, and the study is best performed with the buttocks shifted to the edge of the examination table and the knees and hips flexed and drawn toward the chest. Having patients stand and lean forward over a raised table on their elbows is a position sometimes implemented by urologists and primary care physicians for an examination of the prostate, but it is suboptimal for assessing defecatory disorders. Furthermore, some patients may experience premonitory symptoms or frank vasovagal syncope during the examination, placing them at risk of falling and injuring themselves. We generally have the nurse chaperone position at the head of the examination table to offer reassurance and support the patient through the examination.

Inspection and external maneuvers

The patient is asked to lower their undergarments, allowing an opportunity to subtly inspect for evidence of fecal or urinary seepage or soiling. Thereafter, a careful visual inspection of the perineal and perianal areas is useful to evaluate for anatomic clues relating to the patient's defecatory complaints. The presence of leaked stool, skin erythema, and/or excoriation/maceration may be indicators of fecal seepage or excessive wiping. Other important findings include anal fissures or fistulae, external hemorrhoids, skin tags, scars, perianal abscesses, condylomata acuminata ("anal warts"), or anal neoplasm.

Next, the patient is informed that an examination of the anal area and palpation of the anus and surrounding tissue will be conducted to assess for appreciable tenderness or fluctuance. A Valsalva-like maneuver is conducted wherein the patient is asked to "bear down." The nondominant examining hand can be placed on the abdominal wall anteriorly during this maneuver to determine whether the patient is using excessive abdominal effort in the generation of "push pressure." This maneuver may reveal prolapse of internal hemorrhoids, seepage of stool, or provoke a gaping or patulous anus. Perineal descent, normally around 2 to 3 cm, should also be evident.[17,18] Occasionally this maneuver will precipitate rectal procidentia ("prolapse") with the appearance of a deeper red "mass" descending through the anal verge. Complete (full thickness) rectal procidentia results from the protrusion of all of the rectal layers through the anus, appearing as concentric rings of rectal mucosa. Partial (mucosal) procidentia involves prolapse of only rectal mucosa. Rectal prolapse is more commonly associated with FI, but it can also present as a consequence of straining or act as an anatomic outlet obstruction in association with constipation.

Finally, anocutaneous reflex ("anal wink") testing is performed to determine whether sacral spinal nerve (S2-S5) reflex pathways are intact. Stroking the perineum/perianal area lightly in a 4-quadrant fashion using a cotton swab should lead to involuntary, reflexive contraction of the external anal sphincter.[15] If the cotton tip fails to elicit a sensory response and/or reflex, the test can be repeated with the stick end of the swab. This reflex may be less robust under normal circumstances, but the complete absence of any response is an indication for further, more detailed neurologic evaluation.

Internal maneuvers

Successful completion of an internal examination is predicated on facilitating patient relaxation and comfort. It is essential to detail each step in a relaxed, succinct fashion before initiating each maneuver. Note that the particular order in which internal maneuvers are completed varies by practitioner and no standard protocol has been established. Insertion of the practitioner's index finger (usually of the dominant hand) across the anal sphincter and into the rectum is preceded by application of water-soluble lubrication along the length of the finger. Gentle massage of the posterior ("6 o'clock") margin of the anus with the fingertip will induce relaxation of the anal sphincter, facilitating introduction of the examiner's finger, angled slightly posteriorly, across the anal canal into the rectum. Ideally, the finger should be positioned across the entire length of the anal sphincter (approximately 4 cm), which for most examiners will be at the level just beyond their proximal interphalangeal joint. If a great deal of resistance is met, or in the case of smaller pediatric patients, the fifth ("pinky") finger can be used for this initial portion of the examination. If the patient experiences minor pain, viscous lidocaine can be applied, and the examination should be paused for several minutes to allow it to take effect. If, however, the pain is more extreme, this may be indicative of a deeper anal fissure, which was not identified during the external inspection. In this instance, the examination should be aborted and further investigation via an examination under anesthesia is warranted.

Once the patient is relaxed and has accommodated to the examination, one can gauge resting anal sphincter tone. Resting tone has an important role in the maintenance of fecal continence, with the majority of this tone contributed by the internal anal sphincter.[19] Low resting anal sphincter tone may indicate prior sphincter injury with increased risk of FI, whereas higher resting tone may be indicative of anal hypertension and an anatomic outlet obstruction.[20] Once the resting tone has been established, squeeze maneuvers are pursued. Healthy individuals should be able to demonstrate an increase in external anal sphincter tone and contraction of the puborectalis muscle. Individuals with functional defecation disorders may exhibit an exceedingly robust squeeze, whereas FI patients may have minimal ability to recruit additional musculature. A cough maneuver is another means by which one can assess involuntary squeeze of the anal sphincter complex.

Once these initial studies are completed, the examining finger should palpate the distal most margins of the rectum, noting the presence of hemorrhoids or masses. It is subsequently advanced an additional 2 to 3 cm and rotated to the 12-o'clock position. This allows for palpation of the anterior portion of the rectum where detection of a bulge may indicate the presence of a rectocele. It also allows for palpation of the prostate in men, and the cervix in women. The levator ani muscles should also be assessed as tenderness with traction (especially on the left side) may be indicative of chronic proctalgia or more specifically levator ani syndrome.[21]

Careful attention to the texture of stool in the rectal vault is also essential. In more overt cases of fecal impaction, the presence of a hard scybalous mass (ie, "stool ball") may be apparent. Nonimpacted hard stools (eg, Bristol 1 and 2) are also informative and could factor into the development of "overflow" diarrhea. Even patients with textures in the normal range of the Bristol Stool Form Scale (Bristol 3–5) may experience a functional defecation disorder, particularly if the patient endorses straining to pass softer stools. The presence of loose, watery stool in a patient with FI provides a clinical clue that diarrhea may be the precipitant.

Finally, the function of the pelvic floor unit as a whole can be tested by asking the patient to bear down and attempt to "push out the finger." Under normal circumstances, relaxation of the anal sphincter should be easily discerned and, if the patient generates enough pressure, the finger may be expelled. Appropriate descent of the perineum can also be detected. Paradoxic contraction or failure to relax the anal sphincter and/or puborectalis muscles may be detected in the setting of functional defecation disorders. The tip of the examining finger can be used to discern relaxation of the puborectalis under normal circumstances. Here again, the dyssynergia patient may exhibit further contraction of the puborectalis with a push maneuver, palpable as a "pulling" of the fingertip anteriorly and superiorly.

If there is any concern that the patient did not understand these instructions, we will attempt to repeat any of the maneuvers. Upon completion of these evaluations, the examining finger is withdrawn and the stool on the glove is assessed for the presence of blood or mucus. Performance of fecal occult testing is discouraged because of the potential for false-positive results.[8] Return of anal sphincter tone following withdrawal of the finger should be almost immediate. The appearance of a patulous anus or slow return of tone may be indicative of a sphincter injury or neurologic issue. Facial tissue should be used to remove excess lubrication or externalized stool before the patient is directed to a private setting (ideally a bathroom) to address any hygiene or toileting needs and return to their street clothes. A summary of these maneuvers as well as characteristic findings in patients with FI and functional defecation disorders are provided in **Table 1**. More detailed technical descriptions of the DRE plus video training are provided by Ylitalo and colleagues[21] and Talley and colleagues[15]

Special Patient Populations

Pediatric patients

Though not without controversy, most experts agree that the DRE can be of considerable diagnostic utility in pediatric patients—in particular, those with reported FI or constipation. However, DREs may be deferred by providers to an even greater degree in this patient population.[6,16] A survey of children's hospital patients and their parents revealed that over 75% of children with chronic constipation were referred to a gastroenterologist without the performance of a rectal examination. Indeed, over half of these children were found to have fecal impaction upon completion of DRE.[22] As in all cases, the performance of a DRE should be justified based on its potential diagnostic value. Most of the same technical considerations relevant to DRE in the adult patient also are applicable to this younger population. Depending on the age of the patient, the use of the fifth finger, rather than the index finger, may be necessary to minimize discomfort. There are some additional concerns relating to the potential for psychologically traumatic experiences in pediatric patients. For a very nice review

Table 1
DRE maneuvers and expected findings in healthy individuals and those with defecatory disorders

DRE Component/Maneuver	Expected findings (Normal)	Potential findings in Functional Defecation Disorders	Potential findings in fecal incontinence
Inspection of perineum/perianal area	Healthy skin, good anal tone, hemorrhoids, no soiling of perineum/undergarments	External hemorrhoids, skin tags, anal fissure; normal anal tone; no soiling (minor if prolapsing internal hemorrhoids or overflow diarrhea)	Erythema, excoriation, maceration of skin; fecal soiling/seepage; visually patulous anus
Palpation of anus/perineum	Unremarkable, without pain or fluctuance	Normal, pain if fissure, thrombosed hemorrhoid, or perianal abscess	Usually normal
Anocutaneous reflex	Good sensation and "anal wink" (can be weak and still regarded as normal)	Normal	Normal in most cases; decreased sensation/"wink" if neurologic etiology (diabetes, pudendal neuropathy, Parkinson's, spinal cord compression/injury)
Assessment of resting anal tone	Mild resistance to passage of distal phalange of finger, no pain	Normal, or increased resistance to passage of finger; mild pain with hemorrhoids, extreme pain with fissure	Normal, or decreased resistance to passage of finger (weak)
Palpation of rectum	No findings, internal hemorrhoids	Normal or harder stool content (Bristol 1–5), internal hemorrhoids, rectocele	
Palpation of levator ani	No tenderness	Normal, tenderness if levator ani syndrome/proctalgia fugax	Normal
Push/bear down maneuver	Relaxed abdomen, appropriate lower abdomen tone, anal sphincter and puborectalis relaxation, good (2-3 cm) perineal descent	Breath hold, strain with excess abdominal tension, anal sphincter and/or puborectalis contraction ("pulling of fingertip") or lack of relaxation, excess perineal descent (>4 cm), rare rectal prolapse	Normal or discoordinated push, excess anal sphincter relaxation, minimal (<1 cm) perineal descent, rectal prolapse

Squeeze maneuver	Increased anal/puborectalis tone	Excess anal/puborectalis tone	Minimal increase in anal/puborectalis tone with neuropathy; compensatory strong contraction of external sphincter/puborectalis with internal sphincter injury
Post-DRE inspection	Normal	Normal	Patulous/gaping anus

of special considerations relating to pediatric DRE, please see the review by Orenstein and Wald.[6]

Elderly and chronically ill patients

Older, frail, and chronically ill patients are more susceptible to the development of FI and constipation, including fecal impaction. Such patients generally are less mobile and tend to be prescribed greater numbers of medications. The performance of a DRE may provide sufficient insights into defecatory disorders in this population, thereby precluding the need for more disruptive and invasive testing. Elderly patients may be more susceptible to local trauma with DRE; thus, a particularly gentle approach is warranted. Similarly, these patients may be more likely to suffer from musculoskeletal pain, making left lateral decubitus positioning uncomfortable. The clinician should be sensitive to these considerations and adjust the positioning and approach accordingly. Despite the potential benefit of DRE as a readily accessible, bedside diagnostic tool in this special population, one study of over 160 tertiary, referral palliative care inpatients disappointingly observed that only 4% of these patients had a DRE recorded in their chart (with scant details about the examination findings) in spite of the fact that over 40% of the included individuals had constipation, diarrhea, or incontinence listed as an active medical problem.[23]

DIAGNOSTIC PERFORMANCE OF DRE

Several studies have been conducted to examine the diagnostic yield of DRE, compared to manometric evaluation as the gold standard. In a large study of over 200 constipated patients by Tantiphlachiva and colleagues,[4] 87% of these individuals were found to have dyssynergic defecation based on standard manometric criteria.[24] 73% of these same individuals were found to have a dyssynergia phenotype on DRE. This yielded a good sensitivity (75%) and specificity (87%) for DRE, with an overall positive predictive value of 97% suggesting DRE to be a robust bedside test for the detection of dyssynergic defecation. DRE was also very accurate in detecting normal anal resting tone (86%), squeeze pressure (88%), and impairments in anal sphincter relaxation, that is, "paradoxic contraction" (82%). DRE performed less robustly for detecting reduced resting anal tone (15%) or squeeze pressures (52%) when compared with manometry. It is worth noting that the rectal examinations performed in this study were performed by "a single expert with extensive experience in evaluating patients with constipation and pelvic floor disorders." Whether these results are replicable among general internists or less experienced gastroenterologists requires further study.

An older study comparing DRE to anal sphincter manometry among a cohort of fecally incontinent patients and healthy controls identified good correlations between basal anal sphincter assessment on DRE and manometry (r = 0.56, $P < .001$) and squeeze scores on the DRE compared with manometric assessments of maximal squeeze pressure (r = 0.72, $P < .001$), with similar separation of the continent control and incontinent patients using DRE evaluation or manometry.[25]

A Korean study evaluating a large cohort of patients with chronic constipation (n = 268; 77.2% with dyssynergia via abnormal high-resolution anorectal manometry [HRAM]/balloon expulsion testing) or FI (n = 41) found DRE to have good sensitivity (93.2%), specificity (58.7%), and positive predictive value (91.0%) for dyssynergia using manometry as the gold standard.[26] This led to moderate diagnostic agreement between DRE and HRAM (K = 0.542, $P < .001$). In the FI subset, moderate agreement was detected between anal squeeze pressure measurements on DRE and HRAM (K = 0.418, $P = .006$), but similar to the findings in the Tantiphlachiva study,[4] there was poorer agreement in the two testing methods with regard to anal tone at rest.

Experience with the performance of DRE improves accuracy: in a study of 36 patients with FI or chronic constipation, very high agreements in squeeze and resting anal pressures were detected between ARM and DREs performed by experienced colorectal surgeons (K = 0.96 and 0.7, respectively), whereas junior colorectal surgeon ARM-DRE agreement was considerably lower (K = 0.52 for each measure).[27] Another study reported the results of a DRE examination of FI patients by a single experienced physician and found that DRE findings were concordant with ARM evaluations of anal sphincter pressure. Moreover, the features detected on digital examination correlated with clinical presentations (ie, urge incontinence of feces).[28] Certain clinical scenarios may challenge the diagnostic accuracy of DRE, including the presence of chronic anal fissures. In this setting, one study found that DRE appeared to adequately identify patients with high resting sphincter pressures (sensitivity of 93%) but performed poorly in determining those individuals with low or normal sphincter pressures (specificity of only 16%) yielding a positive predictive value of merely 40% in chronic fissure patients.[29] Also, although DRE performs reasonably well at assessing internal and external anal sphincter function, it is less sensitive to the determination of possible external anal sphincter defects.[30]

Finally, attempts have been made to implement scoring systems for more objective quantification of anal sphincter tone during the DRE. One such approach, the Digital Rectal Examination Scoring System (DRESS), applies a 0 to 5 scoring (3 = normal) to anal tone at rest and with squeeze. A strong positive correlation between the DRESS values and manometry pressures was established (coefficients of 0.82 for resting pressure and 0.81 for squeeze pressure).[31]

SUMMARY

DRE provides reasonably accurate assessments of anal sphincter tone and defecatory function in individuals with FI and functional defecation disorders.[32] In addition, physiologic and structural testing (anorectal manometry, rectal sensation and compliance evaluation, endoanal ultrasound, pudendal nerve terminal motor latency, pelvic magnetic resonance imaging, and anal sphincter electromyography) provides additional, complementary objective information.[18,33] Such additional testing may be useful in determining appropriate therapeutic interventions.

A major obstacle to clinician confidence is the lack of sufficient education and hands-on experience received during medical training. Formal DRE educational programs have been described including the practice of DRE maneuvers on simulated models and the performance of DREs on dedicated rectal teaching associates. These strategies appear to be effective at enhancing global DRE skills on objective structured clinical examinations and enhancing learner confidence in the examination.[34,35] Furthermore, it has been demonstrated that DRE education modules have a direct impact on practice patterns. Direct education of emergency room physicians has resulted in greater utilization and reliance on DRE, with significant decreases in the use of abdominal imaging, even among pediatric populations.[36]

Once clinicians are trained and are more confident in their DRE skills, these techniques will become more refined and an "educated finger" will result. It is then that the clinician can optimally use DRE as a readily available, accurate, and cost-effective tool in the evaluation of patients presenting with defecatory disorders.

Clinical care points

• Mastering the digital rectal examination (DRE) requires dedicated training and hands-on experience.

- The steps of performing a DRE can be developed into a systematic protocol easily implemented in almost any clinical setting.
- Provider hesitation in performing DRE is generally greater than the patient's concerns with regard to undergoing this evaluation.
- The performance of DRE during a clinic visit should not be postponed for future testing (eg, planned imaging or colonoscopy) as this may impose delays in diagnosis.
- With practice and clinical experience, DRE has the potential to achieve comparable accuracy to objective diagnostic testing, including anorectal manometry.

REFERENCES

1. Lawrentschuk N, Bolton DM. Experience and attitudes of final-year medical students to digital rectal examination. Med J Aust 2004;181(6):323–5.
2. Fitzgerald D, Connolly SS, Kerin MJ. Digital rectal examination: national survey of undergraduate medical training in Ireland. Postgrad Med J 2007;83(983): 599–601.
3. Wong RK, Drossman DA, Bharucha AE, et al. The digital rectal examination: a multicenter survey of physicians' and students' perceptions and practice patterns. Am J Gastroenterol 2012;107(8):1157–63.
4. Tantiphlachiva K, Rao P, Attaluri A, et al. Digital rectal examination is a useful tool for identifying patients with dyssynergia. Clin Gastroenterol Hepatol 2010;8(11): 955–60.
5. Duan L, Mukherjee EM, Federman DG. The physical examination: a survey of patient preferences and expectations during primary care visits. Postgrad Med 2020;132(1):102–8.
6. Orenstein SR, Wald A. Pediatric Rectal Exam: Why, When, and How. Curr Gastroenterol Rep 2016;18(1):4.
7. Spence D. Bad medicine: digital rectal examination. BMJ 2011;342:d3421.
8. Longstreth GF. Checking for "the occult" with a finger. A procedure of little value. J Clin Gastroenterol 1988;10(2):133–4.
9. Rockwood TH, Church JM, Fleshman JW, et al. Patient and surgeon ranking of the severity of symptoms associated with fecal incontinence: the fecal incontinence severity index. Dis Colon Rectum 1999;42(12):1525–32.
10. Tabbers MM, DiLorenzo C, Berger MY, et al. Evaluation and treatment of functional constipation in infants and children: evidence-based recommendations from ESPGHAN and NASPGHAN. J Pediatr Gastroenterol Nutr 2014;58(2): 258–74.
11. Beckmann KR, Hennes H, Sty JR, et al. Accuracy of clinical variables in the identification of radiographically proven constipation in children. WMJ 2001; 100(1):33–6.
12. Mathews JM. A Treatise on diseases of the rectum, anus, and Sigmoid flexure. 2nd, revised edition. New York: D. Appleton and Company; 1897.
13. Raizada N, Mittal P, Suri J, et al. Comparative study to evaluate the intersystem association and reliability between standard pelvic organ prolapse quantification system and simplified pelvic organ prolapse scoring system. J Obstet Gynaecol India 2014;64(6):421–4.
14. Joguet E, Robert R, Labat JJ, et al. Anatomical basis of digital rectal examination. Surg Radiol Anat 2012;34(1):73–9.
15. Talley NJ. How to do and interpret a rectal examination in gastroenterology. Am J Gastroenterol 2008;103(4):820–2.

16. Villanueva Herrero JA, Abdussalam A, Kasi A. Rectal exam. *StatPearls*. Treasure Island: FL; 2021.
17. Baek HN, Hwang YH, Jung YH. Clinical Significance of Perineal Descent in Pelvic Outlet Obstruction Diagnosed by using Defecography. J Korean Soc Coloproctol 2010;26(6):395–401.
18. Bharucha AE, Fletcher JG, Seide B, et al. Phenotypic variation in functional disorders of defecation. Gastroenterology 2005;128(5):1199–210.
19. Raizada V, Mittal RK. Pelvic floor anatomy and applied physiology. Gastroenterol Clin North Am 2008;37(3):493–509.
20. Carrington EV, Popa SL, Chiarioni G. Proctalgia Syndromes: Update in Diagnosis and Management. Curr Gastroenterol Rep 2020;22(7):35.
21. Ylitalo AW. Digital Rectal Exam. 2017. Available at: https://emedicine.medscape.com/article/1948001-overview. Accessed April 1, 2021.
22. Gold DM, Levine J, Weinstein TA, et al. Frequency of digital rectal examination in children with chronic constipation. Arch Pediatr Adolesc Med 1999;153(4):377–9.
23. Clark K, Currow DC, Talley NJ. The use of digital rectal examinations in palliative care inpatients. J Palliat Med 2010;13(7):797.
24. Karlbom U, Graf W, Nilsson S, et al. The accuracy of clinical examination in the diagnosis of rectal intussusception. Dis Colon Rectum 2004;47(9):1533–8.
25. Hallan RI, Marzouk DE, Waldron DJ, et al. Comparison of digital and manometric assessment of anal sphincter function. Br J Surg 1989;76(9):973–5.
26. Soh JS, Lee HJ, Jung KW, et al. The diagnostic value of a digital rectal examination compared with high-resolution anorectal manometry in patients with chronic constipation and fecal incontinence. Am J Gastroenterol 2015;110(8):1197–204.
27. Pinto RA, Correa Neto IJF, Nahas SC, et al. Is the Physician Expertise in Digital Rectal Examination of Value in Detecting Anal Tone in Comparison to Anorectal Manometry? Arq Gastroenterol 2019;56(1):79–83.
28. Hill J, Corson RJ, Brandon H, et al. History and examination in the assessment of patients with idiopathic fecal incontinence. Dis Colon Rectum 1994;37(5):473–7.
29. Jones OM, Ramalingam T, Lindsey I, et al. Digital rectal examination of sphincter pressures in chronic anal fissure is unreliable. Dis Colon Rectum 2005;48(2):349–52.
30. Dobben AC, Terra MP, Deutekom M, et al. Anal inspection and digital rectal examination compared to anorectal physiology tests and endoanal ultrasonography in evaluating fecal incontinence. Int J Colorectal Dis 2007;22(7):783–90.
31. Orkin BA, Sinykin SB, Lloyd PC. The digital rectal examination scoring system (DRESS). Dis Colon Rectum 2010;53(12):1656–60.
32. Wald A. Con: Anorectal manometry and imaging are not necessary in patients with fecal incontinence. Am J Gastroenterol 2006;101(12):2681–3.
33. Bharucha AE. Pro: Anorectal testing is useful in fecal incontinence. Am J Gastroenterol 2006;101(12):2679–81.
34. Isherwood J, Ashkir Z, Panteleimonitis S, et al. Teaching digital rectal examination to medical students using a structured workshop-a point in the right direction? J Surg Educ 2013;70(2):254–7.
35. Popadiuk C, Pottle M, Curran V. Teaching digital rectal examinations to medical students: an evaluation study of teaching methods. Acad Med 2002;77(11):1140–6.
36. Kurowski J, Kaur S, Katsogridakis Y, et al. Educational Module Improves Emergency Department Evaluation for Suspected Constipation. J Pediatr 2015;167(3):706–10.e1.

Diagnostic Strategy and Tools for Identifying Defecatory Disorders

Adil E. Bharucha, MBBS, MD[a],*, Enrique Coss-Adame, MD[b,1]

KEYWORDS

- High-resolution anorectal manometry • MRI • Biofeedback therapy • Constipation
- Anal sphincter

KEY POINTS

- Among constipated patients who have not responded to laxatives, anorectal tests are necessary to diagnose defecatory disorders, which should be managed with pelvic floor biofeedback therapy rather than with laxatives.
- In such patients, anal manometry and a rectal balloon expulsion test are initially performed, followed by other tests as necessary. Some centers use defecography in lieu of the rectal balloon expulsion test.
- At a high level, the methods for these tests are standardized. However, the details of methods and normal values vary among techniques.
- Anorectal functions are affected by age and sex. Test results should be interpreted with reference to normal values generated by the same technique.

INTRODUCTION

Based on an assessment of anorectal tests and colonic transit, patients with chronic constipation can be classified into 3 groups: normal transit constipation, slow transit constipation, and defecatory disorders (DD).[1] This review focuses on DD, which are a common cause for chronic constipation and result from a disturbance in the rectoanal functions that facilitate normal defecation.[1,2] Diagnostic tests are necessary because (i) symptoms alone cannot discriminate between DD and other causes of chronic constipation[3] and (ii) DD are optimally managed with pelvic floor biofeedback therapy rather than laxatives.[4,5]

Copyright 2021 Mayo Foundation
[a] Division of Gastroenterology and Hepatology, Mayo Clinic, 200 1st Street SW, Rochester, MN 55905, USA; [b] Department of Gastroenterology, Instituto Nacional de Ciencias Médicas y Nutrición "Salvador Zubirán", México City, Mexico
[1] Present address: Ocaso 51, Interior 105, Col Insurgentes Cuicuilco, Coyoacán, CDMX, Mexico, CP 04530.
* Corresponding author. Division of Gastroenterology and Hepatology, Mayo Clinic, 200 1st Street SW, Rochester, MN 55905, USA.
E-mail address: bharucha.adil@mayo.edu

CLINICAL ASSESSMENT

A meticulous clinical evaluation may suggest the presence of a DD. Before the consultation, the authors ask patients to complete a bowel symptom questionnaire.[1] Thereafter, the symptoms can be confirmed during the interview, aided by pictorial stool form scales. Intuitively, some symptoms (eg, anal digitation, sense of anal blockage during defecation, sense of incomplete evacuation after defecation) suggest a DD. When considered in isolation (ie, not together with the findings of a digital rectal examination), symptoms evaluated with a questionnaire do not discriminate between DD and other causes of constipation.[6,7] Questionnaires provide a snapshot of bowel habits at one point in time. Among patients who have varying stool consistency, they do not disclose whether bowel symptoms are related to the stool consistency. This is an important issue because even healthy people may struggle to evacuate hard stools.[8] It is the authors' perception that difficulty with evacuating soft stools, particularly liquid stools or enemas, strongly suggests disordered defecation. Bowel diaries are extremely useful for characterizing the relationship between stool consistency and ease of defecation.

The onset and history of bowel disturbances should be elicited. Upon inquiry, many patients acknowledge that their symptoms have existed for longer than initially acknowledged, perhaps since childhood.[9] Inadvertent withholding, perhaps secondary to an aversion to using public toilets, or constipation after recent surgery, medication changes, or coexistent urinary symptoms is not uncommon. Not infrequently, irritable bowel syndrome (IBS) and pelvic floor dysfunction will coexist.[10]

A careful digital rectal examination is mandatory.[11] Inspection may disclose an anal fissure or hemorrhoids. A digital rectal examination is useful to assess anal pressure at rest, when patients contract or squeeze their anal sphincter and pelvic floor muscles, and during simulated evacuation.[12,13] Normally, simulated evacuation is accompanied by relaxation of the anal sphincter and puborectalis muscle and perineal descent by 1 to 4 cm. Patients with DD may have anismus (ie, high anal resting pressure), reduced or excessive perineal descent (ie, ballooning of the perineum), and/or rectal prolapse. The puborectalis may not relax normally or paradoxically may contract during simulated evacuation. However, relaxation of the puborectalis may not be perceptible even in patients with normal anorectal functions. Therefore, except for patients who have paradoxical puborectalis contraction, abnormal perineal descent, particularly if markedly reduced or absent, is more useful than impaired puborectalis relaxation for identifying DD.

RATIONALE FOR ANORECTAL TESTS

Although pelvic floor dysfunction can often be excluded or confirmed with reasonable confidence by a careful clinical assessment, anorectal testing is required because studies suggest that a clinical assessment alone does not suffice for identifying DD.[6,7] Moreover, many patients are reassured by objective documentation of a DD, and insurance providers require this before covering pelvic floor retraining by biofeedback therapy. In most patients, anorectal manometry and a rectal balloon expulsion test suffice to confirm or exclude DD. In selected circumstances, additional tests may be necessary as detailed in later discussion.

ANORECTAL MANOMETRY

Anorectal manometry can be performed with conventional catheters that incorporate water-perfused, air-charged, solid-state sensors or with high-resolution catheters (ie, high-resolution manometry [HRM] or 3-dimensional high-resolution anorectal manometry (3D- HR-ARM).[14–18]

Catheter Design

HRM and HDM catheters have 2 benefits over conventional systems. First, because they have more closely spaced sensors that span the entire anal canal, the entire procedure can be performed without moving the catheter (ie, a pull-through maneuver is unnecessary). Hence, each procedure takes less time, perhaps 15 minutes for selected HRM protocols.[19] Second, HRM catheters provide better spatial resolution. There are differences among HRM catheters made by different manufacturers (**Fig. 1**). Conventional and HRM catheters measure anal pressures with comparable precision. Pressures measured with HRM or HDM are much higher, probably because of the manner in which pressures are analyzed.[20]

The HRM catheters made by Medtronic and Medical Measurement Systems are approximately 4 mm in diameter. These catheters provide a single pressure value at each location along the longitudinal axis of the anal canal, that is, they do not measure pressure topography around the catheter circumference. By contrast, the Medtronic HDM catheter measures pressures at specific locations around the circumference and depicts pressures in 3 dimensions.[21,22] Conceptually, this feature may be useful to identify regional weakness of the external anal sphincter and/or to discriminate between squeeze pressures generated by the puborectalis and external anal sphincter.[21] However, more evidence is necessary to substantiate whether HDM enables these

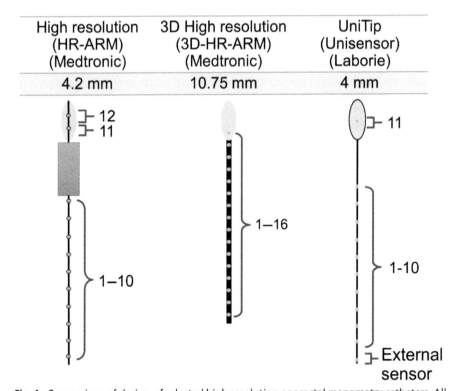

Fig. 1. Comparison of design of selected high resolution anorectal manometry catheters. All 3 catheters have pressure sensors in the rectal balloon and along the shaft. All sensors measure circumferential pressures. The 3D-HR-ARM probe (Medtronic) is much larger (ie, 10.75 mm diameter) than the other 2 catheters shown here. GI, gastrointestinal.

refined assessments. The HDM probe has a diameter of 10.75 mm, which is much larger than other probes.[22] Some patients find this probe uncomfortable. Also, unlike other anorectal manometry probes that are typically 4 to 6 mm in diameter and are flexible, the HDM probe is rigid, does not conform to the anorectal angle, and has to be held by the operator during the test. This "may introduce artifacts, especially if it is not held in the neutral position during maneuvers such as squeeze and bearing down."[22] HRM and HDM catheters are relatively expensive and fragile.

Anorectal Manometry Protocol

Anorectal pressure measurements depend on the methods for assessing and analyzing anorectal pressures. Most centers assess anorectal pressures at rest, during 2 or 3 squeeze maneuvers, and during simulated evacuation, generally with an empty and subsequently with a filled balloon, typically with air. Thereafter, the rectoanal inhibitory reflex and rectal perception of distention are assessed. Some centers also evaluate pressures when patients cough or do a Valsalva maneuver. Although the precise details (eg, number of squeeze maneuvers, duration of measurements) vary among techniques, the International Anorectal Physiology Working Group has suggested approaches to standardize techniques.[23] Pending studies that compare the diagnostic utility of various anorectal manometry techniques, the impact of relatively minor differences in techniques on the diagnostic utility of manometry is unknown.

Analysis of Anorectal Manometry

Arguably, differences in the methods that are used to analyze and summarize pressures are more important than the relatively minor differences in the methods to assess pressures among techniques.[24] For example, ideally, squeeze pressure should consider the distribution of pressures across the anal length and circumference and the duration over which pressures are summarized. Given these differences and the effects of age and sex on anorectal pressures in healthy people,[19] pressures should be compared with normal values derived in age- and sex-matched controls measured with the same technique. Readers are referred to a review[16] and original reports of the largest healthy cohorts of normal anorectal pressures evaluated with the Medtronic HRM catheter (96 women and 47 men),[19] the Medtronic HDM catheter (42 women and 36 men),[22] the Medical Measurements System (now Laborie) HRM catheter (96 women and 29 men),[25] the Sandhill, now Diversatek catheter (27 women and 27 men),[26] and the Medspira portable catheter (74 women and 34 men).[15,18]

The rectoanal gradient during simulated evacuation is the primary criterion for diagnosing DD by manometry. Other features of DD include a higher anal resting pressure (anismus) and/or reduced voluntary augmentation during pelvic floor contraction.[27,28] Intuitively, it would seem that the rectoanal pressure gradient should be positive (ie, rectal pressure is greater than anal pressure) in asymptomatic healthy people with normal rectal evacuation. However, the rectoanal gradient is negative in a substantial proportion of healthy people.[16,19,22,29] Hence, a rectoanal gradient is abnormal only if it is more negative than the lower limit of normal, which, for the Medtronic HRM catheter is −70 mm Hg in women younger than 50 years of age.[19] Using these stringent criteria, patients with DD have lower rectoanal pressure gradients (rectal-anal pressure) during evacuation than healthy people.[30] The rectoanal pressure pattern can also indicate causes of DD, such as decreased propulsive force, paradoxical contraction, or both.[6,7]

The method for analyzing the gradient during evacuation may at least partly explain why the gradient is negative in asymptomatic healthy people. For example, the highest anal pressure at each instant (at 10 Hz) is used to summarize anal pressure. First, because the highest, and not the lowest, anal pressure is used to calculate the gradient, the gradient is generally not the greatest pressure difference between the rectum and the anal canal. Second, "the specific sensor that is used to summarize anal pressure often moves over the 20-second evacuation period."[30] Third, the highest anal pressure measurement is prone to artifact, for example, because of catheter impingement.[31] With the Medtronic HRM and HDM catheters, there is pressure drift, which is typically corrected by the software program.[32] Finally, although the rectoanal gradient (RAG) is a useful metric, it ignores the underlying pressure topography pattern that is evident by careful inspection and is used to classify esophageal motility disorders (eg, subtypes of achalasia).[33]

Newer Approaches to Increase the Diagnostic Utility of High-Resolution Manometry

Three newer approaches may improve the utility of HRM for diagnosing DD: seated HRM, refined approaches to analyze pressure topography during evacuation, and an integrated assessment of pressures during evacuation and a Valsalva maneuver.

Anorectal pressures can be measured in the seated position.[30,34,35] This can be challenging because the catheter may be displaced during evacuation. Catheter displacement can be prevented with a clip attached to the catheter and the inner thigh.[30] A recent study compared existing and newer options to summarize the pressure topography during evacuation in the left lateral and seated positions in 64 healthy and 136 constipated women of whom 52 had a prolonged balloon expulsion time (BET).[30] The gradient was less negative in the seated than the left lateral position. Also, a new approach was used to characterize 4 pressure topography patterns, that is, minimal change, anal relaxation, paradoxical contraction, and transmission (**Fig. 2**). In the seated position, the BET was associated with the pattern, being prolonged in, respectively, 45%, 15%, 53%, and 0% of patients with minimal change, anal relaxation, paradoxical contraction, and transmission. Compared with the existing ManoView RAG in the left lateral position, the integrated analysis (ie, pattern and new gradient) in the left lateral position and the seated ManoView gradient were more effective for discriminating between constipated patients without and with DD. Hence, anorectal HRM ideally should be performed in the more physiologic seated position and analyzed by a 2-tier approach, which incorporates the overall pattern followed by the rectoanal gradient.

It is suggested that patients with DD strain excessively or do a Valsalva maneuver during evacuation, resulting in rectoanal discoordination, which hinders rectal evacuation. A recent study observed that a simultaneous consideration of rectoanal pressures during evacuation and a Valsalva maneuver uncovers rectoanal discoordination and facilitates the diagnosis of DD in selected patients.[36]

RECTAL BALLOON EXPULSION TEST

This simple test is performed in conjunction with an anorectal manometry. The time required to evacuate a balloon filled with warm tap water, typically 50 mL, in the seated position is assessed. The normal values depend on the type of rectal balloon used for the test.[37–39] At most centers, the test is performed with a party or commercial balloon; the upper limit of normal is 1 minute. For a Foley catheter inflated to 50 mL, which is above the manufacturer-recommended limit of 30 mL, the upper limit of normal is 2 minutes.[39] Even with the 2-minute cutoff, 25% of healthy people would be misclassified as abnormal because they require more than 2 minutes.[40]

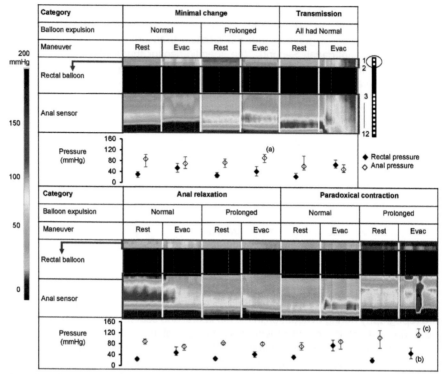

Fig. 2. Median and interquartile values of rectoanal pressures at rest and during evacuation in the seated position in the 4 patterns. Rectoanal pressures were measured by a 12-sensor catheter depicted in the cartoon on the top right. Observe the caudal transmission of pressure from the rectal balloon throughout the anal canal in the transmission pattern. [a] $P < .05$; [b] $P \leq .01$; [c] $P \leq .001$ for comparison of rectal or anal pressure during evacuation in patients with normal versus prolonged BET in the same pattern. Evac, evacuation. (*From* Sharma M, Muthyala A, Feuerhak K, Puthanmadhom Narayanan S, Bailey KR, Bharucha AE. Improving the utility of high-resolution manometry for the diagnosis of defecatory disorders in women with chronic constipation. Neurogastroenterology & Motility. 2020;e13910; with permission.)

Normally, defecation is preceded by the desire to defecate. Some patients with DD have reduced rectal sensation, hence may not perceive the desire to defecate with a balloon inflated to 50 mL.[41] Alternatively, patients can be asked to expel a balloon that is inflated until patients experience the desire to defecate.[42] Further studies are necessary to compare these 2 techniques (ie, fixed vs variable balloon inflation) of assessing rectal evacuation.

Among 106 patients with functional constipation and 24 patients with DD, the BET identified those with DD, documented with defecography, with 88% sensitivity and 89% specificity; positive- and negative-predictive values were 64% and 97% for diagnosis of DD, respectively.[42] However, this uncontrolled study excluded patients with secondary (such as medication-induced) chronic constipation. The rectal balloon was inflated not to a fixed volume but until patients experienced the desire to defecate, averaging 183 mL, which may compensate for reduced rectal sensation identified in some patients with DD.[41] An abnormal rectal balloon expulsion test predicted the response to biofeedback therapy.[4]

BARIUM AND MAGNETIC RESONANCE PROCTOGRAM

After filling the rectum with barium contrast mixed with psyllium or another thickening agent (barium defecography) or gel (magnetic resonance [MR] defecography), lateral images of the anorectum are obtained at rest, during pelvic floor contraction, and during defecation (**Fig. 3**).[43] Abnormalities include inadequate (such as a spastic disorder) or excessive (such as in descending perineum syndrome) widening of the anorectal angle and/or perineal descent during defecation. Internal intussusception, solitary rectal ulcers, rectoceles, and rectal prolapse may also be identified.[43] When the vagina and small intestine are opacified, enteroceles, bladder, and uterovaginal prolapse can be seen.

Introduced more recently, standardized techniques for defecography[44–46] have partly overcome the limited reproducibility of anorectal measurements in older studies.[47] Barium and MR defecography are respectively performed in the seated and the supine position. By comparison to barium defecography, MRI avoids radiation

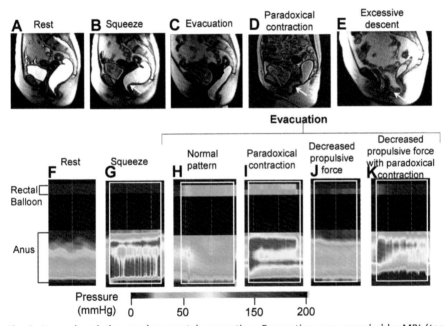

Fig. 3. Normal and abnormal anorectal evacuation. Evacuation was recorded by MRI (*top row*) and HRM (*bottom row*). Relative to rest (*A*), MRI shows increased puborectalis indentation during squeeze (*B, arrow*) and normal relaxation of the puborectalis, perineal descent, opening of the anal canal, and evacuation of ultrasound gel during evacuation (*C*). In patients with constipation, during evacuation, there is paradoxical contraction of the puborectalis (*D, arrow*) and exaggerated perineal descent with an enterocele (*E, arrow*). HRM shows anal pressure at rest (*F*) and increased anal pressure during squeeze (*G*) compared with rest (*F*). The white rectangle demarcates the duration of squeeze (*G*) and evacuation (*H–K*). Note the increased rectal pressure with anal relaxation during evacuation in a healthy person (*H*). By contrast during evacuation in constipated patients, note increased rectal pressure with paradoxical anal contraction (*I*), no change in rectal pressure versus rest (*J*), and no change in rectal pressure with paradoxical anal contraction (*K*). (*From* Bharucha A, Wald A. Chronic Constipation. Mayo Clin Proc. 2019;94(11):2340-2357. https://doi.org/10.1016/j.mayocp.2019.01.031 with permission.)

exposure, more precisely evaluates pelvic organ prolapse and pelvic floor motion,[27,48–50] and is especially useful for uncovering pelvic floor dysfunction in patients who have clinical features of DD with a normal BET; this group includes more than 90% of patients with a large rectocele, enterocele, and/or peritoneocele.[27,51] However, MR defecography is less widely available and more expensive. Most guidelines recommend defecography as a backup test to identify clinically suspected anatomic abnormalities, in patients with persistent symptoms after biofeedback therapy, or when the results of other anorectal tests are inconsistent with clinical findings.[1,52,53] However, some centers where defecography is readily available use this as a first-line test before the BET, perhaps because by contrast to the BET, defecography also depicts structural disturbances and arguably approximates more closely to stool than a rectal balloon.[54]

ASSESSMENT OF RECTAL SENSATION AND DISTENSIBILITY (COMPLIANCE AND CAPACITY)

The awareness of rectal filling is necessary for normal defecation and fecal continence. Some patients with DD have reduced rectal sensation.[55]

Rectal sensation is routinely assessed during anal manometry by manually distending a balloon, secured to a plastic catheter and placed within the rectum with air. In selected patients with DD, for example, when the manometry reveals a profound sensory disturbance, rectal sensation should be evaluated with a barostat, which is not widely available in clinical practice. During balloon inflation, participants are asked about symptoms: first sensation, desire to defecate, urgency, and maximum toleration/pain. The distending volume at each of these sensory thresholds is then recorded. When sensation is evaluated with a barostat, pressure thresholds, and hence compliance is also recorded. Although there is considerable variation between subjects, small studies using manual or barostat techniques suggest that assessments of rectal compliance and sensation within subjects is very reproducible on the same or separate days.[56,57]

Sensory testing may reveal rectal hypersensitivity or hyposensitivity in DD patients. Visceral hypersensitivity, including allodynia and hyperalgesia, abnormal colonic transit, and psychological factors, is associated with IBS symptoms.[58] Among 164 patients with functional gastrointestinal disorders, including 86 IBS patients, rectal barostat distention to 40 mm Hg was 96% sensitive and 72% specific for discriminating IBS patients from normal subjects.[59] Conversely, 18% to 66% of patients with chronic constipation have reduced rectal sensation (rectal *hypo*sensitivity),[9] often allied to an attenuated or absent call to stool; this may be "primary" (owing to direct impairment of afferent pathway function), "secondary," owing to altered biomechanical properties, or both.[60] Biofeedback therapy to correct sensory disturbances is beneficial in fecal incontinence.[61] However, the utility of such therapy in patients with DD has not been evaluated.

Because symptoms alone do not discriminate between DD and other causes of constipation,[6,7] anorectal functions should be evaluated in all patients whose symptoms are refractory to laxatives.[1] Testing should begin with anorectal manometry and a rectal balloon expulsion test.[1] In selected patients, defecography may be necessary as specified above. Some centers use defecography in lieu of the rectal balloon expulsion test.

POTENTIAL FALLACIES IN DIAGNOSTIC TESTING

Several features regarding the interpretation of test results deserve emphasis. First, these tests may be abnormal even in asymptomatic people.[19,49,62] Hence, test results need to be interpreted in the context of the clinical features. Second, there is no gold-standard diagnostic test for DD. Overall, the results of these tests are correlated with each other.[44,51] However, among individual patients, different tests often provide different answers, which confounds the diagnosis of DD.[45] In order to reduce the possibility of a false-positive diagnosis, the Rome IV criteria suggest that 2 or more abnormal tests are required to confirm a diagnosis of DD.[53] Third, although DD are primarily regarded as disorders of function, a subset of patients has structural abnormalities.[1] In some patients (eg, with a large rectocele that fails to empty during defecation and/or is accompanied by a history of anal digitation), the rectocele is probably contributing to symptoms. In other patients, it can be challenging to determine if the rectocele or other abnormalities are contributing to symptoms. Other abnormalities (eg, rectal intussusception) may be secondary to excessive straining rather than the underlying pelvic floor dysfunction. Fourth, it is the authors' perception that some patients with clinical features of pelvic floor dysfunction have seemingly normal rectal evacuation by testing, perhaps because they strain excessively to overcome increased pelvic floor resistance. Thus, an integrated assessment of clinical features and anorectal tests is necessary to confirm or exclude defecation disorders.

ANAL SURFACE ELECTROMYOGRAPHY

Anal electromyography (EMG), which measures the electrical activity of the external anal sphincter, is used to evaluate anal sphincter tone and relaxation during simulated defecation. Initially, anal EMG was performed with needle EMG. An important early study compared needle EMG activity in 16 healthy controls and 194 constipated patients quantified with the strain/squeeze index.[63] Although paradoxical contraction during straining was observed in 83% of patients versus 82% of controls, a mean index of greater than 50 was more common in patients (24%) than in controls (0%), associated with impaired rectal evacuation during defecography, and reduced rectal sensation. The needle EMG indices in the puborectalis muscle and in the external anal sphincter muscle were correlated. Prompted by the finding that EMG activity recorded by intramuscular and surface electrodes, which were placed bilaterally over the subcutaneous portion of the external anal sphincter,[64] is correlated, surface EMG performed with a cylindrical anal probe[39,65] or cutaneous electrodes is used for diagnostic purposes and to provide biofeedback therapy in DD. During straining, relaxation by 20% of baseline values or greater is considered to be normal.[39] Conversely, when activity during evacuation increases by greater than 20% above resting EMG activity, it is considered abnormal. A response that is between 20% above and 20% below baseline values is considered no change. To the authors' knowledge, these normal values are derived from anal manometry but have not been validated in healthy people. In randomized trials, biofeedback therapy provided with anal surface EMG was better than the control arm in constipated patients.[66,67]

COLONIC TRANSIT

Up to 50% of patients with DD have concurrent slow colon transit.[1] Colon transit influences fecal form.[68] Because it is harder to evacuate hard stools,[8] slow colon transit may aggravate the symptoms of difficult defecation.

It is not necessary to prepare the colon before evaluating colonic transit, which can be measured with 3 methods,[69] that is, ingestion of radiopaque markers using abdominal radiographs, scintigraphy, and the wireless motility capsule (WMC).

The radiopaque marker test is typically performed by administering a single capsule (Hinton method) containing 24 plastic markers on day 1 and by obtaining plain abdominal radiographs on day 6 (120 hours later).[69] Retention of 6 or more markers at 120 hours is considered abnormal. A more refined approach (Metcalf method) is to have the patient ingest a capsule containing 24 radiopaque markers on days 1, 2, and 3 and count the markers remaining on abdominal radiographs on days 4 and 7; a total of $\leq$68 markers remaining in the colon is normal, whereas more than 68 markers indicates slow transit.[69]

Colonic transit scintigraphy is a noninvasive and quantitative method of evaluation of total and regional colonic transit.[70,71] Here, a radioisotope (^{111}In or ^{99}Tc) is administered in a coated capsule that dissolves in the colon or terminal ileum or encapsulated in a nondigestible capsule with a test meal. At specific time points, gamma-camera images are obtained to track the isotope as it travels around the colon. The result is summarized by the weighted distribution of the isotope in the colon at 24 hours, and if necessary, at 48 hours.[69] The methods used to summarize colonic transit vary among centers.

The WMC and scintigraphy can noninvasively measure not only colonic but also gastric emptying and small bowel transit.[72] With WMC, these transition points are easily identified. An increase in the pH indicates when the capsule passes into the

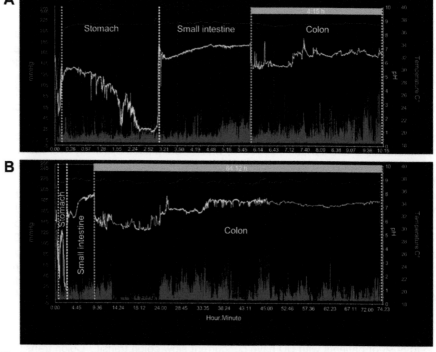

Fig. 4. Representative examples of a WMC in patients with normal (A) and slow colon transit (B). Pressures, temperature, and pH values are respectively shown in red, blue, and green and measure gastric emptying, small bowel transit time, and colonic transit time. Panel A shows a WMC recording with normal colonic transit time (4:15 hours). In contrast, panel B shows a patient with delayed colonic transit time (64:12 hours). Red = pressure (mmHg); green = pH; blue = temperature (°C); X axis = time (hours:minutes). Stomach = between blue and yellow dotted lines; small intestine = between yellow and green dotted lines; colon = after green line.

small bowel, and a subsequent drop of approximately 1.5 units suggests that the capsule is located in the cecum. The WMC is a sensitive and specific test for identifying slow colonic transit, as defined by a colonic transit time of 59 hours or greater (**Fig. 4**). Among patients with chronic constipation, the overall (ie, positive and negative) agreement versus radiopaque markers was 87%.[73] Similar to scintigraphy, the WMC may uncover disturbances of upper gastrointestinal transit in constipated patients.[74]

SUMMARY

Among constipated patients who have not responded to laxatives, anorectal tests are necessary to diagnose DD. At a high level, the methods for these tests are standardized. However, the details of methods and normal values vary among techniques.

Anorectal functions are affected by age and sex. Test results should be interpreted with reference to normal values generated by the same technique. The choice of tests and their interpretation are guided by the clinical features. The results of these tests guide the management of these conditions.

ACKNOWLEDGMENTS

This work was supported in part by USPHS NIH Grant R01 DK78924.

DISCLOSURE

Dr A.E. Bharucha jointly holds patents for the anorectal catheter fixation device, anorectal manometry probe, and an anorectal device for fecal incontinence, respectively, with Medtronic Inc, Medspira Inc, and Minnesota Medical Technologies and receives royalties from Medspira Inc. Dr E. Coss-Adame has nothing to disclose.

REFERENCES

1. Bharucha AE, Lacy BE. Mechanisms, evaluation, and management of chronic constipation. Gastroenterology 2020;158(5):1232–49.e3.
2. Noelting J, Eaton J, Choung RS, et al. The incidence rate and characteristics of clinically diagnosed defecatory disorders in the community. Neurogastroenterol Motil 2016;28(11):1690–7.
3. Rao S, Bharucha AE, Chiarioni G, et al. Functional anorectal disorders. Gastroenterology 2016;150(6):1430–42.
4. Chiarioni G, Salandini L, Whitehead WE. Biofeedback benefits only patients with outlet dysfunction, not patients with isolated slow transit constipation. Gastroenterology 2005;129(1):86–97.
5. Chiarioni G, Whitehead WE, Pezza V, et al. Biofeedback is superior to laxatives for normal transit constipation due to pelvic floor dyssynergia. Gastroenterology 2006;130(3):657–64.
6. Rao SS, Mudipalli RS, Stessman M, et al. Investigation of the utility of colorectal function tests and Rome II criteria in dyssynergic defecation (Anismus). Neurogastroenterology Motil 2004;16(5):589–96.
7. Ratuapli S, Bharucha AE, Noelting J, et al. Phenotypic identification and classification of functional defecatory disorders using high resolution anorectal manometry. Gastroenterology 2013;144:314–22.
8. Bharucha AE, Seide BM, Zinsmeister AR, et al. Insights into normal and disordered bowel habits from bowel diaries. Am J Gastroenterol 2008;103(3):692–8.

9. van Ginkel R, Reitsma JB, Buller HA, et al. Childhood constipation: longitudinal follow-up beyond puberty. Gastroenterology 2003;125(2):357–63.

10. Suttor VP, Prott GM, Hansen RD, et al. Evidence for pelvic floor dyssynergia in patients with irritable bowel syndrome. Dis Colon Rectum 2010;53(2):156–60.

11. Talley NJ. How to do and interpret a rectal examination in gastroenterology. Am J Gastroenterol 2008;103(4):820–2.

12. Tantiphlachiva K, Rao P, Attaluri A, et al. Digital rectal examination is a useful tool for identifying patients with dyssynergia. Clin Gastroenterol Hepatol 2010;8(11): 955–60.

13. Orkin BA, Sinykin SB, Lloyd PC. The digital rectal examination scoring system (DRESS). Dis Colon Rectum 2010;53(12):1656–60.

14. Rao SS, Azpiroz F, Diamant N, et al. Minimum standards of anorectal manometry. Neurogastroenterol Motil 2002;14(5):553–9.

15. Bharucha AE, Stroetz R, Feuerhak K, et al. A novel technique for bedside anorectal manometry in humans. Neurogastroenterol Motil 2015;27(10):1504–8.

16. Lee TH, Bharucha AE. How to perform and interpret a high-resolution anorectal manometry test. J Neurogastroenterol Motil 2016;22(1):46–59.

17. Basilisco G, Bharucha AE. High-resolution anorectal manometry: an expensive hobby or worth every penny? Neurogastroenterol Motil 2017;29(8):e13125.

18. Sharma M, Lowry AC, Rao SS, et al. A multicenter study of anorectal pressures and rectal sensation measured with portable manometry in healthy women and men. Neurogastroenterol Motil 2021;33(6):e14067.

19. Oblizajek NR, Gandhi S, Sharma M, et al. Anorectal pressures measured with high-resolution manometry in healthy people—normal values and asymptomatic pelvic floor dysfunction. Neurogastroenterol Motil 2019;31(7):e13597.

20. Gosling J, Plumb A, Taylor SA, et al. High-resolution anal manometry: repeatability, validation, and comparison with conventional manometry. Neurogastroenterology Motil 2019;31(6):e13591.

21. Raizada V, Bhargava V, Karsten A, et al. Functional morphology of anal sphincter complex unveiled by high definition anal manometery and three dimensional ultrasound imaging. Neurogastroenterol Motil 2011;23(11):1013–9.e460.

22. Coss-Adame E, Rao SS, Valestin J, et al. Accuracy and reproducibility of high-definition anorectal manometry and pressure topography analyses in healthy subjects. Clin Gastroenterol Hepatol 2015;13(6):1143–50.e1.

23. Carrington EV, Heinrich H, Knowles CH, et al. The International Anorectal Physiology Working Group (IAPWG) recommendations: standardized testing protocol and the London classification for disorders of anorectal function. Neurogastroenterol Motil 2020;32(1):e13679.

24. Sharma M, Tirumani-Setty P, Parthasarathy G, et al. Su1604-mechanisms of normal and disordered defecation in women. Gastroenterology 2018;154(6): S543.

25. Carrington EV, Brokjaer A, Craven H, et al. Traditional measures of normal anal sphincter function using high-resolution anorectal manometry (HRAM) in 115 healthy volunteers. Neurogastroenterol Motil 2014;26(5):625–35.

26. Lee HJ, Jung KW, Han S, et al. Normal values for high-resolution anorectal manometry/topography in a healthy Korean population and the effects of gender and body mass index. Neurogastroenterol Motil 2014;26(4):529–37.

27. Bharucha AE, Fletcher JG, Seide B, et al. Phenotypic variation in functional disorders of defecation. Gastroenterology 2005;128:1199–210.

28. Bharucha AE, Croak AJ, Gebhart JB, et al. Comparison of rectoanal axial forces in health and functional defecatory disorders. Am J Physiol Gastrointest Liver Physiol 2006;290(6):G1164–9.
29. Grossi U, Carrington EV, Bharucha AE, et al. Diagnostic accuracy study of anorectal manometry for diagnosis of dyssynergic defecation. Gut 2016;65(3): 447–55.
30. Sharma M, Muthyala A, Feuerhak K, et al. Improving the utility of high resolution manometry for the diagnosis of defecatory disorders in women with chronic constipation. Neurogastroenterol Motil 2020;32(10):e13910.
31. Babaei A, Szabo A, Yorio SD, et al. Pressure exposure and catheter impingement affect the recorded pressure in the Manoscan 360TM system. Neurogastroenterol Motil 2018;09:09.
32. Parthasarathy G, McMaster J, Feuerhak K, et al. Determinants and clinical impact of pressure drift in manoscan anorectal high resolution manometry system. Neurogastroenterology Motil 2016;28(9):1433–7.
33. Pandolfino JE, Fox MR, Bredenoord AJ, et al. High-resolution manometry in clinical practice: utilizing pressure topography to classify oesophageal motility abnormalities. Neurogastroenterology Motil 2009;21(8):796–806.
34. Rao SSC, Kavlock R, Rao S. Influence of body position and stool characteristics on defecation in humans. Am J Gastroenterol 2006;101(12):2790–6.
35. Wu GJ, Xu F, Lin L, et al. Anorectal manometry: should it be performed in a seated position? Neurogastroenterol Motil 2017;29(5):05.
36. Srinivasan SG, Sharma M, Feuerhak K, et al. A comparison of rectoanal pressures during Valsalva maneuver and evacuation uncovers rectoanal discoordination in defecatory disorders. Neurogastroenterol Motil 2021;33(10):e14126.
37. Rao SS, Hatfield R, Soffer E, et al. Manometric tests of anorectal function in healthy adults. Am J Gastroenterol 1999;94(3):773–83.
38. Ratuapli S, Bharucha AE, Harvey D, et al. Comparison of rectal balloon expulsion test in seated and left lateral positions. Neurogastroenterol Motil 2013;25(12): e813–20.
39. Chiarioni G, Kim SM, Vantini I, et al. Validation of the balloon evacuation test: reproducibility and agreement with findings from anorectal manometry and electromyography. Clin Gastroenterol Hepatol 2014;12(12):2049–54.
40. Mazor Y, Prott G, Jones M, et al. Anorectal physiology in health: a randomized trial to determine the optimum catheter for the balloon expulsion test. Neurogastroenterology Motil 2019;31(4):e13552.
41. Gladman MA, Lunniss PJ, Scott SM, et al. Rectal hyposensitivity. Am J Gastroenterol 2006;101(5):1140–51.
42. Minguez M, Herreros B, Sanchiz V, et al. Predictive value of the balloon expulsion test for excluding the diagnosis of pelvic floor dyssynergia in constipation. Gastroenterology 2004;126(1):57–62.
43. Agachan F, Pfeifer J, Wexner SD. Defecography and proctography. Results of 744 patients. Dis Colon Rectum 1996;39(8):899–905.
44. Palit S, Thin N, Knowles CH, et al. Diagnostic disagreement between tests of evacuatory function: a prospective study of 100 constipated patients. Neurogastroenterology Motil 2016;28(10):1589–98.
45. Bordeianou L, Savitt L, Dursun A. Measurements of pelvic floor dyssynergia: which test result matters? Dis Colon Rectum 2011;54(1):60–5.
46. Noelting J, Bharucha AE, Lake DS, et al. Semi-automated vectorial analysis of anorectal motion by magnetic resonance defecography in healthy subjects and fecal incontinence. Neurogastroenterol Motil 2012;24(10):e467–75.

47. Diamant NE, Kamm MA, Wald A, et al. AGA technical review on anorectal testing techniques. Gastroenterology 1999;116(3):735–60.
48. Reiner CS, Tutuian R, Solopova AE, et al. MR defecography in patients with dyssynergic defecation: spectrum of imaging findings and diagnostic value. Br J Radiol 2011;84(998):136–44.
49. Tirumanisetty P, Prichard D, Fletcher JG, et al. Normal values for assessment of anal sphincter morphology, anorectal motion, and pelvic organ prolapse with MRI in healthy women. Neurogastroenterology Motil 2018;30(7):e13314.
50. Puthanmadhom Narayanan S, Sharma M, Fletcher JG, et al. Comparison of changes in rectal area and volume during MR evacuation proctography in healthy and constipated adults. Neurogastroenterology Motil 2019;31(7):e13608.
51. Prichard DO, Lee T, Parthasarathy G, et al. High-resolution anorectal manometry for identifying defecatory disorders and rectal structural abnormalities in women. Clin Gastroenterol Hepatol 2017;15(3):412–20.
52. Wald A, Bharucha AE, Cosman BC, et al. ACG clinical guideline: management of benign anorectal disorders. Am J Gastroenterol 2014;109(8):1141–57 [quiz: 1058].
53. Rao SS, Bharucha AE, Chiarioni G, et al. Functional anorectal disorders. Gastroenterology 2016;25:25.
54. Grossi U, Di Tanna GL, Heinrich H, et al. Systematic review with meta-analysis: defecography should be a first-line diagnostic modality in patients with refractory constipation. Aliment Pharmacol Ther 2018;48(11–12):1186–201.
55. Carrington EV, Scott SM, Bharucha A, et al. Expert consensus document: advances in the evaluation of anorectal function. Nat Rev Gastroenterol Hepatol 2018;15(5):309–23.
56. Hammer HF, Phillips SF, Camilleri M, et al. Rectal tone, distensibility, and perception: reproducibility and response to different distensions. Am J Physiol 1998; 274(3 Pt 1):G584–90.
57. Bharucha AE, Seide B, Fox JC, et al. Day-to-day reproducibility of anorectal sensorimotor assessments in healthy subjects. Neurogastroenterol Motil 2004; 16:241–50.
58. Simren M, Tornblom H, Palsson OS, et al. Cumulative effects of psychologic distress, visceral hypersensitivity, and abnormal transit on patient-reported outcomes in irritable bowel syndrome. Gastroenterology 2019;157(2):391–402.e2.
59. Bouin M, Plourde V, Boivin M, et al. Rectal distention testing in patients with irritable bowel syndrome: sensitivity, specificity, and predictive values of pain sensory thresholds. Gastroenterology 2002;122(7):1771–7.
60. Gladman MA, Aziz Q, Scott SM, et al. Rectal hyposensitivity: pathophysiological mechanisms. Neurogastroenterology Motil 2009;21(5):508–16, e504-505.
61. Deb B, Prichard DO, Bharucha AE. Constipation and fecal incontinence in the elderly. Curr Gastroenterol Rep 2020;22(11):54.
62. Voderholzer WA, Neuhaus DA, Klauser AG, et al. Paradoxical sphincter contraction is rarely indicative of anismus. Gut 1997;41(2):258–62.
63. Karlbom U, Eeg-Olofsson KE, Graf W, et al. Evaluation of the paradoxical sphincter contraction by a strain/squeeze index in constipated patients. Dis Colon Rectum 2005;48(10):1923–9.
64. Axelson HW, Edebol Eeg-Olofsson K. Simplified evaluation of the paradoxical puborectalis contraction with surface electrodes. Dis Colon Rectum 2010;53(6): 928–31.

65. Binnie NR, Kawimbe BM, Papachrysostomou M, et al. The importance of the orientation of the electrode plates in recording the external anal sphincter EMG by non-invasive anal plug electrodes. Int J Colorectal Dis 1991;6(1):5–8.
66. Hart SL, Lee JW, Berian J, et al. A randomized controlled trial of anorectal biofeedback for constipation. Int J colorectal Dis 2012;27(4):459–66.
67. Simon MA, Bueno AM. Efficacy of biofeedback therapy in the treatment of dyssynergic defecation in community-dwelling elderly women. J Clin Gastroenterol 2017;51(10):e90–4.
68. Degen LP, Phillips SF. How well does stool form reflect colonic transit? Gut 1996;39(1):109–13.
69. Bharucha AE, Anderson B, Bouchoucha M. More movement with evaluating colonic transit in humans. Neurogastroenterol Motil 2019;31(2):e13541.
70. van der Sijp JR, Kamm MA, Nightingale JM, et al. Radioisotope determination of regional colonic transit in severe constipation: comparison with radio opaque markers. Gut 1993;34(3):402–8.
71. Nullens S, Nelsen T, Camilleri M, et al. Regional colon transit in patients with dyssynergic defaecation or slow transit in patients with constipation. Gut 2012;61(8):1132–9.
72. Rao SS, Kuo B, McCallum RW, et al. Investigation of colonic and whole gut transit with wireless motility capsule and radiopaque markers in constipation. Clin Gastroenterol Hepatol 2009;7:537–44.
73. Camilleri M, Thorne NK, Ringel R, et al. Wireless pH-motility capsule for colonic transit: prospective comparison with radiopaque markers in chronic constipation. Neurogastroenterology Motil 2010;22:874–82, e233.
74. Rao SS, Mysore K, Attaluri A, et al. Diagnostic utility of wireless motility capsule in gastrointestinal dysmotility. J Clin Gastroenterol 2011;45(8):684–90.

Dyssynergic Defecation and Other Evacuation Disorders

Amol Sharma, MD, MS*, Anam Herekar, MD, Yun Yan, MD, PhD,
Tennekoon Karunaratne, MD, PhD, Satish S.C. Rao, MD, PhD

KEYWORDS

- Constipation • Dyssynergic defecation • Biofeedback therapy • Rectocele
- Levator ani syndrome

KEY POINTS

- Severe, refractory constipation is often due to dyssynergic defecation.
- A thorough digital rectal examination is key in the evaluation of constipated patients.
- No single diagnostic test is sufficient, and therefore, high-resolution anorectal manometry, balloon expulsion testing, and defecography should be used in combination to diagnose dyssynergic defecation.
- Biofeedback therapy is the mainstay of treatment of dyssynergic defecation and may be considered in patients with coexisting rectoceles, slow-transit constipation, and/or irritable bowel syndrome with constipation (IBS-C).
- Levator ani syndrome can be a debilitating cause of anorectal pain, and pelvic neuropathy may be a key pathophysiological disturbance.

INTRODUCTION

Constipation is a common condition that affects 12% to 19% of the worldwide population with a higher predilection for females (estimated ratio of 2.2:1 to males).[1] The prevalence of this condition increases with age and lower socioeconomic status. Constipation is the primary reason for 2.5 million physician office visits annually, and constipation-related emergency room visits and inpatient admissions are increasing in a younger cohort of patients.[2–4] Refractory constipation represents a significant burden to the health care system.[5,6] Constipation is defined by a constellation of symptoms including infrequent bowel movements, excessive straining, hard or lumpy stools, sensations of incomplete evacuation and mechanical obstruction, and/or the use of digital maneuvers for stool evacuation.[7,8] Chronic constipation, defined as symptoms lasting more than 3 months, has been categorized by Rome IV criteria into 4 broad subtypes; (1) functional constipation, (2) irritable bowel syndrome with

Division of Gastroenterology/Hepatology, Medical College of Georgia, Augusta University, Augusta, GA, USA
* Corresponding author. Medical College of Georgia, Augusta University, Augusta University Medical Center, 1120 15th Street, AD-2226, Augusta, GA 30912.
E-mail address: amosharma@augusta.edu

Gastroenterol Clin N Am 51 (2022) 55–69
https://doi.org/10.1016/j.gtc.2021.10.004
0889-8553/22/© 2021 Elsevier Inc. All rights reserved.

constipation (IBS-C), (3) opioid-induced constipation, and (4) functional defecation disorders.[7] Constipation can also be classified as primary, which is due to colonic or anorectal dysfunction, or secondary, associated with intrinsic gastrointestinal (GI) pathology (ie, colonic strictures, malignancies, etc.), in the presence of other medical conditions (metabolic disturbances, thyroid disorders, diabetes mellitus, neuromyopathic disorders) or related to medication use (opioids, anticholinergic agents).[9] Dyssynergic defecation and rectal evacuation disorders are primary functional defecation disorders.

Constipated patients are frequently referred to GI specialists for symptoms refractory to lifestyle modifications and laxatives.[10] Dyssynergic defecation, defined as dyscoordination of rectoanal, abdominal, and pelvic floor muscles to facilitate defecation, is a major cause of refractory primary constipation.[11] Successful understanding of the diagnosis, evaluation, and management of dyssynergic defecation and other evacuation disorders will allow providers to effectively manage these patients. This review focuses on examining the definition, pathophysiology, evaluation, and treatment of dyssynergic defecation and other evacuation disorders.

ANATOMY

A comprehensive understanding of the pelvic floor neuromuscular anatomy is important for diagnosing and treating defecation disorders. The pelvic floor muscles are essential for defecation, sexual function, and micturition. The coccygeus and levator ani muscles combine to form a bowl-shaped pelvic diaphragm through which the rectum passes into the perineum to merge with the anal canal. The iliococcygeus, pubococcygeus, and puborectalis muscles comprise the levator ani complex. The puborectalis muscle forms a U-shaped sling, and its resting tone is responsible for maintaining the anorectal angle, and thus, continence. When the puborectalis relaxes, the anorectal angle straightens, facilitating defecation. The anal canal is composed of internal and external sphincters. The internal anal sphincter (IAS) provides 70% of the resting anal canal tone. The external anal sphincter (EAS) blends superiorly with the puborectalis muscle, and together these muscles maintain fecal continence. The IAS is composed of smooth muscle, whereas both the EAS and puborectalis are skeletal muscles under voluntary control and should relax during defecation attempts. Dyssynergic defecation results from dyscoordination of the rectoanal, abdominal, and pelvic floor muscles. Pelvic floor dysfunction can also result in incomplete rectal evacuation and pain.

The autonomic and somatic innervation of the hindgut and pelvic floor is unique from the rest of the GI tract, as shown in **Fig. 1**. Most of the GI tract receives parasympathetic innervation from the vagus nerve. Pelvic organs, such as the rectum, bladder, and uterus, are innervated by parasympathetic branches from pelvic splanchnic nerves originating from S2-S4 sacral nerves, which send projections through the inferior hypogastric plexus. Sympathetic innervation of the pelvic organs and hindgut originate from thoracolumbar splanchnic nerves T10-L2 coursing through the superior hypogastric plexus to meet the parasympathetic fibers at the inferior hypogastric plexus.

An intact pudendal nerve is crucial to pelvic floor function. The pudendal nerve is a mixed sensorimotor nerve that originates from unmyelinated, parasympathetic projections from Onuf nuclei emanating from sacral branches S2-S4 to innervate the perineal, EAS, and levator ani muscles (also shown in **Fig. 1**).[12] The course of the pudendal nerve can make it susceptible to injury. The sacral nerve roots converge to form the pudendal nerve just proximal to the sacrospinous ligament. The pudendal

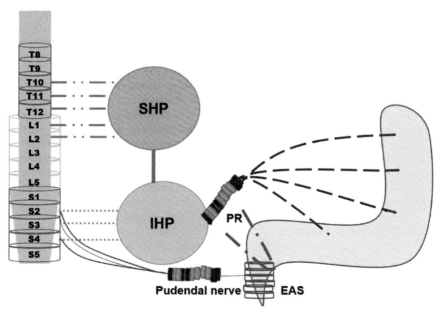

Fig. 1. Diagrammatic representation of sympathetic, parasympathetic, and somatic innervation of the hindgut and pelvic floor. The rectum and distal colon are innervated by parasympathetic branches from pelvic splanchnic nerves originating from S2-S4 sacral nerves, which send projections through the inferior hypogastric plexus (IHP). Sympathetic innervation of the pelvic organs and hindgut originate from thoracolumbar splanchnic nerves T10-L2 coursing through the superior hypogastric plexus (SHP) to meet the parasympathetic fibers at the IHP. The pudendal nerve is a mixed sensorimotor nerve that originates from unmyelinated, parasympathetic projections from Onuf nuclei emanating from sacral branches S2-S4 to innervate the perineal skeletal muscles, external anal sphincter (EAS), and levator ani. PB, puborectalis.

nerve passes between the pyriformis and coccygeus muscles out of the pelvis through the lower greater sciatic foramen and reenters the pelvis through the lesser sciatic foramen.[13] Upon reentering the pelvis, the pudendal nerve, artery, and vein are enveloped by the obturator internus muscle sheath along the ischiorectal fossa in the pudendal canal. Temporary or permanent damage to the pudendal nerve may occur from recurrent stretch injury in the setting of chronic straining during defecation, and abnormal perineal descent, or prolonged or difficult childbirth.[14–16] The perineal branch of the pudendal nerve innervating the EAS is susceptible to the most strain and stretch during perineal descent.[17] Patients with prolonged straining may develop pudendal neuropathy resulting in mixed constipation and fecal incontinence.

DYSSYNERGIC DEFECATION

Dyssynergic defecation is defined as dyscoordination of the rectoanal, abdominal, and pelvic floor muscles necessary for appropriate laxation; it can be characterized by inadequate anal relaxation, paradoxic anal contraction, or inadequate rectal propulsive forces.[18] Evidence suggesting dyssynergic defecation must be present on at least 2 of the 3 tests: balloon expulsion test (BET), anorectal manometry (ARM) or surface electromyography (EMG), and defecography or stool retention on colonic transit study[7] (**Box 1**). Dyssynergic defecation is also often accompanied by altered rectal sensation and/or compliance.[19]

A thorough history and physical examination are essential components of the evaluation of individuals with constipation. It is important to rule out other secondary or coexisting causes via appropriate investigational testing. Prospective stool diaries, either paper or smartphone app based, and validated questionnaires such as the Patient Assessment of Constipation-Quality of Life (PAC-QOL), Patient Assessment of Constipation-Symptoms (PAC-SYM), and Fecal Incontinence and Constipation Assessment (FICA) scale, can also help qualify and quantify bowel patterns, particularly in patients who are neither forthcoming nor precise in their histories.[20–24] In a recent study, 84% of patients described excessive straining, 76% experienced a feeling of incomplete evacuation, and 74% had abdominal bloating.[25] However, these constipation-related symptoms seem to be better predictors of slow transit than pelvic dysfunction, making it difficult to diagnose dyssynergic defecation based on history alone.[26] Environmental and emotional stressors can decrease pain thresholds and perpetuate negative habits, and astute clinicians should explore these precipitating factors with their patients. In subjects with dyssynergic defecation, sexual abuse was reported by 22%.[25]

DIAGNOSTIC TESTING
Digital Rectal Examination

No single test is able to adequately define dyssynergic defecation; thus, diagnostic testing should begin with a detailed digital rectal examination (DRE) (**Fig. 2**).[27] The examiner should first inspect the perianal region and surrounding tissue looking for fissures, hemorrhoids, excoriations, or skin tags. Diminished or lack of perineal sensation and an abnormal anocutaneous reflex can indicate pudendal neuropathy. After the perianal inspection, a lubricated gloved index finger should be inserted into the rectum with the examiner assessing for the presence of stool, strictures, tenderness, or masses. Resting anal tone can also be measured. The patient should be instructed to squeeze, allowing for an assessment of initial and sustained pressures. Pelvic floor coordination can be tested by placing a hand on the abdomen and requesting that the patient bear down or attempt to defecate.[28] It is during this final maneuver that one can best assess rectoanal coordination with a sensitivity and specificity of 75% and

---

Box 1
Rome IV diagnostic criteria for dyssynergic defecation

1. The patient must satisfy diagnostic criteria for functional constipation and/or irritable bowel syndrome with constipation.[a]

2. During repeated attempts to defecate, there must be features of impaired evacuation, as demonstrated by 2 of the following 3 tests:[b]
   a. Abnormal balloon expulsion test
   b. Abnormal anorectal evacuation pattern with manometry or anal surface EMG
   c. Impaired rectal evacuation by imaging

3. Inappropriate contraction of the pelvic floor as measured with anal surface EMG or manometry with adequate propulsive forces during attempted defecation.[b]

[a]Criteria must be fulfilled for the last 3 months with symptom onset at least 6 months before diagnosis.

[b]These criteria are defined by age- and sex-appropriate normal values for each diagnostic technique.

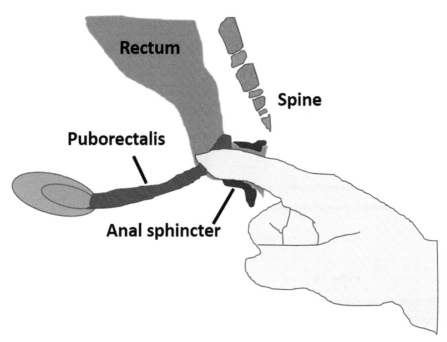

Fig. 2. DRE. The examiner must first inspect the perianal region and surrounding tissue to look for fissures, external hemorrhoids, or skin tags. Diminished or lack of perineal sensation and an abnormal anocutaneous reflex can indicate pudendal neuropathy. A lubricated gloved finger is inserted into the rectum after allowing the anal sphincter to accommodate; the examiner assesses for the presence of stool, stricture, tenderness, or mass and can evaluate the resting anal tone. When the patient is instructed to squeeze, the examiner can gauge the initial and sustained anal squeeze efforts. During the instructed bear down maneuvers with one of the examiner's hands resting on the abdomen, rectoanal coordination can be evaluated.

87%, respectively, for identifying dyssynergia in patients with constipation. A more detailed explanation of the DRE is provided in THE DIGITAL RECTAL EXAM: APPROPRIATE TECHNIQUES FOR THE EVALUATION OF CONSTIPATION AND FECAL INCONTINENCE," in this issue.

Anorectal Manometry

High-resolution ARM (HR-ARM) is useful to define anorectal physiology in patients with suspected defecatory disorders. There is a significant correlation ($P>.001$) between ARM and DRE in identifying patients with inability to relax anal sphincter, paradoxic anal contraction, increased resting tone, and absence of perineal descent.[27] The flexible HR-ARM catheter contains several circumferentially placed sensors that can simultaneously detect pressures longitudinally from the entire anal canal and distal rectum.[8] The spatial-temporal topography of HR-ARM allows for better anatomic and physiologic display than conventional waveforms, previously the gold standard.[29] A rigid 3D high-definition ARM probe is also available allowing for presentation of data in both 2-dimensional and 3-dimensional formats. Regardless of the probe used, anorectal pressures at rest, with squeeze, and during simulated evacuation can be measured. Four types of dyssynergic patterns have been described with manometric profiles as shown in **Fig. 3**.[30] The results of ARM can be influenced by external factors, including body positioning.[31] Therefore, providers need to be cognizant of the

Normal

Rectum: adequate intrarectal propulsion

Anal sphincter: normal relaxation

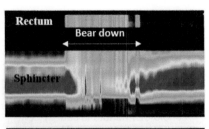

Type I

Rectum: adequate intrarectal propulsion

Anal sphincter: paradoxical contraction

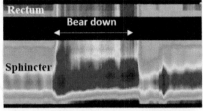

Type II

Rectum: inadequate intrarectal propulsion

Anal sphincter: paradoxical contraction

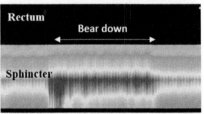

Type III

Rectum: adequate intrarectal propulsion

Anal sphincter: absent or inadequate relaxation

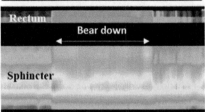

Type IV

Rectum: inadequate intrarectal propulsion

Anal sphincter: absent or inadequate relaxation

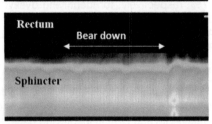

Fig. 3. Manometric subtypes of dyssynergic defecation.

potential for overdiagnosis of dyssynergic defecation when studies are only performed in the left lateral decubitus position.

ARM probes also have an attached balloon around the rectal sensors that can be inflated to assess rectal sensory function. Rectal sensation is evaluated in response to gradual intermittent balloon distension to identify initial, constant desire to defecate and maximum tolerable sensations. Rectal hyposensitivity has been associated with patients with spinal cord injury and fecal incontinence and is more common in patients with functional rather than structural defecatory disorders (ie, rectal prolapse, excessive perineal descent, or rectocele).[32] Severe rectal hyposensitivity may also be associated with fecal seepage, especially in children and adolescents. Alternatively, rectal hypersensitivity is a hallmark of IBS-C.

Balloon Expulsion Test

BET is a simple, adjunctive test to ARM.[18] BET is most often performed when a balloon attached to a catheter is inserted into the rectum and filled with 50 mL warm water. The patient is then asked to sit on a commode and attempt to evacuate the balloon. A threshold of 1 minute is usually considered normal,[19] but there is considerable variation across clinical practice with some centers considering cutoffs of 2 or 3 minutes abnormal. When compared with ARM and defecography, BET has a high specificity and negative predictive value, but poor positive predictive value and a low sensitivity around 50% for dyssynergic defecation.[33]

Defecography

Defecography can be used to evaluate pelvic floor disorders including rectoceles, rectal prolapse, solitary rectal ulcer, descending perineum syndrome, and intussusception.[34] Barium defecography (evacuation proctography) involves instillation of radiopaque barium paste into the rectum. The anatomy and function of the pelvic floor is then fluoroscopically assessed as a patient attempts to defecate. Dynamic imaging is used to record the structural and functional changes of the anal canal and rectum. Magnetic resonance (MR) defecography also visualizes the anterior (bladder and urethra) and middle (vagina and uterus) pelvic structures in addition to the anorectum, which may allow for a more comprehensive evaluation of patients with multiorgan involvement or those who have previously undergone pelvic surgeries.[35] MR defecography has the advantage of using intrinsic soft tissue contrast, multiplanar imaging capability, and absence of ionizing radiation and is well tolerated by most patients.[36] A prospective comparative study, however, showed that barium proctography was more sensitive in detecting trapping rectoceles (75% versus 31%, $P<.001$) and intussusception (56% versus 35%, $P = .023$).[37] This observation was likely attributable to body position given that barium proctography is performed in the seated position, whereas MR defecography is performed in the semirecumbent position.

Biofeedback Therapy

Biofeedback therapy is the foundation of any treatment approach to dyssynergic defecation. An effective biofeedback therapy program should take into account patient symptoms, underlying pathophysiology, age, comorbid conditions, and patient expectations. Neuromuscular or biofeedback training is an instrument-based "operant-conditioning" technique that corrects the dyssynergia between abdominal, rectal, and anal muscles for coordinated evacuation and corrects impaired rectal sensation. Treatment efficacy ranges from 70% to 80% among randomized controlled trials (RCTs).[38] Biofeedback therapy is more effective than sham treatment, polyethylene glycol, or diazepam.[39,40] Long-term studies have shown that the efficacy of biofeedback therapy after completion of treatment is maintained for more than 2 years.[41,42] Home biofeedback therapy using handheld monitoring devices, which may increase access to care to patients with dyssynergic defecation, was recently found to be noninferior to office therapy with significantly lower median cost.[43]

The purpose of biofeedback therapy is to train patients to generate effective abdominal push efforts that are reflected on a visual monitor as increased intrarectal pressure synchronized with decreased anal sphincter pressure corresponding to relaxation to promote successful and complete defecation.[44] Three main phases of the biofeedback therapy for constipation, established as the Rao protocol, are shown in **Fig. 4.**[45,46] The first phase involves patient evaluation and education. The therapist reviews the patient's stool diary, assesses the patient-reported symptoms using visual analog scales, and educates the patient on the purpose of anorectal function (ARM) testing, normal physiology of defecation, and pathology of dyssynergic defecation. The biofeedback therapy protocol and treatment goals are also reviewed, including instruction on diaphragmatic breathing exercises and timed toilet training. The second or active phase of biofeedback therapy involves both verbal feedback from the therapist and visual/auditory feedback from the visual monitor. While sitting on a commode with a manometry probe inserted into the rectum patients visualize the pressure changes of the rectum and anal canal with real-time feedback, as shown in **Fig. 5.**[44,47] The duration of training sessions lasts 30 to 60 minutes, approximately 1 to 2 weeks apart with a total of 4 to 6 sessions. The therapist should encourage the patient to practice training at home. In the third or reinforcement phase, follow-up biofeedback therapy sessions should occur at 6 weeks and 3, 6, and 12 months after completion of the active phase. Rectal sensory training can also be provided by intermittent, ramp rectal balloon inflation for patients with dyssynergia with impaired rectal sensation.[44]

Alternative treatment options for dyssynergic defecation include botulinum toxin injection, intrarectal diazepam, myectomy, or ileostomy. However, these treatments are associated with mixed results,[48,49] For example, injection of botulinum toxin into the anal sphincter may result in fecal incontinence.[50] In patients with other overlapping types of constipation, such as slow-transit constipation or IBS-C, appropriate pharmacologic treatments such as secretagogues or prokinetic serotonergic agents may be added.

Functional Anorectal Pain

Functional anorectal pain is subdivided into 3 diagnoses depending on the symptom duration and presence of anorectal tenderness. Patients with levator ani syndrome (LAS) experience ongoing anorectal pain with tenderness upon palpation of levator ani muscles. Patients with unspecified anorectal pain have persistent anorectal pain without tenderness of the levator ani muscles. With proctalgia fugax, patients endure brief episodes of pain lasting a few seconds to minutes with longer pain-free

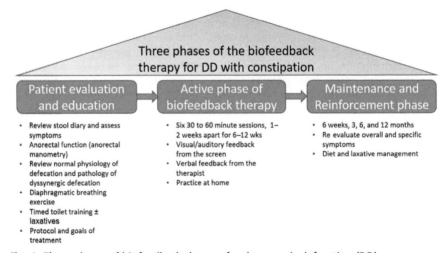

Fig. 4. Three phases of biofeedback therapy for dyssynergic defecation (DD).

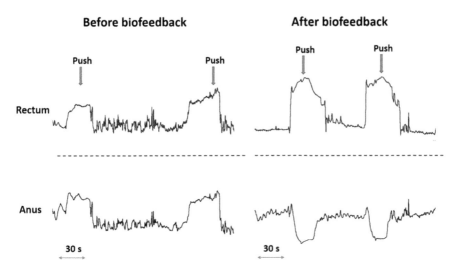

Before biofeedback   **After biofeedback**

Fig. 5. Manometric changes observed during biofeedback therapy. This example of successful biofeedback therapy demonstrates a patient with type I dyssynergic defecation (*left*). After biofeedback therapy, the patient is able to maintain adequate rectal propulsion with relaxation of the anal sphincter (*right*).

intervals.[7,51] It is important to exclude structural or other organic causes of rectal pain. DRE and anoscopy allow examiners to rule out anal fissures, fistulas, and hemorrhoids. Flexible sigmoidoscopy can identify other causes including inflammatory bowel disease, intramuscular abscesses, and solitary rectal ulcers.

Levator Ani Syndrome

Chronic, recurrent rectal pain in patients with LAS usually lasts greater than 30 minutes.[7,51] On physical examination, tenderness occurs with traction on puborectalis muscle. In a US householder survey conducted to assess for functional GI disorders, 6.6% among 5430 participants were estimated to have LAS.[52]

Translumbosacral anorectal magnetic stimulation (TAMS), a novel noninvasive neurophysiological test, can be used to detect lumbosacral neuropathy that is present in patients with LAS. TAMS uses a magnetic coil placed on the skin in 4 regions over the lumbosacral plexi and single magnetic pulses measure the latencies of motor evoked potentials (MEP) of anal and rectal muscles. In a study of 251 patients with anorectal disorders, patients with LAS were found to have bilateral, prolonged lumboanal, sacroanal, and sacrorectal MEPs ($P<.02$), suggesting significant anorectal neuropathy.[53]

Comparative uncontrolled studies have shown that sitz baths, muscle relaxants, diathermy, tricyclic antidepressants, and sacral nerve stimulation may be helpful.[54] In a randomized controlled study comparing biofeedback therapy, electrogalvanic stimulation, and massage, biofeedback therapy was found to be superior with reduction of rectal pain lasting for 1 year after treatment.[55] Botulinum toxin injection has been ineffective in relieving anal pain.[56] Recently, a pilot open-label study demonstrated that translumbosacral neuromodulation therapy (TNT), a novel and noninvasive treatment similar to TAMS, but using repetitive magnetic stimulation (600–900 pulses each of 4 sites), significantly improved anorectal pain in patients with LAS.[57]

Proctalgia Fugax

Pain in proctalgia fugax locates to the rectum and is unrelated to defecation. Episodes of pain in patients with proctalgia fugax may last up to 30 minutes.[7,51] Proctalgia fugax is twice as common in females with a mean age of 51 years.[58] In two-thirds of cases, pain in proctalgia fugax is stabbing, cramping, or spasmlike.[59]

As episodes of pain in proctalgia fugax are brief and infrequent, no specific treatment recommendations are endorsed.[60] A conservative approach includes patient reassurance and warm sitz baths. If symptoms persist for greater than 3 months, topical treatments with glyceryl trinitrate (0.2%) or diltiazem (2%) may be considered. Salbutamol inhalation (200 μg), warm water enemas, clonidine (150 μg, twice a day), local anesthetic blocks, or botulinum toxin injection into the IAS have also been suggested.[61]

Rectocele

A rectocele is an outpouching of the rectal wall either anteriorly toward the vagina or posteriorly through the sacrum.[62] Small rectoceles (<2 cm) are common in healthy individuals.[62] Advanced age, vaginal deliveries, obesity, constipation, and previous pelvic surgeries, such as hemorrhoidectomy or episiotomy, are associated with rectoceles. Patients with rectoceles commonly present with symptoms similar to dyssynergic defecation. Approximately 9 of 10 patients with significant rectoceles have other associated defecatory conditions, such as intussusception, dyssynergic defecation, and abnormal perineal descent.[63]

Patients with rectoceles may experience constipation, fecal incontinence, or vaginal symptoms such as dyspareunia or anterior bulging, with "splinting" (digital manipulation of vaginal wall to allow passage of stool) used to reduce the latter anatomic variant. In such patients, a thorough physical examination includes a vaginal examination in addition to a DRE to assess rectocele length and width as well as to evaluate the perineal body.

HR-ARM and BET should be performed in patients with functional constipation and rectoceles who fail conservative management. If the results are equivocal, dynamic barium or MR defecography can quantify the size of the rectocele and identify other underlying anatomic abnormalities such as intussusception, solitary rectal ulcer syndrome, or descending perineum syndrome.

Initial treatment consists of conservative medical management, such as fiber, increased water consumption, and laxatives. Biofeedback therapy also provides relief in patients with both dyssynergic defecation and large rectoceles (greater than 2 cm).[64] Seventy percent of patients respond to medical management and biofeedback therapy.[65] Surgical repairs, most commonly posterior colporrhaphy or the STARR (stapled transanal rectal resection) procedure are considered for refractory, large rectoceles. Posterior colporrhaphy involves transvaginal repair of the rectovaginal septum. The addition of a biological or prosthetic graft to the repair has not been shown to afford further durability or significant benefits when compared with conventional surgery and is not recommended.[66] Several transanal surgical approaches have been tested aiming to resect redundant rectal mucosa resulting in obstructive defecatory symptoms.[66] The STARR procedure uses a stapler device for endorectal resection of the distal rectum in patients with obstructive defecatory symptoms attributable to rectocele or rectal intussusception. However, a high rate of symptom recurrence and decline in quality of life after the STARR procedure has been reported in long-term follow-up.[67]

Descending Perineum Syndrome

Descending perineum syndrome (DPS) is characterized by excessive perineal descent during straining with the perineum falling below the pubococcygeal line (a line drawn from the coccyx to the pubic symphysis). Risk factors for DPS include female gender, age, multiple vaginal deliveries, and underlying rectocele. Repetitive straining can result in a weak pelvic floor and cause rectal ballooning into the anal canal. Symptoms include feelings of incomplete evacuation, straining or overt fecal incontinence.

Defecography is an essential test to diagnose DPS with MR defecography allowing better visualization of surrounding soft tissues of the pelvis. Counseling against excessive straining during defecation, medical management, and biofeedback therapy should be considered in cases of DPS to prevent further exacerbation. There is no consensus on the appropriate surgical treatment of DPS. In a small case series, 9 female patients underwent isolated retroanal levator plate myorrhaphy, which resulted in a mean reduction of perineal descent of 1.08 cm (extremes: 0–1.5). Further studies integrating defecography are needed to validate this surgical option.[68]

SUMMARY

Constipation is a common disorder with increasing prevalence and severity that impairs the quality of life for many patients. Laxative-refractory constipation is often due to underlying dyssynergic defecation. A diagnosis of dyssynergic defecation cannot be made by history alone. A thorough DRE is a key initial step in the evaluation of patients with constipation and anorectal symptoms. No single diagnostic test can define anorectal pathology, and therefore, HR-ARM, BET, and defecography should be considered in combination. Biofeedback therapy is the mainstay for treatment of dyssynergic defecation and may be considered in patients with rectoceles, slow-transit constipation, and IBS-C. Biofeedback therapy is safe, effective, and durable in the appropriate patient. Home biofeedback therapy should increase access to care for many patients. LAS can be a debilitating cause of anorectal pain, and lumbosacral neuropathy may be a key pathophysiological disturbance. TNT is an emerging treatment of LAS that targets lumbosacral neuropathy.

CLINICS CARE POINTS

- DRE should be performed in routine clinical practice for the evaluation of anorectal disorders. Digital palpation should be used to assess for tenderness, spasm, mass, or stricture and bear down to assess pelvic floor coordination, perineal descent, and rectal mucosal intussusception or prolapse.

- Dyssynergic defecation should be diagnosed by fulfilling criteria for functional constipation or IBS-C with the presence of at least 2 of 3 abnormal test results: BET, anorectal pressure profile by manometry or surface EMG, and/or defecography.

- Biofeedback therapy is the mainstay for treatment of dyssynergic defecation. Patient expectations, age, and comorbidities should be taken into account to ensure optimal participation, and referral to an experienced biofeedback therapist is essential to ensure successful treatment.

- Most patients with significant rectoceles have other associated conditions including intussusception, dyssynergic defecation, and abnormal perineal descent. Biofeedback therapy should be considered in patients with rectoceles before surgical referral.

- The presence, location, and duration of anorectal tenderness can be used to differentiate between the different causes of functional anorectal pain

AUTHOR CONTRIBUTIONS

A. Sharma was involved with the concept and design of the article; drafting of the article; critical revision of the article for important intellectual talent content, including figures and tables; and approved the final draft for submission. A. Herekar was involved with writing the article, developing figures and tables, and critical revision. Y. Yan was involved with writing the article and developing figures and tables. S.S.C. Rao was involved with critical revision of the article for important intellectual talent content, including figures and tables.

ACKNOWLEDGMENTS

The authors would like to thank Helen Smith, who provided secretarial and administrative assistance.

DISCLOSURE

Dr. Sharma serves on advisory board of Takeda and Phathom Pharmaceuticals.

REFERENCES

1. Higgins PD, Johanson JF. Epidemiology of constipation in North America: a systematic review. Am J Gastroenterol 2004;99:750–9.
2. Singh G, Lingala V, Wang H, et al. Use of health care resources and cost of care for adults with constipation. Clin Gastroenterol Hepatol 2007;5:1053–8.
3. Sethi S, Mikami S, LeClair J, et al. Inpatient burden of constipation in the United States: an analysis of national trends in the United States from 1997 to 2010. Am J Gastroenterol 2014;109:250–6.
4. Sommers T, Corban C, Sengupta N, et al. Emergency department burden of constipation in the United States from 2006 to 2011. Am J Gastroenterol 2015;110: 572–9.
5. Suares NC, Ford AC. Prevalence of, and risk factors for, chronic idiopathic constipation in the community: systematic review and meta-analysis. Am J Gastroenterol 2011;106:1582–91 [quiz 1581, 1592].
6. Nellesen D, Yee K, Chawla A, et al. A systematic review of the economic and humanistic burden of illness in irritable bowel syndrome and chronic constipation. J Manag Care Pharm 2013;19:755–64.
7. Rao SS, Bharucha AE, Chiarioni G, et al. Anorectal disorders. Gastroenterology 2016;150:1430–42.e4.
8. Sharma A, Rao S. Constipation: pathophysiology and current therapeutic approaches. Gastrointest Pharmacol 2016;239:59–74.
9. Serra J, Mascort-Roca J, Marzo-Castillejo M, et al. Clinical practice guidelines for the management of constipation in adults. Part 1: Definition, aetiology and clinical manifestations. Gastroenterol Hepatol 2017;40:132–41.
10. Basilisco G, Coletta M. Chronic constipation: a critical review. Dig Liver Dis 2013; 45:886–93.
11. Rao SS, Camilleri M. Approach to the patient with constipation. Yamadas Textbook Gastroenterol 2015;20:757–80.
12. Sharma A, Rao S, Harrison JH. Anorectal Function. 2020.
13. Gray H, Standring S. Gray's anatomy: the anatomical basis of clinical practice. London: Churchill Livingstone; 2008.

14. Jones P, Lubowski D, Swash M, et al. Relation between perineal descent and pudendal nerve damage in idiopathic faecal incontinence. Int J Colorectal Dis 1987; 2:93–5.
15. Sultan AH, Kamm MA, Hudson CN. Pudendal nerve damage during labour: prospective study before and after childbirth. BJOG 1994;101:22–8.
16. Lubowski D, Swash M, Nicholls R, et al. Increase in pudendal nerve terminal motor latency with defaecation straining. Br J Surg 1988;75:1095–7.
17. Lien K-C, Morgan DM, Delancey JO, et al. Pudendal nerve stretch during vaginal birth: a 3D computer simulation. Am J Obstet Gynecol 2005;192:1669–76.
18. Rao SS, Ozturk R, Laine L. Clinical utility of diagnostic tests for constipation in adults: a systematic review. Am J Gastroenterol 2005;100:1605–15.
19. Rao SS, Hatfield R, Soffer E, et al. Manometric tests of anorectal function in healthy adults. Am J Gastroenterol 1999;94:773–83.
20. Yan Y, Jimenez E, Karunaratne T, et al. Assessment of mobile APP for constipation and incontinence: randomized crossover study in healthy subjects. Am J Gastroenterol 2019;114:S1578.
21. Yan Y, Jimenez E, Sharma A, et al. How useful is constipation stool APP compared to paper stool diary-randomized study of constiaption and healthy subjects. Gastroenterology 2020;158:S400.
22. Marquis P, De La Loge C, Dubois D, et al. Development and validation of the Patient Assessment of Constipation Quality of Life questionnaire. Scand J Gastroenterol 2005;40:540–51.
23. Frank L, Kleinman L, Farup C, et al. Psychometric validation of a constipation symptom assessment questionnaire. Scand J Gastroenterol 1999;34:870–7.
24. Bharucha AE, Locke G III, Seide B, et al. A new questionnaire for constipation and faecal incontinence. Aliment Pharmacol Ther 2004;20:355–64.
25. Rao SS, Tuteja AK, Vellema T, et al. Dyssynergic defecation: demographics, symptoms, stool patterns, and quality of life. J Clin Gastroenterol 2004;38:680–5.
26. Curtin B, Jimenez E, Rao SS. Clinical Evaluation of a Patient With Symptoms of Colonic or Anorectal Motility Disorders. J Neurogastroenterol Motil 2020;26:423.
27. Tantiphlachiva K, Rao P, Attaluri A, et al. Digital rectal examination is a useful tool for identifying patients with dyssynergia. Clin Gastroenterol Hepatol 2010;8: 955–60.
28. Rao SS. Dyssynergic defecation and biofeedback therapy. Gastroenterol Clin North Am 2008;37:569–86, viii.
29. Lee TH, Bharucha AE. How to Perform and Interpret a High-resolution Anorectal Manometry Test. J Neurogastroenterol Motil 2016;22:46–59.
30. Rao SS, Patcharatrakul T. Diagnosis and Treatment of Dyssynergic Defecation. J Neurogastroenterol Motil 2016;22:423–35.
31. Rao SS, Kavlock R, Rao S. Influence of body position and stool characteristics on defecation in humans. Am J Gastroenterol 2006;101:2790–6.
32. Gladman MA, Lunniss PJ, Scott SM, et al. Rectal hyposensitivity. Am J Gastroenterol 2006;101:1140–51.
33. Minguez M, Herreros B, Sanchiz V, et al. Predictive value of the balloon expulsion test for excluding the diagnosis of pelvic floor dyssynergia in constipation. Gastroenterology 2004;126:57–62.
34. Karasick S, Karasick D, Karasick SR. Functional disorders of the anus and rectum: findings on defecography. AJR Am J Roentgenol 1993;160:777–82.
35. Colaiacomo MC, Masselli G, Polettini E, et al. Dynamic MR imaging of the pelvic floor: a pictorial review. Radiographics 2009;29:e35.

36. Piloni V, Tosi P, Vernelli M. MR-defecography in obstructed defecation syndrome (ODS): technique, diagnostic criteria and grading. Tech Coloproctol 2013;17: 501–10.

37. Zafar A, Seretis C, Feretis M, et al. Comparative study of magnetic resonance defaecography and evacuation proctography in the evaluation of obstructed defaecation. Colorectal Dis 2017;19:O204–9.

38. Heymen S, Scarlett Y, Jones K, et al. Randomized, controlled trial shows biofeedback to be superior to alternative treatments for patients with pelvic floor dyssynergia-type constipation. Dis Colon Rectum 2007;50:428–41.

39. Rao SS, Seaton K, Miller M, et al. Randomized controlled trial of biofeedback, sham feedback, and standard therapy for dyssynergic defecation. Clin Gastroenterol Hepatol 2007;5:331–8.

40. Chiarioni G, Whitehead WE, Pezza V, et al. Biofeedback is superior to laxatives for normal transit constipation due to pelvic floor dyssynergia. Gastroenterology 2006;130:657–64.

41. Lee HJ, Boo SJ, Jung KW, et al. Long-term efficacy of biofeedback therapy in patients with dyssynergic defecation: results of a median 44 months follow-up. Neurogastroenterol Motil 2015;27:787–95.

42. Rao SS, Valestin J, Brown CK, et al. Long term efficacy of biofeedback therapy for dyssynergia-randomized controlled trial The. Am J Gastroenterol 2010;105:890.

43. Rao SS, Valestin JA, Xiang X, et al. Home-based versus office-based biofeedback therapy for constipation with dyssynergic defecation: a randomised controlled trial. Lancet Gastroenterol Hepatol 2018;3:768–77.

44. Rao SS, Welcher KD, Pelsang RE. Effects of biofeedback therapy on anorectal function in obstructive defecation. Dig Dis Sci 1997;42:2197–205.

45. Rao SS. Biofeedback therapy for constipation in adults. Best Pract Res Clin Gastroenterol 2011;25:159–66.

46. Patcharatrakul T, Pitisuttithum P, Rao S, et al. Biofeedback therapy. In: Rao SS, Lee YY, Ghoshal UC, editors. Clinical and basic neurogastroenterology and motility. 1st edition. Cambridge (MA): Academic Press; 2020. p. 517–32.

47. Rao SS, Benninga MA, Bharucha AE, et al. ANMS-ESNM position paper and consensus guidelines on biofeedback therapy for anorectal disorders. Neurogastroenterol Motil 2015;27:594–609.

48. Ron Y, Avni Y, Lukovetski A, et al. Botulinum toxin type-A in therapy of patients with anismus. Dis Colon Rectum 2001;44:1821–6.

49. Podzemny V, Pescatori LC, Pescatori M. Management of obstructed defecation. World J Gastroenterol 2015;21:1053–60.

50. Hallan R, Melling J, Womack N, et al. Treatment of anismus in intractable constipation with botulinum A toxin. Lancet 1988;332:714–7.

51. Bharucha AE, Lee TH. Anorectal and Pelvic Pain. Mayo Clin Proc 2016;91: 1471–86.

52. Drossman DA, Li Z, Andruzzi E, et al. U.S. householder survey of functional gastrointestinal disorders. Prevalence, sociodemography, and health impact. Dig Dis Sci 1993;38:1569–80.

53. Yan Y, Herekar A, Gu G, et al. Clinical utility of translumbosacral anorectal magnetic stimulation (TAMS) test in anorectal disorders. Gastroenterology 2019;156. S-354-S-355.

54. Atkin GK, Suliman A, Vaizey CJ. Patient characteristics and treatment outcome in functional anorectal pain. Dis colon rectum 2011;54:870–5.

55. Chiarioni G, Nardo A, Vantini I, et al. Biofeedback is superior to electrogalvanic stimulation and massage for treatment of levator ani syndrome. Gastroenterology 2010;138:1321–9.
56. Rao SS, Paulson J, Mata M, et al. Clinical trial: effects of botulinum toxin on Levator ani syndrome–a double-blind, placebo-controlled study. Aliment Pharmacol Ther 2009;29:985–91.
57. Rao SS, Yan Y, Erdogan A, et al. Translumbosacral neuromodulation theraphy (TNT): a novel treatment for levator ani syndrome (LAS). Gastroenterology 2020;158:S–145.
58. de Parades V, Etienney I, Bauer P, et al. Proctalgia fugax: demographic and clinical characteristics. What every doctor should know from a prospective study of 54 patients. Dis colon rectum 2007;50:893–8.
59. Chiarioni G, Popa S-L. Anorectal pain. Clinical and basic neurogastroenterology and motility. London: Elsevier; 2020. p. 505–15.
60. Wald A, Bharucha AE, Cosman BC, et al. ACG clinical guideline: management of benign anorectal disorders. Official J Am Coll Gastroenterol 2014;109:1141–57.
61. Jeyarajah S, Chow A, Ziprin P, et al. Proctalgia fugax, an evidence-based management pathway. Int J Colorectal Dis 2010;25:1037–46.
62. Mustain WC. Functional Disorders: Rectocele. Clin Colon Rectal Surg 2017;30: 63–75.
63. Rotholtz N, Efron J, Weiss E, et al. Anal manometric predictors of significant rectocele in constipated patients. Tech Coloproctol 2002;6:73–7.
64. Mimura T, Roy AJ, Storrie JB, et al. Treatment of impaired defecation associated with rectocele by behavioral retraining (biofeedback). Dis colon rectum 2000;43: 1267–72.
65. Hicks CW, Weinstein M, Wakamatsu M, et al. In patients with rectoceles and obstructed defecation syndrome, surgery should be the option of last resort. Surgery 2014;155:659–67.
66. Schey R, Cromwell J, Rao SS. Medical & surgical management of pelvic floor disorders affecting defecation. Am J Gastroenterol 2012;107:1624.
67. Adams K, Papagrigoriadis S. Stapled transanal rectal resection (STARR) for obstructive defaecation syndrome: patients with previous pelvic floor surgery have poorer long-term outcome. Colorectal Dis 2013;15:477–80.
68. Beco J. Interest of retro-anal levator plate myorrhaphy in selected cases of descending perineum syndrome with positive anti-sagging test. BMC Surg 2008; 8:13.

Fecal Incontinence
Pathogenesis, Diagnosis, and Updated Treatment Strategies

Stacy Menees, MD, MS[a,b,]*, William D. Chey, MD[a]

KEYWORDS

- Fecal incontinence • Accidental bowel leakage • Anal sphincter • Sphincter injury

KEY POINTS

- FI is common and often goes underreported to health care providers. Physicians should inquire about these symptoms.
- FI is commonly associated with older age; GI diseases and symptoms, such as change in bowel habits (typically loose and/or frequent stools, fecal urgency); and debility.
- First-line treatment involves a combination of dietary and lifestyle modifications. Second-line treatment involves the use of medications that help modify bowel habits, and biofeedback training. If conservative methods fail to improve FI symptoms, then other surgical options are considered, such as sacral nerve stimulation and anal sphincter augmentation.

INTRODUCTION

Fecal incontinence (FI) is defined as the involuntary loss or passage of solid or liquid stool in patients. It is important to point out that the definition of FI does not include flatus incontinence nor fecal soilage. Fecal soilage is defined as the staining or streaking of underwear with fecal material or mucus. Additionally, anal incontinence (AI) and FI are often used interchangeably; however, AI comprises liquid and stool incontinence along with flatus incontinence in its definition.

With the publication of the Rome IV diagnostic criteria for FI in 2016, there were two key changes in the diagnosis of FI.[1] Rome IV does not distinguish structural or neurogenic causes from functional FI. With this change, the leaders from the Rome Foundation acknowledge that there are multiple, overlapping factors that lead to FI and that this prior distinction in Rome III had no impact in guiding treatment. With the Rome IV diagnostic criteria, the definition for the frequency of FI has also changed, from an

[a] Division of Gastroenterology and Hepatology, Department of Internal Medicine, Michigan Medicine Health System, Ann Arbor, MI, USA; [b] Veterans Affairs Ann Arbor Healthcare System, Ann Arbor, MI, USA
* Corresponding author. Department of Internal Medicine, Division of Gastroenterology and Hepatology, University of Michigan Health System, 3912 Taubman Center, 1500 East Medical Center Drive, SPC 5362, Ann Arbor, MI 48109.
E-mail address: sbartnik@med.umich.edu

Gastroenterol Clin N Am 51 (2022) 71–91
https://doi.org/10.1016/j.gtc.2021.10.005
0889-8553/22/Published by Elsevier Inc.
gastro.theclinics.com

occurrence once per month in Rome III to an occurrence of two times or greater per month in Rome IV.

Because of the disparate populations and definitions used in different studies, the prevalence of FI has varied widely, ranging from 2.0% to 20.7%.[2–6] The largest population-based survey using the National Institutes of Health Patient Reported Outcomes Measurement Information System gastrointestinal (GI) questionnaires found that one in seven people suffered from FI in their lifetime and approximately 1 in 20 had an FI episode in the last 7 days.[2] The prevalence of FI varies by age with the youngest participants having the lowest prevalence at 2.6% for those aged 20 to 29 years with increasing prevalence to 15.3% in subjects 70 years or older. The highest prevalence of FI is found in those living in nursing homes or other institutionalized settings, with a prevalence among this population between 46% and 67%.[7,8]

The true prevalence of FI is still likely underestimated because FI is significantly underreported by patients to their physicians.[9,10] Because of its embarrassing nature, patients are often reluctant to discuss their symptoms.[11–13] In a recent analysis of the Mature Women's Health Study, Brown and colleagues[9] found that two-thirds of women with FI do not seek care for their symptoms even though 40% of them had symptoms severe enough to impact their quality of life. Additionally, practitioners also bear some responsibility for the underdiagnosis of FI. Studies have demonstrated that all types of practitioners routinely fail to inquire about FI during outpatient visits.[14,15]

Quality of life is significantly negatively impacted in patients with FI. Patients report significant psychological stress with FI, causing anxiety and depression.[16,17] FI symptoms impact social activities, travel, and physical recreation.[12,18,19] For some, it leads to social isolation because of the fear and embarrassment of accidental bowel leakage.[20] To understand the burden of FI on patients, Rubin and colleagues[21] surveyed a cohort of severely ill, hospitalized subjects, of which 70% believed that bowel or bladder incontinence was as bad or worse than death. Among geriatricians, FI is a significant risk factor that increases the likelihood of referral of elderly patients to a nursing home.[22–24] Lastly, FI is associated with substantial economic costs to society.[14,25] Xu and colleagues[25] examined the direct and indirect costs of FI within the United States and found an average cost of $4110 per patient annually.

PATHOGENESIS

Continence is a complex process that involves the interaction of a neurologically intact levator ani complex (puborectalis muscle), internal anal sphincter (IAS), external anal sphincter (EAS), and compliant rectum. FI often occurs from one or more insults to the continence process including altered bowel motility, anal sphincter muscle damage or weakening, etiologies for poor rectal compliance, which includes rectal inflammation, abnormal rectal sensation, and dysfunctional pelvic floor musculature. In 80% of patients, findings suggest more than one pathophysiologic factor that causes FI.[26] Aging impacts the mechanisms of continence in multiple ways. Both sphincters can be affected with fibrosis and thickening leading to decreased resting tone, with thinning of the EAS producing a weak squeeze pressure.[27,28] Additionally, decreased rectal sensation, rectal compliance, and rectal capacity all cause impairment of colorectal sensorimotor and rectal reservoir function.[29]

RISK FACTORS

Multiple studies have been performed that have described risk factors for FI (**Table 1**).[8–11,13,23,30–33] Major risk factors for FI include advancing age, GI symptoms and GI diseases that cause changes in stool consistency, and nursing home

Table 1	
Risk factors for FI	
Patient-Level Factors	**Medical Comorbidities**
Increasing age	Dementia
Latino	Diabetes mellitus
Obesity	HIV
Gender (controversial female > male)	Multiple chronic illnesses
Active tobacco use	Urinary incontinence
Non-Hispanic African American (protective)	Decreased mobility/debility
Asian (protective)	Neurologic diseases/prior stroke
Postmenopause	History of pelvic radiation
Nursing home resident	Multiple sclerosis
	History of prostate cancer
GI symptoms and diseases	Scleroderma
Diarrhea	Spinal cord injury
Rectal urgency	
Irritable bowel syndrome	Prior surgery
Inflammatory bowel disease	Cholecystectomy
Celiac disease	Hysterectomy
Chronic intermittent constipation	Anorectal surgery
Constipation/fecal impaction	Sphincterotomy
Rectal sensation disorders	Hemorrhoidectomy
Rectal hypersensitivity	Anterior resection of the rectum
Rectal hyposensitivity	Colectomy with/out ileoanal pouch anastomosis
Obstetric history	Drugs (see **Table 2**)
Multiparity	
Episiotomy	Pelvic floor disorders
Sphincter laceration	Rectocele
Operative delivery (forceps/vacuum)	Descending perineum syndrome
Prolonged second stage of labor	Rectal prolapse
Birthweight >8.8 lb	

residency. The GI symptoms that are most strongly associated with FI are diarrhea and urgency.[2,3,30,31,34] However, any GI disease that can cause loose/watery stools or frequent bowel movements (more than 21 stools per week) can lead to FI.[2,3,15,32,34] Sometimes, FI may actually be caused by underlying constipation with or without fecal impaction, causing overflow diarrhea.[2,8] The mechanism of incontinence with diarrhea is multifactorial, but is likely caused by the increased difficulty of retaining loose/watery stool, which can overwhelm the anal sphincter as high volumes of effluent are delivered to the rectum under a short interval of time, reflex inhibition of the IAS, and/or interactions between the consistency of the stool and sphincter defects. Other major risk factors include diabetes mellitus, prior anorectal surgery, prostate cancer therapy, urinary incontinence, episiotomy, prior operative vaginal delivery or severe vaginal laceration, hysterectomy, anal intercourse, spinal injuries, and multiple chronic comorbidities.[2,3,33–40]

DIAGNOSIS

The first step in identifying affected patients is to ask about FI. Patients prefer the term "accidental bowel leakage" over "fecal incontinence" or "bowel incontinence."[41] To start the conversation, your practice can add "accidental bowel leakage" to the GI review of systems for new or return-visit paperwork. It is important to obtain a detailed history. One must determine whether the patient has symptoms of fecal soilage or FI by the amount of leakage and characterizing stool consistency, FI frequency, and timing of episodes. Patients should be queried if the episodes are passive/insensate versus active/urge incontinence. It is these questions that can help elucidate the underlying mechanisms for their symptoms. If patients report passive incontinence, it indicates that there is more likely to be an issue with the IAS or peripheral neuropathy, whereas those with urge incontinence are more likely to have a problem with the EAS/puborectalis muscle, a noncompliant rectum, or diarrhea. In patients who report fecal soilage, there may be incomplete defecation, structural (ie, rectal prolapse), or rectal sensation issues. Current medications should be reviewed to identify any medication that can exacerbate FI (**Table 2**). It is also important to consider constipating medications as a cause for overflow diarrhea/overflow incontinence. The physical examination must include a digital rectal examination to assess for rectal prolapse, sphincter defects, rectal tone, and fecal impaction. If fecal impaction is present, then treatment should focus on the management of constipation. An algorithm for the evaluation and management of FI is described in **Fig. 1**.

Fecal Soilage

An initial work-up for patients with fecal soilage should include anorectal manometry to evaluate for dyssynergic defecation. If present, the patient should be referred for

Table 2	
Medications that can exacerbate FI	
Drugs that cause loose stools	Bariatric: orlistat
	Cardiovascular: ACE inhibitors, ARB inhibitors, β-blockers, hydralazine, methyldopa, digoxin, procainamide, quinidine, statine, gemfibrozil, clofibrate, furosemide, acetazolamide, ethacrynic acid
	Endocrine: metformin, GLP-1 receptor agonists, levothyroxine
	GI: laxatives (sorbitol, lactulose), H2RAs, PPIs, magnesium-containing antacids, misoprostol, aminosalicylic acids, chenodeoxycholic acid, ursodeoxycholic acid
	Heme/oncologic: chemotherapeutic agents, immune checkpoint inhibitors, epidermal growth factor receptor inhibitors
	Infectious disease: broad-spectrum antibiotics
	Neurologic: levodopa, benzodiazepines
	Psychiatry: SSRIs, bupropion, nefazodone, trazadone, vortioxetine, lithium,
	Rheumatologic: colchicine, NSAIDS
	Random: magnesium supplements, bisphosphonates
Topical drugs applied to anus	Diltiazem gel, botulinum toxin A, glyceryl trinitrate ointment, bethanechol cream
Drugs that alter sphincter tone	SSRIs, β-blockers, nitrates, calcium channel antagonists, sildenafil, α_1-adrenoreceptor blockers

ACE, angiotensin-converting enzyme; ARB, angiotensin receptor blocker; NSAID, nonsteroidal anti-inflammatory drug; PPI, proton pump inhibitor; SSRI, selective serotonin reuptake inhibitor.

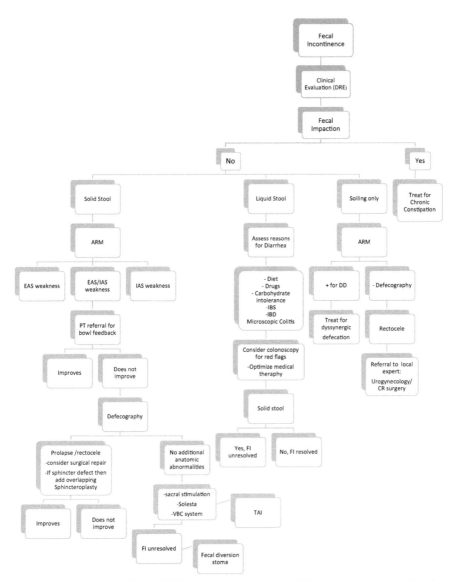

Fig. 1. FI treatment algorithm. ARM, anorectal manometry; CR, colorectal surgery; DD, dyssynergic defecation; DRE, digital rectal examination; IBD, inflammatory bowel disease; IBS, irritable bowel syndrome; PT, physical therapy; TAI, transanal irrigation; VBC, vaginal bowel control.

physical therapy and biofeedback training (BFT) and nonpharmacologic treatment options described next are considered (**Fig. 1**). Postvoid enemas are considered to remove residual stool in the rectum and anal canal.

Liquid Stool Incontinence

If the patient is incontinent with liquid stool only, then evaluation for causes of diarrhea should be pursued. If there is GI bleeding or diarrhea is persistent and not meal-related or occurs during the nighttime hours, colonoscopy should be performed to rule out organic diseases. Common causes of diarrhea include caffeine consumption, medication side effects, carbohydrate intolerance, microscopic colitis, irritable bowel syndrome, small intestinal bacterial overgrowth, bile acid malabsorption, and inflammatory bowel disease. Management generally focuses on dietary and lifestyle interventions and antidiarrheal pharmacologic options described next (see **Fig. 1**), but varies based on cause.

Solid Stool Incontinence

The approach for the patient with solid stool incontinence should begin with anorectal manometry to evaluate for weakness in the EAS, IAS, or both. If present, then referral to physical therapy for BFT is appropriate. If incontinence does not improve, then functional imaging with either fluoroscopic defecography or MRI defecography should be performed to evaluate for concomitant anatomic abnormalities.[35,36] If pelvic organ prolapse or rectocele is identified, then referral for surgical intervention should be considered, with or without sphincter repair as indicated. If surgical options are being considered, then an endoscopic ultrasound or transanal ultrasound is needed to assess sphincter integrity. If no anatomic abnormalities are identified, minimally invasive approaches, such as injectable bulking agents or vaginal bowel control system, is attempted. If these methods fail, surgical intervention with implantation of a sacral nerve stimulator is used. Definitive treatment with fecal diversion via colostomy or ileostomy is considered when all other treatments fail (see **Fig. 1**).

TREATMENT OF FECAL INCONTINENCE

Treatment of FI varies from noninvasive strategies, such as dietary and lifestyle changes, physical therapy with BFT, pharmacologic agents, sphincter augmentation methods with injectable bulking agents, and bowel control systems, to minimally invasive options, such as sacral nerve stimulation (SNS), to more invasive surgical interventions of sphincteroplasty or fecal diversion surgery. These options are listed in **Fig. 1**.

Dietary Interventions

Dietary interventions should focus on foods and beverages that are known to cause loose stools or urgency. Some 50% to 70% of participants report dietary triggers including caffeine, dairy, and fat-free substitutes.[42,43] Additionally, foods that are high in fermentable oligo-, di-, and mono-saccharides and polyols (FODMAP) can cause symptoms of diarrhea and urgency. Therefore, avoidance or reduction of these triggers is helpful by reducing FI symptoms.[44,45] Dietary fiber and/or stool bulking agents, such as psyllium, can improve symptoms of FI. Patients with the highest amount of fiber in their diets are least likely to experience FI.[46] In a pilot trial comparing psyllium versus gum arabic versus placebo, Bliss and colleagues[47] demonstrated a significant decrease in FI episodes after 1 month of either psyllium (49% of stools at baseline associated with FI to 17% with psyllium) or gum arabic (66% of stools at baseline associated with FI to 18% with gum arabic) as compared with placebo. In a much larger follow-up trial of 189 patients, Bliss and colleagues[48] compared psyllium versus gum arabic versus carboxymethylcellulose versus placebo on FI frequency. Psyllium was associated with a 50% decrease in FI episodes, whereas carboxymethylcellulose increased FI episodes by 32%. Minimal change was noted in the gum arabic and placebo arms. The recommended daily fiber intake for adults is 25 to 35 g. Slow introduction of fiber of no more than 5 g/wk is suggested to avoid bloating.

Lifestyle Modifications

Potentially modifiable risk factors, such as obesity, inactivity, and smoking, should be addressed.[49] Weight loss has been shown to improve FI in obese women.[50,51] Behavioral techniques for FI should also be implemented. This includes bowel-retraining techniques, such as toileting scheduling, particularly after meals to counter the gastrocolic reflex, and performing a few Kegel exercises between wiping to reduce episodes of incontinence.[52] People with FI should also be taught to pause and perform Kegel exercises when they feel an episode coming on rather than rush to the bathroom. Rushing to the toilet increases abdominal wall pressure, which can overwhelm a weak sphincter complex and increase the likelihood of incontinence.

Some patients may also benefit from vaginal splinting and/or techniques, such as anal wicking or postvoid enemas, to prevent fecal soilage or mild incontinence. Vaginal splinting is used in patients with an identified rectocele and involves the insertion of their finger into the vagina with pressure applied posteriorly toward the rectum.[53] Anal wicking is the technique of placing a long piece of cotton or a cotton ball shaped into a wick between the buttocks, resting directly on the anus so that mild seepage of fecal material is contained.[53] Lastly, patients may also benefit from perianal barrier creams to prevent skin excoriation and incontinence-associated dermatitis.[54]

Pharmacologic Therapy

Up to two-thirds of FI episodes are associated with diarrhea or loose stool. Medications that decrease motility should be used in patients with FI.[3] These include antidiarrheal/antimotility agents, bile acid resins, tricyclic antidepressants, and others that can enhance anal sphincter tone.

Loperamide has been evaluated as a single agent or in combination with other treatments in three randomized controlled studies. The Fecal Incontinence Prescription (Rx) Management (FIRM) randomized, crossover study of 80 adults (68% male) by Markland and colleagues,[55] compared daily loperamide versus psyllium in the treatment of FI. Both groups demonstrated improvement in number of FI episodes per week (loperamide: 7.9–4.1, $P < .001$; psyllium: 7.3–4.8, $P = .008$) and quality of life, but there was no difference between loperamide and psyllium among these end points. Loperamide was associated with higher rates of constipation (29%) and abdominal pain (17%) than psyllium, and psyllium had higher rates of diarrhea (17.1%), but no other adverse effects were noted. One participant died while taking loperamide during the second intervention, although further commentary on this was not provided. In the CAPABLE trial by Jelovsek and colleagues,[56] 300 participants were randomly assigned to four groups: (1) oral placebo plus education, (2) placebo plus anorectal manometry–assisted biofeedback, (3) loperamide plus education, or (4) loperamide plus anorectal manometry–assisted biofeedback. All four groups demonstrated some improvement in St. Mark's score, although there was no significant difference between groups at 24 weeks. Similar to Markland and colleagues, constipation was the most common adverse event reported, occurring in 2% of the groups receiving loperamide. Sjodahl and colleagues[57] randomized 64 female patients to either biofeedback (4–6 months) or medical treatment with loperamide and a stool bulking agent (2 months) and then added the other therapy to provide a course of combination therapy. When used alone, both single treatments failed to significantly decrease FI episodes. However, the number of FI episodes decreased significantly with combination treatment (median, 6 episodes/2 weeks to 2.5 episodes/2 weeks; $P < .0001$).

It is estimated that 1% of the population has bile acid diarrhea, thus putting individuals at risk for FI.[58] Remes-Troche and coworkers[59] compared the use of BFT with cholestyramine matched to a group who underwent BFT only. Subjects in the combination therapy group showed decreased stool frequency ($P < .01$), improved stool consistency ($P = .001$), and a reduced number of incontinent episodes ($P < .04$). In contrast, in the BFT group, stool frequency ($P = .8$) and stool consistency (0.23) did not improve compared with baseline.

In another small, open trial of 20 mg of amitriptyline in 18 patients compared with 24 control subjects, 89% in the amitriptyline group reported reduction of FI episodes.[60] Amitriptyline also led to significant improvement in median incontinence score ($P < .001$) and anal pressure ($P < .001$) compared with baseline. However, general use is limited in the elderly population because of anticholinergic, orthostatic hypotension and sedating side effects.

In a Cochrane Review, Omar and Alexander[61] identified 16 trials evaluating the efficacy of various medications for the treatment of FI in heterogenous subjects including the elderly, postsurgical, and diarrhea cohorts. This review included seven antidiarrheal medication trials (loperamide, codeine, diphenoxylate plus atropine), six trials for medications that enhance anal sphincter tone (phenylephrine gel or sodium valproate), one trial of zinc aluminum ointment, and two trials of laxatives in patients with FI caused by constipation and overflow diarrhea. No studies that compared a medication with another treatment modality were included. Although the data are limited, these studies showed improvement in FI but most reported side effects (only zinc-aluminum ointment had no reported adverse effects). There were insufficient data to recommend any one type of medication over another.

Biofeedback Therapy

Pelvic floor muscle training alone has been shown to be effective for the treatment of urinary incontinence, but outcomes for FI seem to be improved with the addition of BFT in uncontrolled studies.[62,63] BFT is a form of physical therapy that uses electronic instruments to monitor unconscious, physiologic activities and then use a visual or auditory signal to "feedback" the information to the patient. Although BFT techniques vary, the methods, which may be used independently or in combination, include: strength training to improve the striated muscles of the pelvic floor, rectal sensory training to enhance the ability to perceive and respond to rectal distentions, and then integrating the coordination of strength and sensory training for the anal sphincters.[64] In addition to pelvic floor exercises (PFE), BFT modalities include surface and/or intra-anal electromyography, manometric pressures, electrical stimulation, rectal distention balloons, and transanal ultrasound.[65] The success of BFT is variable with reports of 50% continence rates and up to 75% decrease in FI episodes in uncontrolled studies.[64] The first landmark trial by Norton and colleagues[66] randomized 171 patients with FI to one of four treatment groups: (1) standard care including advice from experienced specialist nurses for 3 to 6 months, (2) standard care plus anal sphincter exercises taught verbally and by digital examinations, (3) the above plus computer-assisted biofeedback involving coordination techniques with visual feedback of sphincter contractions, and (4) all of the above plus the daily use of a home biofeedback device. BFT was not superior to standard care with advice (53% improved in BFT group vs 54% in standard care + advice). These findings suggest that BFT does not offer any added benefit over standard care alone. However, this study did not evaluate the efficacy of BFT in patients who did not respond to conservative measures. To address this limitation, Heymen and colleagues[67] randomized 108 patients (after excluding 60 subjects who were adequately treated with medication, education, and behavioral strategies) to either PFE alone or manometric biofeedback plus PFE. Manometric biofeedback was more effective than PFE taught by verbal instructions with an intention-to-treat analysis demonstrating 77% achieving adequate relief. Additionally, instrumented biofeedback and PFE were more effective than conservative management alone. In reviewing the aforementioned CAPABLE trial, which had two arms that offered BFT singly and in combination with loperamide, the change in the FI severity relative to baseline was not significantly different among these groups versus the placebo plus education group. In the most recent Cochrane Review, Norton and Cody[63] did not find any evidence that specific types of biofeedback or exercise were more beneficial than the other, but found that BFT or electrical stimulation was more efficacious than PFE alone in patients that have failed to respond to other conservative measures. In aggregate, the data suggest that a structured course of education and medical management should initially be offered to patients with FI and if this fails, BFT should be considered.

Anal Augmentation

Perianal injection of bulking agents

The use of an injectate to augment the native anal sphincter is considered in patients with mild to moderate FI and those who have failed conservative medical therapies. At present, the most common injectable medication is dextranomer microspheres stabilized with hyaluronic acid (NASHA/Dx, Solesta, Palette Life Sciences, Santa Barbara, CA), although other injectable materials have been used (eg, autologous fat, carbon-coated beads, collagen, glutaraldehyde and silicone). A multicenter, randomized, sham-controlled study found that approximately half of the subjects receiving NASHA/Dx had a greater than 50% reduction in the number of FI events compared with 30% of patients with the sham injections (odds ratio, 2.36; 95% confidence interval [CI], 1.24–4.27; P = .0089).[68] An earlier, open-label trial demonstrated similar effectiveness results that lasted at least 12 months after treatment.[69] A later, randomized, controlled, evaluator-blinded trial comparing NASHA/Dx with BFT of 126 patients with AI demonstrated similar improvements in St. Mark's score between both arms (NASHA/Dx baseline 12.9 [95% CI, 11.8–14.0] to 8.3 [95% CI, 6.7–9.8]; BFT baseline 12.6 [95% CI, 11.4–13.8] to 7.2 [95% CI, 7.2–8.8]).[70] Adverse events that have been reported include pain (14%) and bleeding (7%) with serious rare complications of rectal or prostate abscess.

Radiofrequency Energy

The use of radiofrequency energy to the IAS to stimulate increased collagen deposition in the IAS and improve continence and sphincter tone has been approved by the Food and Drug Administration (FDA) since 2002.[71] A recent review found 11 studies with a total of 220 patients. The authors concluded that radiofrequency energy may be useful for the carefully selected patient (those with adequate muscle mass and collagen in the sphincter at baseline) to reduce the number of incontinence episodes and improve quality of life.[72] However, the results from the available studies have been variable, including two small recent studies.[73,74] Lam and colleagues[73] performed a small prospective cohort trial that failed to show any significant clinical response or durability up to 3 years following the procedure and also failed to show any improvement in anorectal pressures or rectal compliance, as measured by rectal endoscopic ultrasound and anorectal manometry. Visscher and colleagues[74] performed a randomized, sham-controlled trial of 40 subjects using a change in Vaizey incontinence score as the primary outcome. Both arms showed a small improvement in the Vaizey incontinence score, although with a negligible clinical impact. Because of these disappointing results, this therapy is not widely available in clinical practice.

Neuromodulation

Sacral nerve stimulation

In patients with moderate to severe FI who have failed to respond to more conservative measures, SNS is considered. SNS (Interstim, Medtronic, Minneapolis, MN) has been used for the last 20 years and is thought to improve FI by chronically stimulating the sacral nerves, and therefore the corresponding muscles, by applying a low-voltage electrical current via an implanted electrode through the corresponding sacral foramen.[75] Patton and colleagues[76] found that SNS induces colonic retrograde propagated contractions thus delaying colonic transit and delivery of stool to rectum. SNS placement is performed in a two-stage process with permanent device implantation if there is a reduction in FI in the trial period.

A recent Cochrane Review found that SNS is effective in improving FI.[75] In multiple small crossover studies, with the SNS device turned on, FI episodes were reduced 59% to 88% compared with conventional medical therapy.[77–79] FI symptom improvement seems to be durable, with Hull and colleagues[80] reporting 89% of patients reporting continued significant reduction in weekly episodes of FI at 5 years postimplantation compared with baseline (mean, 9.1 episodes of FI per week at baseline compared with 1.7 per week at 5 years), and about a third of patients continent. Multiple studies have shown impressive results with SNS even in patients with known sphincter defects, noting that the degree of defect did not impact results.[81–84]

Percutaneous Tibial Nerve Stimulation

The tibial nerve shares nerve fibers with the sacral nerve and stimulation of the tibial nerve is comparable with SNS in the treatment of urinary incontinence.[85–87] Uncontrolled trials and one small randomized controlled trial demonstrated 44% to 82% efficacy using the criteria of success of greater than 50% reduction in FI episodes.[88] Thin and colleagues[89] showed that percutaneous tibial nerve stimulation and SNS had comparable results in the treatment of FI, at least in the short term. However, when percutaneous tibial nerve stimulation was compared with a sham electrical stimulation procedure in two large randomized controlled trials, no difference was seen in FI clinical outcomes between the two groups.[90,91] Therefore, enthusiasm for this noninvasive treatment as a primary treatment of FI alone has dampened, but it provides a viable treatment option in patients with concurrent urge incontinence.

Insertion Devices

Anal inserts

Anal inserts that temporarily occlude the anal canal and prevent stool leakage are an option in patients with FI. Approved in the United States, Renew inserts (Renew Medical, Foster City, CA) are a single-use, disposable silicone device that is expelled at defecation. In a multicenter, open-label study of 73 patients, 78% had a 50% or greater reduction of FI and were very or extremely satisfied, with a median reduction of 0.9 episode/day to 0.2 episode/day.[92] However, there was a 35% drop out rate because of complaints of constant rectal pressure, because the device sits below the dentate line. In a small study of patients with familial adenomatous polyposis who had undergone restorative proctocolectomy with ileal pouch–anal anastomosis, the device was effective in 6/15 (40%) and acceptable to 8/15 (53%) of patients.[93]

This device could be considered for patients with low-grade FI and soilage but at present is no longer commercially available in the United States because of FDA import restrictions.

Vaginal Bowel Control System

The vaginal bowel control system (Eclipse System, Pelvalon Inc, Sunnyvale CA) is a vaginally placed device that was approved by the FDA in 2015 for women with FI. The device is fitted like a vaginal pessary with a posteriorly directed inflatable balloon. With balloon inflation, it occludes the rectal vault and prevents incontinence. At time for defecation, the patient then temporarily deflates the system. The major advantage of this device is that it is easily reversible and controlled by the patient. Richter and colleagues[94] were able to successfully fit 61 of 110 participants with 86% of women enrolled in the trial achieving treatment success and 41% reporting continence. A follow-up open-label study followed 73 participants who were successfully fitted with the system for 12 months.[95] The authors found that close to half reported lasting continence and 80% of the remaining participants had more than a 75% reduction in incontinence episodes. The most common adverse event was vaginal wall injury, with most adverse events (90/134%; 67%) occurring during the fitting period. Per Eclipse System instructions, practitioners are to evaluate for vaginal atrophy and "continue any existing prescription of vaginal estrogen cream, and consider the prescription of vaginal estrogen cream for patients with mild or moderate atrophy."[96]

Transanal Irrigation

Transanal irrigation is where large-volume water is introduced into the distal colon through the anus, facilitating emptying of the rectosigmoid and the left colon. There are various systems in use for this, including Biotrol (Biotrol International, Earth City, MO), Peristeen (Coloplast Inc, Humlebaek, Denmark), and Navina (Wellspect Health-Care, Mölndal, Sweden). With the performance of regular irrigations, control of bowel function is accomplished.[97] Studies available to assess the efficacy of transanal irrigation in FI are heterogenous with most enrolling patients with constipation, and only a single study enrolling individuals with isolated FI.[98] Efficacy rates vary, from complete continence in 9% to 38%, to 75% reporting improvement. Discontinuation rates have been reported as high as 57% because of a lack of efficacy, pain, and the lengthy nature of the irrigation procedure.

Surgical Options

More invasive surgical options are considered when conservative therapies have failed. Besides SNS, other options include sphincteroplasty, muscle transposition, antegrade continence enema (ACE), and fecal diversion. The transobturator posterior anal sling and artificial bowel sphincter are no longer available in the United States.

Sphincteroplasty

Repair of the anal sphincter with an anterior overlapping technique has long been used to treat FI caused by EAS injury when conservative therapies have failed. Most women with FI caused by anal sphincter injury have a history of vaginal delivery, and the most common risk factors include multiple vaginal deliveries, need for vaginal instrumentation during labor, third- or fourth-degree tear, pudendal nerve injury, and failed prior sphincteroplasty.[99,100] In the short-term, the median rate of either good or excellent fecal continence with sphincteroplasty is 70%, ranging from 30% to 83%.[101,102] However, numerous recent long-term studies have failed to confirm the durability of sphincteroplasty.[101,103–107] Long-term continence decreases from 0% to 60% in most studies. Although many studies have suggested that advanced age at the time of the surgery was a risk factor for long-term failure, a recent systematic review did not find any consistent risk factors predictive of failure.[107] Additionally, a large retrospective review of 321 women did not show any significant difference in long-term severity of FI, quality of life, or postoperative satisfaction between younger and older women.[108] Based on these findings, sphincteroplasty is no longer considered a primary treatment option for patients with FI.

Muscle transposition
Transposition of the gracilis muscle is another surgical technique that was used more commonly in the past for medically refractory FI, but it is rarely used now because of the high rate of adverse events associated with this procedure and availability of less invasive but equally effective treatment options.[102]

Antegrade continence enema
ACE for the treatment of FI has long been used in the pediatric population with good success.[109] However, this technique is rarely used in the adult population. The surgery involves the creation of a stoma from the appendix, terminal ileum, cecum, or another proximal access point, with water or enema solution instillation via this access point, which allows fecal material to be flushed from the colon in an antegrade manner. A recent systematic review found that most adults (47%–100%) were still performing ACE at 6 to 55 months follow-up, and at least a third of patients achieved full continence.[110] In the most recent observational study of 30 Dutch patients with FI or constipation, using the Malone continence scale (success rate is calculated by combining the full and partial success rates, using the number of subjects [n = 30] in the intention-to-treat group as denominator), ACE resulted in a disappointing overall success rate of 37%.[111]

Fecal Diversion
Use of colostomy or ileostomy for fecal diversion is considered when all other modalities of treatment have failed.[112,113] This is considered a last option for patients with FI, but for some can dramatically improve quality of life.[114] Physicians may consider this in patients with severe perianal trauma, severe neurogenic incontinence, severe radiation-induced incontinence, or complete pelvic floor denervation. Norton and colleagues[115] found that 83% of patients who had undergone colostomy placement for their FI had minimal to no restrictions in their life with their ostomy, and that 84% would choose to have the stoma placement again.

Potential Future Treatments

Translumbosacral neuromodulation therapy
Using the translumbosacral anorectal magnetic stimulation test, there is evidence for neurogenic disturbances with prolongation of the latency and amplitude of motor-evoked potentials in 88% of subjects with FI.[116] With these findings, Rao and colleagues[117] studied the efficacy of repetitive magnetic stimulation or translumbosacral neuromodulation therapy delivered at 1, 5, or 15 Hz at two lumbar and two sacral sites over 6 weeks in 33 patients with FI who had failed conservative measures. In all arms, FI improved using the end point of greater than or equal to a 50% reduction in the number of FI episodes. After 6 weeks of treatment, 1 Hz (10 of 11 patients; 91%) was more effective than 5 Hz (4 of 11 responders; 36%) and 15 Hz (6 of 11 responders; 54%), with a pooled responder rate of 61% (20 of 33 responders). Future, sham-controlled studies of translumbosacral neuromodulation therapy in men and women with FI are necessary to evaluate this promising modality.

Magnetic anal sphincter
The magnetic anal sphincter (MAS; Fenix, Torax Medical, Inc, St. Paul, MN) is a newer therapeutic option that was approved by the FDA as a humanitarian use device. The device is composed of a band of small, interlinked titanium beads with magnetic cores. This MAS is surgically implanted around the EAS. It functions to reinforce and improve competence of the sphincter. The magnets separate with Valsalva maneuver, thus allowing for defecation.

In a feasibility study, Lehur and colleagues[118] implanted MAS in 14 women, all of whom had previously failed other treatments. Only 5 of 14 were followed for at least 6 months, but among this group, there was a 91% mean reduction in average weekly FI episodes and a significant improvement in quality of life. Two of the 14 patients had the device explanted because of infection, and one had spontaneous passage of the device. Other observed adverse events included bleeding, pain, and obstructed defecation. This pilot group plus additional participants (35 total) were implanted with MAS between 2008 and 2011 and followed for a median period of 5.0 years (range, 0–5.6 years).[119] There was a 31% drop out rate because of device removal. In patients who retained their MAS device, 79%, 91%, and 73% reported treatment success at 1, 3, and 5 years. There were 30 adverse events reported in 20 patients, most commonly defecatory dysfunction (20%), pain (14%), erosion (11%), and infection (11%).

In a separate single-center study, Pakravan and Helmes[120] reported the results of 18 patients implanted with MAS for FI, followed up to 2 years (mean follow-up, 607 days). Because of an intraoperative rectal perforation in one subject, the procedure was aborted. Of the 17 remaining subjects, 76% of patients demonstrated at least a 50% reduction in number of weekly FI events. None of their patients required surgical removal of MAS, but 29% had pain and/or swelling.

Stem cell therapy
Both animal and human studies in which local injections of mesenchymal (bone marrow– or adipose-derived) or muscle-derived (muscle-derived stem cells or myoblasts derived from them) stem cells have been reported. These studies have demonstrated some encouraging functional results by stimulating the repair of acute and subacute anal sphincter injuries.[121] Stem cells combined with normal cells on bioengineered scaffolds have achieved the successful creation and implantation of intrinsically innervated anal sphincter constructs.[122] The clinical evidence, based on adipose-derived stem cells and myoblasts, is extremely limited yet has yielded some promising results, and seems to be safe.[123–125] Although there may be promise for this method in the future, much more research into the utility of autologous or stem cell transplant must be undertaken before it is ready for use in clinical practice.

SUMMARY

FI is a common and debilitating condition that often goes underreported to health care providers. As a provider, it is important to ask patients about FI symptoms and to identify risk factors. Although there are many possible risk factors associated with FI, the most significant seem to be advancing age, diarrhea or loose stool, GI diseases stool, fecal urgency, and generalized debility.

A therapeutic algorithm is presented in **Fig. 1**. Evaluation and management are tailored to specific symptoms and characteristics of the incontinence. Work-up often begins with a detailed digital rectal examination and in many cases, anorectal manometry. Depending on the patient's symptoms, other procedures (eg, colonoscopy, dynamic pelvic floor imaging) may also be needed. Once the burden of illness and cause of FI has been characterized, conservative treatments should be pursued.

Typically, initial therapies involve a combination of lifestyle and dietary modifications, pharmacologic agents, and BFT. If these treatments fail to improve FI symptoms, then other interventions are considered. Generally, less invasive options should be tried first, such as SNS, before other surgical options are explored.

CLINICS CARE POINTS

- Patients with gI symptoms and diseases associated with diarrhea at a marked increased risk for FI.
- Patients will not freely volunteer that they have FI-you must ask.
- Reverse the reversible (loose stool/diarrhea).Look for dietary causes-osmotics in their diets, caffeine, and lack of fiber.
- Start low and slow with psyllium and increase it gradually weekly.Toileting schedule after each meal can reduce episodes of FI.
- Rushing to the toilet will increase the likelihood of FI by increasing the intra-abdominal pressure and overwhelming the sphincter complex.
- Utilizing a physical therapist trained in pelvic floor is essential for effective biofeedback training.
- Sacral stimulation demonstrates the highest efficacy of continence.

DISCLOSURE

S. Menees discloses the following: Consultant for Takeda. W.D. Chey discloses the following: Consultant for AbbVie, Alfasigma, Allakos, Alnylam, Arena, Biomerica, Ferring, Gemelli, Ironwood, Nestle, Phathom, Progenity, Redhill, Ritter, Salix/Valeant, QOL Medical, Takeda, Urovant, and Vibrant; grants from Commonwealth Diagnostics International, Biomerica, Salix, QOL Medical, and Vibrant; and Stock Options from GI on Demand, Modify Health, and Ritter.

REFERENCES

1. Drossman DA, Hasler WL. Rome IV-functional GI disorders: disorders of gut-brain interaction. Gastroenterology 2016;150(6):1257–61.
2. Menees SB, Almario CV, Spiegel BMR, et al. Prevalence of and factors associated with fecal incontinence: results from a population-based survey. Gastroenterology 2018;154(6):1672–81.e3.
3. Whitehead WE, Borrud L, Goode PS, et al. Fecal incontinence in US adults: epidemiology and risk factors. Gastroenterology 2009;137(2):512–7, 517.e1-512.
4. Ditah I, Devaki P, Luma HN, et al. Prevalence, trends, and risk factors for fecal incontinence in United States adults, 2005-2010. Clin Gastroenterol Hepatol 2014;12(4):636–43, e1-2.
5. Koloski NA, Talley NJ, Boyce PM. Epidemiology and health care seeking in the functional GI disorders: a population-based study. Am J Gastroenterol 2002; 97(9):2290–9.
6. Botlero R, Bell RJ, Urquhart DM, et al. Prevalence of fecal incontinence and its relationship with urinary incontinence in women living in the community. Menopause 2011;18(6):685–9.
7. Bliss DZ, Harms S, Garrard JM, et al. Prevalence of incontinence by race and ethnicity of older people admitted to nursing homes. J Am Med Dir Assoc 2013;14(6):451.e1–7.

8. Nelson R, Furner S, Jesudason V. Fecal incontinence in Wisconsin nursing homes: prevalence and associations. Dis Colon Rectum 1998;41(10):1226–9.
9. Brown HW, Wexner SD, Lukacz ES. Factors associated with care seeking among women with accidental bowel leakage. Female Pelvic Med Reconstr Surg 2013;19(2):66–71.
10. Whitehead WE. Diagnosing and managing fecal incontinence: if you don't ask, they won't tell. Gastroenterology 2005;129(1):6.
11. Norton C. Nurses, bowel continence, stigma, and taboos. J Wound Ostomy Continence Nurs 2004;31(2):85–94.
12. Bharucha AE, Zinsmeister AR, Locke GR, et al. Symptoms and quality of life in community women with fecal incontinence. Clin Gastroenterol Hepatol 2006; 4(8):1004–9.
13. Bharucha AE, Zinsmeister AR, Locke GR, et al. Prevalence and burden of fecal incontinence: a population-based study in women. Gastroenterology 2005; 129(1):42–9.
14. Dunivan GC, Heymen S, Palsson OS, et al. Fecal incontinence in primary care: prevalence, diagnosis, and health care utilization. Am J Obstet Gynecol 2010; 202(5):493.e1–6.
15. Hosmer AE, Saini SD, Menees SB. Prevalence and severity of fecal incontinence in Veterans. J Neurogastroenterol Motil 2019;25(4):576–88.
16. Smith TM, Menees SB, Xu X, et al. Factors associated with quality of life among women with fecal incontinence. Int Urogynecol J 2013;24(3):493–9.
17. Melville JL, Fan MY, Newton K, et al. Fecal incontinence in US women: a population-based study. Am J Obstet Gynecol 2005;193(6):2071–6.
18. Perry S, Shaw C, McGrother C, et al. Prevalence of faecal incontinence in adults aged 40 years or more living in the community. Gut 2002;50(4):480–4.
19. Brown HW, Wexner SD, Segall MM, et al. Quality of life impact in women with accidental bowel leakage. Int J Clin Pract 2012;66(11):1109–16.
20. Miner PB Jr. Economic and personal impact of fecal and urinary incontinence. Gastroenterology 2004;126(1 Suppl 1):S8–13.
21. Rubin EB, Buehler AE, Halpern SD. States Worse Than Death Among Hospitalized Patients With Serious Illnesses. JAMA Intern Med 2016;176(10):1557–9.
22. Talley NJ, O'Keefe EA, Zinsmeister AR, et al. Prevalence of gastrointestinal symptoms in the elderly: a population-based study. Gastroenterology 1992; 102(3):895–901.
23. Grover M, Busby-Whitehead J, Palmer MH, et al. Survey of geriatricians on the effect of fecal incontinence on nursing home referral. J Am Geriatr Soc 2010; 58(6):1058–62.
24. Tsuji I, Whalen S, Finucane TE. Predictors of nursing home placement in community-based long-term care. J Am Geriatr Soc 1995;43(7):761–6.
25. Xu X, Menees SB, Zochowski MK, et al. Economic cost of fecal incontinence. Dis Colon Rectum 2012;55(5):586–98.
26. Rao SS. Fecal incontinence in a 56-year-old female executive. Clin Gastroenterol Hepatol 2007;5(4):422–6.
27. Fox JC, Fletcher JG, Zinsmeister AR, et al. Effect of aging on anorectal and pelvic floor functions in females. Dis Colon Rectum 2006;49(11):1726–35.
28. Lewicky-Gaupp C, Hamilton Q, Ashton-Miller J, et al. Anal sphincter structure and function relationships in aging and fecal incontinence. Am J Obstet Gynecol 2009;200(5):559.e1–5.
29. Yu SW, Rao SS. Anorectal physiology and pathophysiology in the elderly. Clin Geriatr Med 2014;30(1):95–106.

30. Kalantar JS, Howell S, Talley NJ. Prevalence of faecal incontinence and associated risk factors; an underdiagnosed problem in the Australian community? Med J Aust 2002;176(2):54–7.
31. Menees SB, Smith TM, Xu X, et al. Factors associated with symptom severity in women presenting with fecal incontinence. Dis Colon Rectum 2013;56(1): 97–102.
32. Markland AD, Goode PS, Burgio KL, et al. Incidence and risk factors for fecal incontinence in black and white older adults: a population-based study. J Am Geriatr Soc 2010;58(7):1341–6.
33. Markland AD, Dunivan GC, Vaughan CP, et al. Anal intercourse and fecal incontinence: evidence from the 2009-2010 National Health and Nutrition Examination Survey. Am J Gastroenterol 2016;111(2):269–74.
34. Bharucha AE, Zinsmeister AR, Schleck CD, et al. Bowel disturbances are the most important risk factors for late onset fecal incontinence: a population-based case-control study in women. Gastroenterology 2010;139(5):1559–66.
35. Christoforidis D, Bordeianou L, Rockwood TH, et al. Faecal incontinence in men. Colorectal Dis 2011;13(8):906–13.
36. Nelson R, Norton N, Cautley E, et al. Community-based prevalence of anal incontinence. JAMA 1995;274(7):559–61.
37. Bharucha AE, Zinsmeister AR, Locke GR, et al. Risk factors for fecal incontinence: a population-based study in women. Am J Gastroenterol 2006;101(6): 1305–12.
38. Quander CR, Morris MC, Melson J, et al. Prevalence of and factors associated with fecal incontinence in a large community study of older individuals. Am J Gastroenterol 2005;100(4):905–9.
39. Geynisman-Tan J, Kenton K, Leader-Cramer A, et al. Anal penetrative intercourse as a risk factor for fecal incontinence. Female Pelvic Med Reconstr Surg 2018;24(3):252–5.
40. Wu JM, Matthews CA, Vaughan CP, et al. Urinary, fecal, and dual incontinence in older U.S. adults. J Am Geriatr Soc 2015;63(5):947–53.
41. Brown HW, Wexner SD, Segall MM, et al. Accidental bowel leakage in the mature women's health study: prevalence and predictors. Int J Clin Pract 2012;66(11):1101–8.
42. Andy UU, Ejike N, Khanijow KD, et al. Diet modifications in older women with fecal incontinence: a qualitative study. Female Pelvic Med Reconstr Surg 2020;26(4):239–43.
43. Hansen JL, Bliss DZ, Peden-McAlpine C. Diet strategies used by women to manage fecal incontinence. J Wound Ostomy Continence Nurs 2006;33(1): 52–61 [discussion: 61-52].
44. Menees SB, Chandhrasekhar D, Liew EL, et al. A low FODMAP diet may reduce symptoms in patients with fecal incontinence. Clin Transl Gastroenterol 2019; 10(7):e00060.
45. Menees SB, Jackson K, Fenner D, et al. A randomized pilot study to compare the effectiveness of a low FODMAP diet vs. psyllium in patients with fecal incontinence and loose stools. Gastroenterology 2020;158(6):S4.
46. Joh HK, Seong MK, Oh SW. Fecal incontinence in elderly Koreans. J Am Geriatr Soc 2010;58(1):116–21.
47. Bliss DZ, Jung HJ, Savik K, et al. Supplementation with dietary fiber improves fecal incontinence. Nurs Res 2001;50(4):203–13.
48. Bliss DZ, Savik K, Jung HJ, et al. Dietary fiber supplementation for fecal incontinence: a randomized clinical trial. Res Nurs Health 2014;37(5):367–78.

49. Townsend MK, Matthews CA, Whitehead WE, et al. Risk factors for fecal incontinence in older women. Am J Gastroenterol 2013;108(1):113–9.

50. Markland AD, Richter HE, Burgio KL, et al. Weight loss improves fecal incontinence severity in overweight and obese women with urinary incontinence. Int Urogynecol J 2011;22(9):1151–7.

51. Burgio KL, Richter HE, Clements RH, et al. Changes in urinary and fecal incontinence symptoms with weight loss surgery in morbidly obese women. Obstet Gynecol 2007;110(5):1034–40.

52. Norton C, Whitehead WE, Bliss DZ, et al. Conservative management of Fecal Incontinence in Adults Committee of the International Consultation on I. Management of fecal incontinence in adults. Neurourol Urodyn 2010;29(1):199–206.

53. Program MMMBC. Available at: http://www.med.umich.edu/1libr/MBCP/Splinting.pdf. March 18, 2021.

54. Kon Y, Ichikawa-Shigeta Y, Iuchi T, et al. Effects of a skin barrier cream on management of incontinence-associated dermatitis in older women: a cluster randomized controlled trial. J Wound Ostomy Continence Nurs 2017;44(5):481–6.

55. Markland AD, Burgio KL, Whitehead WE, et al. Loperamide Versus Psyllium Fiber for Treatment of Fecal Incontinence: The Fecal Incontinence Prescription (Rx) Management (FIRM) Randomized Clinical Trial. Dis Colon Rectum 2015; 58(10):983–93.

56. Jelovsek JE, Markland AD, Whitehead WE, et al. Controlling faecal incontinence in women by performing anal exercises with biofeedback or loperamide: a randomised clinical trial. Lancet Gastroenterol Hepatol 2019;4(9):698–710.

57. Sjodahl J, Walter SA, Johansson E, et al. Combination therapy with biofeedback, loperamide, and stool-bulking agents is effective for the treatment of fecal incontinence in women: a randomized controlled trial. Scand J Gastroenterol 2015;50(8):965–74.

58. Camilleri M. Bile acid diarrhea: prevalence, pathogenesis, and therapy. Gut Liver 2015;9(3):332–9.

59. Remes-Troche JM, Ozturk R, Philips C, et al. Cholestyramine: a useful adjunct for the treatment of patients with fecal incontinence. Int J Colorectal Dis 2008; 23(2):189–94.

60. Santoro GA, Eitan BZ, Pryde A, et al. Open study of low-dose amitriptyline in the treatment of patients with idiopathic fecal incontinence. Dis Colon Rectum 2000; 43(12):1676–81, discussion: 1681-1672].

61. Omar MI, Alexander CE. Drug treatment for faecal incontinence in adults. Cochrane Database Syst Rev 2013;6:CD002116.

62. Dumoulin C, Hay-Smith J. Pelvic floor muscle training versus no treatment, or inactive control treatments, for urinary incontinence in women. Cochrane Database Syst Rev 2010;(1):CD005654.

63. Norton C, Cody JD. Biofeedback and/or sphincter exercises for the treatment of faecal incontinence in adults. Cochrane Database Syst Rev 2012;7:CD002111.

64. Chiarioni G, Ferri B, Morelli A, et al. Bio-feedback treatment of fecal incontinence: where are we, and where are we going? World J Gastroenterol 2005; 11(31):4771–5.

65. Van Koughnett JA, Wexner SD. Current management of fecal incontinence: choosing amongst treatment options to optimize outcomes. World J Gastroenterol 2013;19(48):9216–30.

66. Norton C, Chelvanayagam S, Wilson-Barnett J, et al. Randomized controlled trial of biofeedback for fecal incontinence. Gastroenterology 2003;125(5):1320–9.

67. Heymen S, Scarlett Y, Jones K, et al. Randomized controlled trial shows biofeedback to be superior to pelvic floor exercises for fecal incontinence. Dis Colon Rectum 2009;52(10):1730–7.

68. Graf W, Mellgren A, Matzel KE, et al. Efficacy of dextranomer in stabilised hyaluronic acid for treatment of faecal incontinence: a randomised, sham-controlled trial. Lancet 2011;377(9770):997–1003.

69. Dodi G, Jongen J, de la Portilla F, et al. An open-label, noncomparative, multicenter study to evaluate efficacy and safety of NASHA/Dx gel as a bulking agent for the treatment of fecal incontinence. Gastroenterol Res Pract 2010;2010: 467136.

70. Dehli T, Stordahl A, Vatten LJ, et al. Sphincter training or anal injections of dextranomer for treatment of anal incontinence: a randomized trial. Scand J Gastroenterol 2013;48(3):302–10.

71. Efron JE. The SECCA procedure: a new therapy for treatment of fecal incontinence. Surg Technol Int 2004;13:107–10.

72. Frascio M, Mandolfino F, Imperatore M, et al. The SECCA procedure for faecal incontinence: a review. Colorectal Dis 2014;16(3):167–72.

73. Lam TJ, Visscher AP, Meurs-Szojda MM, et al. Clinical response and sustainability of treatment with temperature-controlled radiofrequency energy (Secca) in patients with faecal incontinence: 3 years follow-up. Int J Colorectal Dis 2014; 29(6):755–61.

74. Visscher AP, Lam TJ, Meurs-Szojda MM, et al. Temperature-controlled delivery of radiofrequency energy in fecal incontinence: a randomized sham-controlled clinical trial. Dis Colon Rectum 2017;60(8):860–5.

75. Thaha MA, Abukar AA, Thin NN, et al. Sacral nerve stimulation for faecal incontinence and constipation in adults. Cochrane Database Syst Rev 2015;8: CD004464.

76. Patton V, Wiklendt L, Arkwright JW, et al. The effect of sacral nerve stimulation on distal colonic motility in patients with faecal incontinence. Br J Surg 2013;100(7): 959–68.

77. Leroi AM, Parc Y, Lehur PA, et al. Efficacy of sacral nerve stimulation for fecal incontinence: results of a multicenter double-blind crossover study. Ann Surg 2005;242(5):662–9.

78. Vaizey CJ, Kamm MA, Roy AJ, et al. Double-blind crossover study of sacral nerve stimulation for fecal incontinence. Dis Colon Rectum 2000;43(3):298–302.

79. Kahlke V, Topic H, Peleikis HG, et al. Sacral nerve modulation for fecal incontinence: results of a prospective single-center randomized crossover study. Dis Colon Rectum 2015;58(2):235–40.

80. Hull T, Giese C, Wexner SD, et al. Long-term durability of sacral nerve stimulation therapy for chronic fecal incontinence. Dis Colon Rectum 2013;56(2):234–45.

81. Ratto C, Litta F, Parello A, et al. Sacral nerve stimulation is a valid approach in fecal incontinence due to sphincter lesions when compared to sphincter repair. Dis Colon Rectum 2010;53(3):264–72.

82. Brouwer R, Duthie G. Sacral nerve neuromodulation is effective treatment for fecal incontinence in the presence of a sphincter defect, pudendal neuropathy, or previous sphincter repair. Dis Colon Rectum 2010;53(3):273–8.

83. Iachetta RP, Cola A, Villani RD. Sacral nerve stimulation in the treatment of fecal incontinence - the experience of a pelvic floor center: short term results. J Interv Gastroenterol 2012;2(4):189–92.

84. Ratto C, Litta F, Parello A, et al. Sacral nerve stimulation in faecal incontinence associated with an anal sphincter lesion: a systematic review. Colorectal Dis 2012;14(6):e297–304.
85. Bosch JL, Groen J. Sacral (S3) segmental nerve stimulation as a treatment for urge incontinence in patients with detrusor instability: results of chronic electrical stimulation using an implantable neural prosthesis. J Urol 1995;154(2 Pt 1): 504–7.
86. MacDiarmid SA, Siegel SW. Posterior tibial nerve stimulation before a trial of sacral nerve stimulation for refractory urge incontinence. J Urol 2014;191(6): 1652–4.
87. Vandoninck V, Van Balken MR, Finazzi Agro E, et al. Posterior tibial nerve stimulation in the treatment of urge incontinence. Neurourol Urodyn 2003;22(1):17–23.
88. van der Wilt AA, Giuliani G, Kubis C, et al. Randomized clinical trial of percutaneous tibial nerve stimulation versus sham electrical stimulation in patients with faecal incontinence. Br J Surg 2017;104(9):1167–76.
89. Thin NN, Taylor SJ, Bremner SA, et al. Randomized clinical trial of sacral versus percutaneous tibial nerve stimulation in patients with faecal incontinence. Br J Surg 2015;102(4):349–58.
90. Knowles CH, Horrocks EJ, Bremner SA, et al. Percutaneous tibial nerve stimulation versus sham electrical stimulation for the treatment of faecal incontinence in adults (CONFIDeNT): a double-blind, multicentre, pragmatic, parallel-group, randomised controlled trial. Lancet 2015;386(10004):1640–8.
91. Leroi AM, Siproudhis L, Etienney I, et al. Transcutaneous electrical tibial nerve stimulation in the treatment of fecal incontinence: a randomized trial (CONSORT 1a). Am J Gastroenterol 2012;107(12):1888–96.
92. Lukacz ES, Segall MM, Wexner SD. Evaluation of an anal insert device for the conservative management of fecal incontinence. Dis Colon Rectum 2015; 58(9):892–8.
93. Segal JP, Leo CA, Hodgkinson JD, et al. Acceptability, effectiveness and safety of a Renew((R)) anal insert in patients who have undergone restorative proctocolectomy with ileal pouch-anal anastomosis. Colorectal Dis 2019;21(1):73–8.
94. Richter HE, Matthews CA, Muir T, et al. A vaginal bowel-control system for the treatment of fecal incontinence. Obstet Gynecol 2015;125(3):540–7.
95. Richter HE, Dunivan G, Brown HW, et al. A 12-month clinical durability of effectiveness and safety evaluation of a vaginal bowel control system for the nonsurgical treatment of fecal incontinence. Female Pelvic Med Reconstr Surg 2019; 25(2):113–9.
96. Pelvalon I. Eclipse™ system instructions for use. Available at: http://eclipsesystem. com/wp-content/uploads/2017/09/IFU615-Rev-D-Physician-Instructions-for-Use-170831.pdf. March 21, 2021.
97. Emmanuel A. Neurogenic bowel dysfunction. F1000Res 2019;8:F1000.
98. Mekhael M, Kristensen HO, Larsen HM, et al. Transanal irrigation for neurogenic bowel disease, low anterior resection syndrome, faecal incontinence and chronic constipation: a systematic review. J Clin Med 2021;10(4):753.
99. Johnson E, Carlsen E, Steen TB, et al. Short- and long-term results of secondary anterior sphincteroplasty in 33 patients with obstetric injury. Acta Obstet Gynecol Scand 2010;89(11):1466–72.
100. Dudding TC, Vaizey CJ, Kamm MA. Obstetric anal sphincter injury: incidence, risk factors, and management. Ann Surg 2008;247(2):224–37.
101. Bravo Gutierrez A, Madoff RD, Lowry AC, et al. Long-term results of anterior sphincteroplasty. Dis Colon Rectum 2004;47(5):727–31 [discussion: 731-722].

102. Wexner SD, Bleier J. Current surgical strategies to treat fecal incontinence. Expert Rev Gastroenterol Hepatol 2015;9(12):1577–89.

103. Oom DM, Gosselink MP, Schouten WR. Anterior sphincteroplasty for fecal incontinence: a single center experience in the era of sacral neuromodulation. Dis Colon Rectum 2009;52(10):1681–7.

104. Zutshi M, Tracey TH, Bast J, et al. Ten-year outcome after anal sphincter repair for fecal incontinence. Dis Colon Rectum 2009;52(6):1089–94.

105. Halverson AL, Hull TL. Long-term outcome of overlapping anal sphincter repair. Dis Colon Rectum 2002;45(3):345–8.

106. Maslekar S, Gardiner AB, Duthie GS. Anterior anal sphincter repair for fecal incontinence: good long-term results are possible. J Am Coll Surg 2007;204(1):40–6.

107. Glasgow SC, Lowry AC. Long-term outcomes of anal sphincter repair for fecal incontinence: a systematic review. Dis Colon Rectum 2012;55(4):482–90.

108. El-Gazzaz G, Zutshi M, Hannaway C, et al. Overlapping sphincter repair: does age matter? Dis Colon Rectum 2012;55(3):256–61.

109. Sinha CK, Grewal A, Ward HC. Antegrade continence enema (ACE): current practice. Pediatr Surg Int 2008;24(6):685–8.

110. Patel AS, Saratzis A, Arasaradnam R, et al. Use of antegrade continence enema for the treatment of fecal incontinence and functional constipation in adults: a systematic review. Dis Colon Rectum 2015;58(10):999–1013.

111. Sturkenboom R, van der Wilt AA, van Kuijk SMJ, et al. Long-term outcomes of a Malone antegrade continence enema (MACE) for the treatment of fecal incontinence or constipation in adults. Int J Colorectal Dis 2018;33(10):1341–8.

112. Meurette G, Duchalais E, Lehur PA. Surgical approaches to fecal incontinence in the adult. J Visc Surg 2014;151(1):29–39.

113. Hocevar B, Gray M. Intestinal diversion (colostomy or ileostomy) in patients with severe bowel dysfunction following spinal cord injury. J Wound Ostomy Continence Nurs 2008;35(2):159–66.

114. Colquhoun P, Kaiser R Jr, Efron J, et al. Is the quality of life better in patients with colostomy than patients with fecal incontinence? World J Surg 2006;30(10):1925–8.

115. Norton C, Burch J, Kamm MA. Patients' views of a colostomy for fecal incontinence. Dis Colon Rectum 2005;48(5):1062–9.

116. Rao SS, Coss-Adame E, Tantiphlachiva K, et al. Translumbar and transsacral magnetic neurostimulation for the assessment of neuropathy in fecal incontinence. Dis Colon Rectum 2014;57(5):645–52.

117. Rao SSC, Xiang X, Sharma A, et al. Translumbosacral neuromodulation therapy for fecal incontinence: a randomized frequency response trial. Am J Gastroenterol 2021;116(1):162–70.

118. Lehur PA, McNevin S, Buntzen S, et al. Magnetic anal sphincter augmentation for the treatment of fecal incontinence: a preliminary report from a feasibility study. Dis Colon Rectum 2010;53(12):1604–10.

119. Sugrue J, Lehur PA, Madoff RD, et al. Long-term experience of magnetic anal sphincter augmentation in patients with fecal incontinence. Dis Colon Rectum 2017;60(1):87–95.

120. Pakravan F, Helmes C. Magnetic anal sphincter augmentation in patients with severe fecal incontinence. Dis Colon Rectum 2015;58(1):109–14.

121. Trebol J, Carabias-Orgaz A, Garcia-Arranz M, et al. Stem cell therapy for faecal incontinence: current state and future perspectives. World J Stem Cells 2018; 10(7):82–105.

122. Dadhich P, Bohl JL, Tamburrini R, et al. BioSphincters to treat fecal incontinence in nonhuman primates. Sci Rep 2019;9(1):18096.

123. Frudinger A, Pfeifer J, Paede J, et al. Autologous skeletal-muscle-derived cell injection for anal incontinence due to obstetric trauma: a 5-year follow-up of an initial study of 10 patients. Colorectal Dis 2015;17(9):794–801.
124. Sarveazad A, Newstead GL, Mirzaei R, et al. A new method for treating fecal incontinence by implanting stem cells derived from human adipose tissue: preliminary findings of a randomized double-blind clinical trial. Stem Cell Res Ther 2017;8(1):40.
125. Boyer O, Bridoux V, Giverne C, et al. Autologous myoblasts for the treatment of fecal incontinence: results of a phase 2 randomized placebo-controlled study (MIAS). Ann Surg 2018;267(3):443–50.

Neurogenic Bowel Dysfunction

The Impact of the Central Nervous System in Constipation and Fecal Incontinence

Seifeldin Hakim, MD[a], Tanmay Gaglani, MD[b], Brooks D. Cash, MD[a],*

KEYWORDS

- Neurogenic bowel dysfunction • Spinal cord injury • Constipation
- Fecal incontinence

KEY POINTS

- Neurogenic bowel dysfunction is a consequence of spinal cord disorders resulting in chronic constipation, fecal incontinence, abdominal pain, and gut dysmotility.
- Although the musculoskeletal sequelae of spinal cord disorders are the most visible outward signs of these conditions, the gastrointestinal symptoms of spinal cord disorders, most notably neurogenic bowel dysfunction, are highly prevalent and debilitating.
- Treatment strategies for neurogenic bowel dysfunction include lifestyle modification, pharmacologic management, rectal stimulation, biofeedback, colonic irrigation, and surgical management.

INTRODUCTION AND EPIDEMIOLOGY OF NEUROGENIC BOWEL DYSFUNCTION

The spinal cord is a component of the central nervous system (CNS) that plays a significant role in many physiologic functions including movement, sensation, and multiple subconscious processes, including digestion. Patients who suffer from spinal cord disorders experience significant morbidity not only physically, but also socially, psychologically, and economically. One of the many sequelae of spinal cord disorders is neurogenic bowel dysfunction (NBD). This broad term encompasses a constellation of symptoms including chronic constipation, fecal incontinence, abdominal pain, and gut dysmotility. Symptoms of NBD occur as a result of spinal cord lesions that disrupt autonomic and enteric reflexes. NBD typically occurs in patients suffering from

[a] Division of Gastroenterology, Hepatology and Nutrition, The University of Texas Health Science Center at Houston, 6431 Fannin, MSB 4.234, Houston, TX 77030, USA; [b] Department of Internal Medicine, The University of Texas Health Science Center at Houston, 6431 Fannin, Houston, TX 77030, USA
* Corresponding author.
E-mail address: brooks.d.cash@uth.tmc.edu

Gastroenterol Clin N Am 51 (2022) 93–105
https://doi.org/10.1016/j.gtc.2021.10.006
0889-8553/22/© 2021 Elsevier Inc. All rights reserved.

traumatic spinal cord injury (SCI), multiple sclerosis (MS), spina bifida particularly mye-lomeningocele, cauda equina syndrome, Parkinson's disease, and stroke.

SCI, both traumatic and nontraumatic, has an estimated prevalence of 2.5 million cases globally. The estimated prevalence of NBD in patients with SCI is as high as 80%.[1–4] In 2010, the National Spinal Cord Injury Statistical Center indicated that 265,000 people are living with traumatic SCI in the United States, translating to a prev-alence of 855 per million. The annual US incidence of SCI is approximately 54 per million people.[5,6] It was estimated that 2.3 million patients have MS globally and MS is considered the most prevalent nontraumatic cause of disability in young adults.[7] Parkinson's disease affects over 3 million people globally and it is the second most common neurodegenerative disease.[8] SCI has a male predominance and a bimodal distribution with the first peak at age 15 to 29 years and the second peak in those aged over 65 years. The various etiologies of SCI explain the bimodal distribution pattern with traumatic causes, motor vehicle accidents and falls, accounting for over 50% of new cases, followed by nontraumatic causes.[9,10] Although the musculo-skeletal sequelae of SCI are the most visible outward signs of these conditions, the gastrointestinal symptoms of SCI, most notably NBD, are also highly prevalent and debilitating.

NEUROANATOMY AND NEUROPHYSIOLOGY

Normal bowel function is a complex and incompletely understood process that is dependent on anatomic integrity, intact innervation, adequate nutrition, hormonal ho-meostasis, and behavioral components. Colonic transit is important for final digestive processing, fluid and electrolyte balance, the formation of final stool consistency, and solid waste elimination. In health, colonic contractions and peristalsis facilitate the transport of stool to the rectum, which acts as a reservoir for stool until evacuation oc-curs in a socially and hygienically acceptable fashion.[11] To understand the pathophys-iology of NBD, we must understand the neuroanatomy and neurophysiology that control voluntary and involuntary gut function.

The intrinsic enteric nervous system involves Auerbach's myenteric plexus as well as Meissner's submucosal plexus and regulates peristalsis, secretions, and absorp-tion of luminal contents. Auerbach's plexus lies between the inner circular and outer longitudinal layers of the muscularis propria and extends throughout the entire length of the gut, providing secretomotor innervation. Meissner's submucosal plexus is located in the submucosa between the circular muscle layer and the muscularis mu-cosa and plays an important part in secretory control.[12]

The extrinsic innervation pathway of the bowel is composed of sensory and visceral innervation from the spinal cord, which conducts bidirectional signals between the gut and various CNS centers in the brain through the dorsal column and the spinothalamic tracts.[12,13] Somatic nerve fibers provide somatic sensation through the pudendal nerve, which supplies the anal canal distal to the dentate line, including the external anal sphincter. These somatic fibers originate from the S2-S4 root levels and are under voluntary control. The vagus nerve innervates the gut proximally and extends distally to the splenic flexure, providing visceral sensation and parasympathetic innervation. The spinal cord provides parasympathetic supply to the remaining colon and rectum via the sacral plexus, whereas the thoracolumbar spinal cord (T5-L2) provides the sympathetic supply.[12,14,15] In general, parasympathetic nervous activity enhances contractions and stimulates secretions, whereas the sympathetic nervous system suppresses these functions.[15,16] Brain areas involved in gut function include the cingulate cortex, insula, thalamus, and the somatosensory and prefrontal cortices.

The act of defecation is a result of coordinated reflexes at the spinal cord level, which is controlled and influenced by the brain cortex, and some of the most striking pathophysiologies in NBD arises from impaired neural function affecting not only gut transit but also the sensory and motor process of colorectal evacuation.[13]

CLINICAL PRESENTATION OF NBD

NBD is frequently described as colonic and/or pelvic floor dysfunction that presents as reduced colonic contractions, abnormal colonic transit, severe constipation, disordered evacuation reflexes, stool impaction, and fecal overflow incontinence or flatus incontinence.[17,18] NBD presentation varies according to the level and severity of neurologic lesions and there are 2 primary types of NBD, upper motor neuron (UMN) bowel syndrome and lower motor neuron (LMN) bowel syndrome. The division of these syndromes occurs in the spinal cord at the level of the conus medullaris. Supraconus SCI (T12 and above) results in UMN NBD and is manifested by hyperreflexia of the bowels with increased rectal and sigmoid compliance, increased anal sphincter tone, disruption of external anal sphincter control, with preserved reflex coordination and propulsion through the colorectum. These lesions tend to promote stool retention and constipation. Stool evacuation in individuals with these types of SCI usually occurs by means of reflex activation through stimulant laxatives or digital stimulation introduced to the rectum.[19,20] In contrast, LMN lesions typically result in an areflexic bowel with loss of peristalsis, slower stool propulsion, reduced rectal compliance, diminished anal tone, and in some cases a completely atonic anal sphincter. LMN lesions can significantly prolong colonic transit times and patients usually experience constipation and incontinence.[19,21] However, patients with incomplete LMN injury can retain the sensation of rectal fullness and the ability to evacuate their bowels. The pathophysiologic mechanisms of fecal incontinence and constipation in patients with incomplete SCI are similar to patients with complete SCI with preserved sacral reflexes. Furthermore, individual variations in bowel habits and preexisting conditions can affect the phenotypic bowel pattern in NBD.[22]

Approximately 80% of SCI patients experience NBD, making it more prevalent than urinary and sexual dysfunction in these patients. The most common manifestation of NBD is constipation; however, the exact incidence is contested in the literature as clinical definitions vary from study to study.[20] De Looze and colleagues reported an incidence of constipation of 58% in SCI, whereas Stone and colleagues reported only 20% of patients are having "difficulty with bowel evacuation."[23,24] It was estimated that 61% to 75% of SCI patients have experienced one-time fecal incontinence and at least 45% to 56% experience monthly incontinence.[20] Podnar showed that 80% of patients with cauda equina syndrome reported constipation and reported higher fecal incontinence rates.[20,25] Abdominal pain is another common symptom in NBD patients; however, it remains unclear if the abdominal pain in NBD is inherently due to SCI injury and neuropathy or is a sequela of NBD-related complications such as constipation.[26]

Lesions of the spinal cord above the T6 sympathetic outflow tract, generally associated with tetraplegia or high-level paraplegia, can be complicated by autonomic dysreflexia. In such cases, afferent stimuli including those associated with severe constipation, urinary retention, manual evacuation of stool, or use of stimulant laxatives can trigger the sympathetic nervous system. The resultant increased sympathetic activity, without regulation from typical autonomic pathways, can lead to significant elevations in blood pressure through vasoconstriction while the cardiac vagus reacts to baroreflex mediated increases in vagal stimulation. Patients with these patterns of SCI and NBD may experience palpitations, hypertension, headaches, and flushing accompanied by bradycardia and shortness of breath. In extreme instances, if left untreated, autonomic dysreflexia can result in seizures, strokes, or even death.[15,27–30]

Although abdominal pain can be a common symptom in patients with NBD, it is also possible that somatic sensation of visceral organs can be impaired in NBD, such that abdominal pain sensation may also be attenuated. Patients with NBD tend to have more frequent hospitalizations for acute abdominal pathologies such as volvulus, megacolon, or impaction presenting atypically and later than patients with intact innervations. As a result, patients with NBD tend to have increased morbidity and mortality from such conditions. In one small study, only 2 of 9 patients with NBD due to SCI presenting with these acute abdominal emergencies demonstrated typical findings.[9,31,32]

It is also important to consider the psychological aspects of SCI arising as a result of paralysis, functional impairments, relative loss of independence, and persistent somatic pain. SCI patients encounter challenges to their daily lives such as disruption to their work, family, social relationships, and community participation. It has been estimated that up to 30% of patients with SCI report long-term clinical depression and anxiety.[33–37]

Although the life expectancy of patients with tetraplegia is 10 years shorter than the general population, the life expectancy of patients with paraplegia is comparable to that of the general population. Hence, individuals with paraplegia may live to an older age with complications related to their SCI, particularly NBD, as demonstrated in a prospective follow-up study over 19 years of patients with SCI by Nielsen and colleagues[16] In this study, a validated questionnaire was sent initially in 1996 to 589 Danish SCI association members and the same questionnaire was sent to all surviving members in 2006 and again in 2015. A total of 109 SCI patients responded to all 3 questionnaires. The proportion of respondents needing more than 40 minutes for each bowel movement increased from 21% to 39%, the use of laxatives increased and the proportion of patients considering themselves very constipated increased from 19% to 31%. Interestingly, although self-assessed severity of constipation increased with time, quality of life and the methods of bowel care reported by patients remained stable, despite a sizable proportion of patients undergoing stoma surgery during the study period.

DIAGNOSTIC APPROACH TO PATIENTS WITH NBD
Clinical Assessment

A detailed history and physical pertaining to the patient's bowel habits, neurologic and medical conditions and treatments, and specifics regarding the patient's SCI including the level of injury should be obtained in all cases. These clinical components are imperative for understanding the patient's symptoms pertaining to their bowel function. All abdominal symptoms should be investigated thoroughly, and a bowel diary can be used to track bowel function including the frequency of bowel movements, stool consistency, time spent toileting, episodes of incontinence, and episodes of fecal impaction. History of hospitalizations for bowel-related problems, physical maneuvers used for bowel management, and the impact of NBD and SCI symptoms on quality of life should also be documented.[38,39] Several scoring systems have been implemented for assessing the severity of NBD symptoms. One commonly used system is the Cleveland Clinic scoring system to simplify evaluation and management of constipated patients as well as the St. Mark's scoring system for fecal incontinence grading.[40,41] The NBD score is a 10-item score developed and validated among patients with SCI and NBD that has been translated into multiple languages and contains the most cited endpoints in clinical trials.[42,43] A recent score called Monitoring Efficacy of Neurogenic bowel dysfunction Treatment On Response (MENTOR) can be used to monitor the treatment of NBD patients.[2,43] In addition to the historical aspects of evaluation, a detailed physical examination should be performed including abdominal examination, digital rectal examination to assess rectal filling, anal sphincter tone, sensation, voluntary contraction, and to evaluate for anorectal pathology such as fissures, hemorrhoids, or rectal prolapse.[39]

Imaging

As in non-NBD patients, appropriate abdominal imaging should be performed whenever there are alarm symptoms such as weight loss, acute changes in bowel habits, or gastrointestinal bleeding. However, it may be challenging to detect some alarm symptoms in patients with NBD due to comorbid conditions associated with SCI such as depression and neurologic disease progression. Commonly obtained abdominal imaging studies in patients with NBD include abdominal plain film series and computed tomography to assess stool burden and colonic dilation and colonic marker studies to assess colonic transit time.[44] Providers should have a low threshold to obtain the necessary imaging to evaluate abdominal emergencies given their often delayed presentations in this population.[45]

Anorectal Manometry

Biofeedback is a therapeutic process in which a rectal manometer is used to assess rectal muscular activation when the patient is conducting various maneuvers and breathing techniques. The physiologic responses to the patient's efforts can be visualized through anorectal pressures measured by the manometer and patient-specific techniques for facilitating bowel movements can be developed. Although not a primary modality for diagnosing NBD, anorectal manometry can be used in conjunction with pelvic floor biofeedback therapy and baseline evaluation before treatment should be considered.

Health Maintenance

Patients with NBD should undergo the typical colorectal cancer (CRC) age-based screening/surveillance process based on age, family history, and personal history of colorectal neoplasia. A recent study showed that despite SCI patients having suboptimal rates of preventative care screenings, they did not have an increased risk of CRC incidence or mortality.[46] Additional time and effort should be used for colonoscopy preparation in patients with SCI and suboptimal preparation should be anticipated. A case series of 440 colonoscopies in SCI patients showed that most colonoscopies performed in these patients were for diagnostic purposes rather than for CRC screening or polyp surveillance.[47] The same study showed that unsatisfactory bowel preparation was recorded more often in SCI patients with a lower rate of complete examination. Hospitalization for assistance with bowel preparation may improve satisfactory completion rates.

TREATMENT OF PATIENTS WITH NBD

The goals of therapy for NBD are multiple and include ensuring that toileting occurs in an efficient manner, reduction in fecal incontinence, and minimization of quality-of-life impairment due to bowel management. Usually, the treatment of NBD requires a multifaceted approach to achieve adequate bowel function.[37]

Diet and Lifestyle Modification

A high fiber diet is widely recommended for health; however, there is very limited data on dietary supplementation in the management of NBD. A high fiber diet can lead to increased bloating and flatulence; however, these symptoms can be minimized by decreasing insoluble fiber content and increasing soluble, nonfermentable fiber content gradually. Caffeine and alcohol should be minimized, and patients should be encouraged to establish a routine for bowel care by attempting to schedule bowel movements at consistent times in an effort to minimize fecal impaction and incontinence risk. Modification of body position during bowel movements can also be used to enhance the efficiency of content evacuation for some patients. The optimal position for rectal evacuation is seated with knees above waist level. Assistive devices can be used to maintain specific positions during defecation.[21,48,49] Anal plugs or pledgets can also be used to prevent leakage of flatus and small volumes of feces in NBD patients with passive incontinence and are best tolerated in patients with reduced rectal sensation.[38]

Rectal Stimulation/Evacuation

Korsten and colleagues showed in a small study that digital rectal stimulation was associated with increased left-sided colonic activity.[50] Digital rectal stimulation via a circular motion of the finger for 20 to 30 seconds stimulates the anorectal colonic reflex, which results in enhanced contractions of the descending colon and rectum that may promote rectal evacuation in patients with SCI. Digital evacuation of stool is another option for rectal evacuation. It does not depend on contractions, but rather involves physical removal of stool present in the rectum with a finger using a hooking motion. These 2 maneuvers should be used with caution in patients with SCI above the T6 sympathetic outflow tract because they can elicit autonomic dysreflexia, which can be life-threatening.[51] This condition is due to the segregation of spinal sympathetic neurons from supraspinal modulation and is characterized by episodic hypertension and baroflex-mediated bradycardia. Immediate actions to mitigate autonomic dysreflexia include changing posture to an upright position, raising the head and lowering the legs, loosening or removing any tight clothing or accessories such as braces, catheter tape, socks or stockings, shoes, and bandages, and emptying the urinary bladder. If conservative measures are ineffective, pharmaceutical therapy with organic nitrates (most often in paste form applied above the level of the SCI) and nifedipine can be used for immediate therapy.[52]

Abdominal Massage

Limited data exist on the role of abdominal massage in patients with NBD. It may have some role in the management of chronic constipation in patients with neurologic diseases, but no large study has evaluated its role in NBD. Ayas and colleagues showed in a small study of 24 patients that abdominal massage helped to improve abdominal distention and fecal incontinence, led to higher mean frequencies of defecation, and decreased total colonic transit time.[53] However, Janssen and colleagues used an electromechanical device for abdominal massage in a study of 21 patients and failed to demonstrate the improvement of bowel function in NBD.[54]

Biofeedback

A small study showed improvement in patient symptoms of NBD following biofeedback therapy.[55] Wiesel and colleagues showed a beneficial effect of biofeedback in MS patients with limited disability.[56] Wald showed in a small case series that biofeedback was associated with good response in children with meningomyelocele and NBD.[57]

Rectally Administered Medications/Enema

Rectally administered suppositories may aid in stimulating reflex contraction. Bisacodyl and glycerin suppositories are commonly used to assist with stool evacuation, but suppository use can be challenging due to difficulty with placement in patients with impaired anal tone. Enemas can also be attempted, but large volume enemas may be challenging due to difficulty with retention and the possibility of triggering autonomic dysreflexia.[38]

Oral Pharmacologic Therapy

Oral prokinetics can be used to help with gut dysmotility in NBD. Rajendran showed that cisapride can reduce mouth to cecum transit time and Geders showed that it was able to reduce colonic transit time in patients with NBD. However, cisapride is not available because of its association with cardiac dysrhythmia.[58,59] Prucalopride is a selective serotonin (5-HT4) receptor agonist that facilitates cholinergic and excitatory nonadrenergic noncholinergic neurotransmission. A pilot study by Krogh showed that prucalopride increased the frequency of bowel movements per week and reduced the median colonic transit time in SCI patients with NBD.[60] Korsten and colleagues showed that infusion of neostigmine alone as well as neostigmine/glycopyrrolate combination infusion improved bowel evacuation in NBD compared with placebo.[61] However, it was also observed that infusion of neostigmine alone resulted in more parasympathomimetic adverse effects than the combination therapy. Rosman and colleagues showed that intramuscular injection of neostigmine/glycopyrrolate in NBD improved bowel evacuation by reducing colonic transit time and had comparable adverse effects to placebo.[62] Oral secretagogues are a relatively new class of medications that have been shown to be effective in managing chronic constipation, but they have not been studied in NBD.[63,64]

Transanal Irrigation

Transanal irrigation (TAI) was first described for NBD in 1987 by Shandling and Gilmour[65] and a commercially available version was approved in the United States in 2012. TAI has emerged as an effective and cost-effective method for the management of NBD. This technique involves introducing a large volume of water into the colon and rectum through the anus to induce reflex colorectal voiding and bowel emptying. The water is introduced using a single-use device, which can be either cone or catheter, the choice of which depends on the patient's choice, hand strength and dexterity, and anal sphincter integrity. After instilling fluid, the device is removed and the contents of the rectum and some of the more distal colon are evacuated.[66–68] Most TAI products recommend using 10 to 20 mL/kg of fluid during each use and they are typically prescribed for daily or every other day use.[69] Christensen and colleagues showed that TAI was associated with a lower Cleveland Clinic constipation score, St. Mark's fecal incontinence score, and NBD score compared with conservative bowel management.[66] Another study by Christensen showed that TAI reduced symptoms of NBD and resulted in lower total health care costs compared with conservative bowel management.[67] Emmanuel and colleagues demonstrated that TAI is cost-saving and associated with reduced risk of stoma surgery, urinary tract infections, episodes of fecal incontinence, and improved the quality of life for patients with NBD.[68] The challenge of TAI is that most devices require a manual compression of the pump to introduce water from a reservoir into the bowel and this can be challenging for individuals with SCI. TAI may be better applied to adult patients with NBD. Blair showed in his study that the pediatric dropout rate with TAI was 16% due to noncompliance or balloon extrusion.[70] Recently, an electronic TAI system was made available, consisting of a control unit, pump, and smartphone application. This device has been shown in a recent clinical trial to be effective for patients with NBD.[71]

Antegrade Colonic Irrigation

The Malone Antegrade Continence Enema (MACE) was initially described in 1990. The procedure entails using a small segment of the intestine (typically the appendix) to create a stoma with a valve mechanism that allows catherization of the bowel but avoids leakage of stool.[72,73] Several studies demonstrated a success rate of MACE up to 80% and it is associated with decreased constipation, fecal incontinence, and enhanced quality of life.[69,74–76] A recent meta-analysis showed that MACE is an effective long-term treatment option in patients with fecal incontinence and constipation and recommended that it be considered before performing a definitive colostomy.[77] An analysis from the National Spina Bifida Patient Registry of 5209 individuals from 2009 to 2015 showed that MACE was used by 17.7% of adults and 27.2% of adolescents with NBD in this cohort.[78] In 1996, Shandling and colleagues described the creation of a cecostomy through the placement of a percutaneous tube or button which allowed antegrade enemas to be instilled into the colon. The tube needs to be exchanged periodically, typically by interventional radiology practitioners.[69,79] The benefit of cecostomy over MACE is that the appendix can be used as a urinary stoma for catheterization among patients who also have atonic urinary bladders as a result of their SCI. Bevill and colleagues showed that 88% of patients with cecostomy were satisfied and 92% indicated that they would have the cecostomy tube placed again.[80] A retrospective study of 49 patients comparing outcomes of patients with MACE versus cecostomy reported similar fecal continence and complication rates, but each group had unique challenges with stomal stenosis being most common for the MACE group and tube dislodgement for the cecostomy group.[81]

Colostomy

Bowel diversion through stoma formation is considered the last option for patients with NBD because it is invasive and not easily reversible. It may be most helpful in patients with intact use of their upper limbs.[19] Left-sided colostomy is an option for patients who have perianal wounds and fecal incontinence; however, it is not a good option for colonic emptying unless the patient has adequate colonic motility. Some patients may still require laxatives or irrigation with left-sided colostomy. Right-sided colostomy or ileostomy are both less likely to cause colonic emptying problems; however, they are also both associated with more liquid stool that requires more committed bowel and stoma care.[38,82] Complications after bowel diversion include diversion colitis, surgical adhesions, and stomal complications. When indicated, colostomy reduces the number of hours spent on bowel care and reduces the number of hospitalizations caused by NBD. It is also associated with increased independence, and improved quality of life in some series, but must be individualized.[82–84]

Neurostimulation

Stimulation of the nervous pathway affecting bowel motility has been a subject of interest for a large number of studies. Most of these studies are retrospective or pilot studies with small numbers of patients and short follow-up periods. Sacral anterior root stimulation triggers micturition and at the same time, stimulates peristalsis in the distal colon and rectum.[85] Sacral nerve stimulation has been suggested with limited data available to date. Other proposed forms of neurostimulation include nerve rerouting, posterior tibial nerve stimulation, dorsal genital nerve stimulation, peripheral electrical stimulation, and magnetic stimulation, but there is insufficient data in the literature to recommend one technique over the other or over the previously mentioned treatment modalities.[86]

SUMMARY

SCI and NBD are life-changing events for affected patients. The clinical manifestations of NBD vary depending on the level and severity of the spinal cord lesion. Managing patients with NBD can be challenging because of comorbidities such as immobility, bladder dysfunction, progressive neurologic decline, psychological factors, loss of independence, and social withdrawal. Management of NBD is best done in a multimodal, multidisciplinary fashion and should be individualized, depending on the residual neurologic capabilities of the patient and their predominant gastrointestinal symptoms.

CLINICS CARE POINTS

- The gastrointestinal symptoms of SCI, most notably NBD, are highly prevalent and debilitating.

- A detailed history and physical pertaining to the patient's bowel habits, neurologic and medical conditions and treatments, and specifics regarding the patient's SCI including the level of injury should be obtained in all cases.

- The goals of therapy for NBD are to achieve efficient toileting and require a multifaceted approach to achieve adequate bowel function.

- Management of NBD commonly involves lifestyle modifications, physical therapy, laxative medications, and surgical interventions.

DISCLOSURE

The authors have nothing to disclose.

REFERENCES

1. Saunders LL, Selassie AW, Hill EG, et al. Traumatic spinal cord injury mortality, 1981-1998. J Trauma 2009;66(1):184–90.
2. Emmanuel A, Krogh K, Kirshblum S, et al. Creation and validation of a new tool for the monitoring efficacy of neurogenic bowel dysfunction treatment on response: the MENTOR tool. Spinal Cord 2020;58(7):795–802.
3. Kelly MS, Wiener JS, Liu T, et al. Neurogenic bowel treatments and continence outcomes in children and adults with myelomeningocele. J Pediatr Rehabil Med 2020;13(4):685–93.
4. Brochard C, Peyronnet B, Dariel A, et al. Bowel Dysfunction related to spina bifida: keep it simple. Dis Colon Rectum 2017;60(11):1209–14.
5. National Spinal Cord Injury Statistical Center. Spinal cord injury facts and figures at a glance. J Spinal Cord Med 2010;33(4):439–40.
6. Frontera JE, Mollett P. Aging with spinal cord injury: an update. Phys Med Rehabil Clin N Am 2017;28(4):821–8.
7. Browne P, Chandraratna D, Angood C, et al. Atlas of multiple sclerosis 2013: a growing global problem with widespread inequity. Neurology 2014;83(11): 1022–4.

8. Lang AE, Lozano AM. Parkinson's disease. First of two parts. N Engl J Med 1998; 339(15):1044–53.

9. Qi Z, Middleton JW, Malcolm A. Bowel dysfunction in spinal cord injury. Curr Gastroenterol Rep 2018;20(10):47.

10. van den Berg MEL, Castellote JM, Mahillo-Fernandez I, et al. Incidence of spinal cord injury worldwide: a systematic review. Neuroepidemiology 2010;34(3): 184–92 [discussion: 192].

11. Rapps N, van Oudenhove L, Enck P, et al. Brain imaging of visceral functions in healthy volunteers and IBS patients. J Psychosom Res 2008;64(6):599–604.

12. Goyal RK, Hirano I. The enteric nervous system. N Engl J Med 1996;334(17): 1106–15.

13. Preziosi G, Gordon-Dixon A, Emmanuel A. Neurogenic bowel dysfunction in patients with multiple sclerosis: prevalence, impact, and management strategies. Degener Neurol Neuromuscul Dis 2018;8:79–90.

14. Schweiger M. Method for determining individual contributions of voluntary and involuntary anal sphincters to resting tone. Dis Colon Rectum 1979;22(6):415–6.

15. Goetz LL, Emmanuel A, Krogh K. International standards to document remaining autonomic Function in persons with SCI and neurogenic bowel dysfunction: Illustrative cases. Spinal Cord Ser Cases 2018;4:1.

16. Nielsen SD, Faaborg PM, Finnerup NB, et al. Aging with neurogenic bowel dysfunction. Spinal Cord 2017;55(8):769–73.

17. Coggrave M, Norton C. Management of faecal incontinence and constipation in adults with central neurological diseases. Cochrane Database Syst Rev 2013; 12:CD002115.

18. Lynch AC, Antony A, Dobbs BR, et al. Bowel dysfunction following spinal cord injury. Spinal Cord 2001;39(4):193–203.

19. Krassioukov A, Eng JJ, Claxton G, et al. Neurogenic bowel management after spinal cord injury: a systematic review of the evidence. Spinal Cord 2010;48(10):718–33.

20. Trivedi PM, Kumar L, Emmanuel AV. Altered colorectal compliance and anorectal physiology in upper and lower motor neurone spinal injury may explain bowel symptom pattern. Am J Gastroenterol 2016;111(4):552–60.

21. Martinez L, Neshatian L, Khavari R. Neurogenic bowel dysfunction in patients with neurogenic bladder. Curr Bladder Dysfunct Rep 2016;11(4):334–40.

22. Vallès M, Mearin F. Pathophysiology of bowel dysfunction in patients with motor incomplete spinal cord injury: comparison with patients with motor complete spinal cord injury. Dis Colon Rectum 2009;52(9):1589–97.

23. De Looze D, Van Laere M, De Muynck M, et al. Constipation and other chronic gastrointestinal problems in spinal cord injury patients. Spinal Cord 1998;36(1):63–6.

24. Stone JM, Nino-Murcia M, Wolfe VA, et al. Chronic gastrointestinal problems in spinal cord injury patients: a prospective analysis. Am J Gastroenterol 1990; 85(9):1114–9.

25. Podnar S. Bowel dysfunction in patients with cauda equina lesions. Eur J Neurol 2006;13(10):1112–7.

26. Faaborg PM, Finnerup NB, Christensen P, et al. Abdominal pain: a comparison between neurogenic bowel dysfunction and chronic idiopathic constipation. Gastroenterol Res Pract 2013;2013:365037.

27. Inskip JA, Lucci V-EM, McGrath MS, et al. A community perspective on bowel management and quality of life after spinal cord injury: the influence of autonomic dysreflexia. J Neurotrauma 2018;35(9):1091–105.

28. Walter M, Knüpfer SC, Cragg JJ, et al. Prediction of autonomic dysreflexia during urodynamics: a prospective cohort study. BMC Med 2018;16(1):53.

29. Krassioukov A, Warburton DE, Teasell R, et al. Spinal cord injury rehabilitation evidence research team a systematic review of the management of autonomic dysreflexia after spinal cord injury. Arch Phys Med Rehabil 2009;90(4):682–95.
30. Krassioukov AV, Furlan JC, Fehlings MG. Autonomic dysreflexia in acute spinal cord injury: an under-recognized clinical entity. J Neurotrauma 2003;20(8):707–16.
31. Ebert E. Gastrointestinal involvement in spinal cord injury: a clinical perspective. J Gastrointestin Liver Dis 2012;21(1):75–82.
32. Sarıfakıoğlu B, Afşar SI, Yalbuzdağ ŞA, et al. Acute abdominal emergencies and spinal cord injury; our experiences: a retrospective clinical study. Spinal Cord 2014;52(9):697–700.
33. van Leeuwen CMC, Kraaijeveld S, Lindeman E, et al. Associations between psychological factors and quality of life ratings in persons with spinal cord injury: a systematic review. Spinal Cord 2012;50(3):174–87.
34. Phillips BN, Smedema SM, Fleming AR, et al. Mediators of disability and hope for people with spinal cord injury. Disabil Rehabil 2016;38(17):1672–83.
35. Migliorini CE, New PW, Tonge BJ. Comparison of depression, anxiety and stress in persons with traumatic and non-traumatic post-acute spinal cord injury. Spinal Cord 2009;47(11):783–8.
36. Aaby A, Ravn SL, Kasch H, et al. The associations of acceptance with quality of life and mental health following spinal cord injury: a systematic review. Spinal Cord 2020;58(2):130–48.
37. Dibley L, Coggrave M, McClurg D, et al. "It's just horrible": a qualitative study of patients' and carers' experiences of bowel dysfunction in multiple sclerosis. J Neurol 2017;264(7):1354–61.
38. Emmanuel A. Neurogenic bowel dysfunction. F1000Res 2019;8. https://doi.org/10.12688/f1000research.20529.1.
39. Tate DG, Wheeler T, Lane GI, et al. Recommendations for evaluation of neurogenic bladder and bowel dysfunction after spinal cord injury and/or disease. J Spinal Cord Med 2020;43(2):141–64.
40. Agachan F, Chen T, Pfeifer J, et al. A constipation scoring system to simplify evaluation and management of constipated patients. Dis Colon Rectum 1996;39(6):681–5.
41. Vaizey CJ, Carapeti E, Cahill JA, et al. Prospective comparison of faecal incontinence grading systems. Gut 1999;44(1):77–80.
42. Krogh K, Christensen P, Sabroe S, et al. Neurogenic bowel dysfunction score. Spinal Cord 2006;44(10):625–31.
43. Studsgaard Slot SD, Baunwall SMD, Emmanuel A, et al. The monitoring efficacy of neurogenic bowel dysfunction treatment on response (MENTOR) in a non-hospital setting. J Clin Med 2021;10(2):263.
44. Evans RC, Kamm MA, Hinton JM, et al. The normal range and a simple diagram for recording whole gut transit time. Int J Colorectal Dis 1992;7(1):15–7.
45. Preziosi G, Emmanuel A. Neurogenic bowel dysfunction: pathophysiology, clinical manifestations and treatment. Expert Rev Gastroenterol Hepatol 2009;3(4):417–23.
46. Koblinski JE, DeVivo MJ, Chen Y, et al. Colorectal cancer mortality after spinal cord injury. J Spinal Cord Med 2020;1–6. https://doi.org/10.1080/10790268.2020.1808294.
47. Morris BP, Kucchal T, Burgess AN. Colonoscopy after spinal cord injury: a case-control study. Spinal Cord 2015;53(1):32–5.
48. Vande Velde S, Van Biervliet S, Van Renterghem K, et al. Achieving fecal continence in patients with spina bifida: a descriptive cohort study. J Urol 2007;178(6):2640–4.

49. Cameron KJ, Nyulasi IB, Collier GR, et al. Assessment of the effect of increased dietary fibre intake on bowel function in patients with spinal cord injury. Spinal Cord 1996;34(5):277–83.

50. Korsten MA, Singal AK, Monga A, et al. Anorectal stimulation causes increased colonic motor activity in subjects with spinal cord injury. J Spinal Cord Med 2007;30(1):31–5.

51. Faaborg PM, Christensen P, Krassioukov A, et al. Autonomic dysreflexia during bowel evacuation procedures and bladder filling in subjects with spinal cord injury. Spinal Cord 2014;52(6):494–8.

52. Eldahan KC, Rabchevsky AG. Autonomic dysreflexia after spinal cord injury: systemic pathophysiology and methods of management. Auton Neurosci 2018;209: 59–70.

53. Ayaş S, Leblebici B, Sözay S, et al. The effect of abdominal massage on bowel function in patients with spinal cord injury. Am J Phys Med Rehabil 2006; 85(12):951–5.

54. Janssen TWJ, Prakken ES, Hendriks JMS, et al. Electromechanical abdominal massage and colonic function in individuals with a spinal cord injury and chronic bowel problems. Spinal Cord 2014;52(9):693–6.

55. Mazor Y, Jones M, Andrews A, et al. Anorectal biofeedback for neurogenic bowel dysfunction in incomplete spinal cord injury. Spinal Cord 2016;54(12):1132–8.

56. Wiesel PH, Norton C, Roy AJ, et al. Gut focused behavioural treatment (biofeedback) for constipation and faecal incontinence in multiple sclerosis. J Neurol Neurosurg Psychiatry 2000;69(2):240–3.

57. Wald A. Use of biofeedback in treatment of fecal incontinence in patients with meningomyelocele. Pediatrics 1981;68(1):45–9.

58. Rajendran SK, Reiser JR, Bauman W, et al. Gastrointestinal transit after spinal cord injury: effect of cisapride. Am J Gastroenterol 1992;87(11):1614–7.

59. Geders JM, Gaing A, Bauman WA, et al. The effect of cisapride on segmental colonic transit time in patients with spinal cord injury. Am J Gastroenterol 1995; 90(2):285–9.

60. Krogh K, Jensen MB, Gandrup P, et al. Efficacy and tolerability of prucalopride in patients with constipation due to spinal cord injury. Scand J Gastroenterol 2002; 37(4):431–6.

61. Korsten MA, Rosman AS, Ng A, et al. Infusion of neostigmine-glycopyrrolate for bowel evacuation in persons with spinal cord injury. Am J Gastroenterol 2005; 100(7):1560–5.

62. Rosman AS, Chaparala G, Monga A, et al. Intramuscular neostigmine and glycopyrrolate safely accelerated bowel evacuation in patients with spinal cord injury and defecatory disorders. Dig Dis Sci 2008;53(10):2710–3.

63. Sarosiek I, Bashashati M, Alvarez A, et al. Lubiprostone accelerates intestinal transit and alleviates small intestinal bacterial overgrowth in patients with chronic constipation. Am J Med Sci 2016;352(3):231–8.

64. Jamal MM, Adams AB, Jansen J-P, et al. A randomized, placebo-controlled trial of lubiprostone for opioid-induced constipation in chronic noncancer pain. Am J Gastroenterol 2015;110(5):725–32.

65. Shandling B, Gilmour RF. The enema continence catheter in spina bifida: successful bowel management. J Pediatr Surg 1987;22(3):271–3.

66. Christensen P, Bazzocchi G, Coggrave M, et al. A randomized, controlled trial of transanal irrigation versus conservative bowel management in spinal cord-injured patients. Gastroenterology 2006;131(3):738–47.

67. Christensen P, Andreasen J, Ehlers L. Cost-effectiveness of transanal irrigation versus conservative bowel management for spinal cord injury patients. Spinal Cord 2009;47(2):138–43.

68. Emmanuel A, Kumar G, Christensen P, et al. Long-term cost-effectiveness of transanal irrigation in patients with neurogenic bowel dysfunction. PLoS One 2016;11(8):e0159394.

69. Kelly MS. Malone antegrade continence enemas vs. cecostomy vs. transanal irrigation-what is new and how do we counsel our patients? Curr Urol Rep 2019;20(8):41.

70. Blair GK, Djonlic K, Fraser GC, et al. The bowel management tube: an effective means for controlling fecal incontinence. J Pediatr Surg 1992;27(10):1269–72.

71. Emmanuel A, Kurze I, Krogh K, et al. An open prospective study on the efficacy of Navina Smart, an electronic system for transanal irrigation, in neurogenic bowel dysfunction. PLoS One 2021;16(1):e0245453.

72. Malone PS, Curry JI, Osborne A. The antegrade continence enema procedure why, when and how? World J Urol 1998;16(4):274–8.

73. Malone PS, Ransley PG, Kiely EM. Preliminary report: the antegrade continence enema. Lancet 1990;336(8725):1217–8.

74. Christensen P, Kvitzau B, Krogh K, et al. Neurogenic colorectal dysfunction - use of new antegrade and retrograde colonic wash-out methods. Spinal Cord 2000; 38(4):255–61.

75. Teichman JMH, Zabihi N, Kraus SR, et al. Long-term results for Malone antegrade continence enema for adults with neurogenic bowel disease. Urology 2003;61(3): 502–6.

76. Worsøe J, Christensen P, Krogh K, et al. Long-term results of antegrade colonic enema in adult patients: assessment of functional results. Dis Colon Rectum 2008;51(10):1523–8.

77. Chan DSY, Delicata RJ. Meta-analysis of antegrade continence enema in adults with faecal incontinence and constipation. Br J Surg 2016;103(4):322–7.

78. Wiener JS, Suson KD, Castillo J, et al. Bowel management and continence in adults with spina bifida: Results from the National Spina Bifida Patient Registry 2009-15. J Pediatr Rehabil Med 2017;10(3–4):335–43.

79. Shandling B, Chait PG, Richards HF. Percutaneous cecostomy: a new technique in the management of fecal incontinence. J Pediatr Surg 1996;31(4):534–7.

80. Bevill MD, Bonnett K, Arlen A, et al. Outcomes and satisfaction in pediatric patients with Chait cecostomy tubes. J Pediatr Urol 2017;13(4):365–70.

81. Hoy NY, Metcalfe P, Kiddoo DA. Outcomes following fecal continence procedures in patients with neurogenic bowel dysfunction. J Urol 2013;189(6):2293–7.

82. Safadi BY, Rosito O, Nino-Murcia M, et al. Which stoma works better for colonic dysmotility in the spinal cord injured patient? Am J Surg 2003;186(5):437–42.

83. Rosito O, Nino-Murcia M, Wolfe VA, et al. The effects of colostomy on the quality of life in patients with spinal cord injury: a retrospective analysis. J Spinal Cord Med 2002;25(3):174–83.

84. Munck J, Simoens C, Thill V, et al. Intestinal stoma in patients with spinal cord injury: a retrospective study of 23 patients. Hepatogastroenterology 2008; 55(88):2125–9.

85. Rasmussen MM, Kutzenberger J, Krogh K, et al. Sacral anterior root stimulation improves bowel function in subjects with spinal cord injury. Spinal Cord 2015; 53(4):297–301.

86. Worsøe J, Rasmussen M, Christensen P, et al. Neurostimulation for neurogenic bowel dysfunction. Gastroenterol Res Pract 2013;2013:563294.

Opioid-Related Constipation

Joy J. Liu, MD, Darren M. Brenner, MD*

KEYWORDS

- Constipation • Opioid • PAMORA • Pharmacotherapy

KEY POINTS

- Opioid-related constipation (ORC) refers to constipation that is caused or exacerbated by opioid therapy and should be differentiated from other forms of chronic constipation.
- Opioids affect not only intestinal transit but also pelvic floor function, which may be reflected by abnormal pelvic floor dynamic testing.
- Over-the-counter laxatives may be efficacious for opioid-induced constipation (OIC) and should be considered first-line agents. When these fail, peripherally acting μ-opioid receptor antagonists (PAMORAs) are suitable alternatives.
- More research is needed to determine the impact of secretagogues and prokinetics, which may be more efficacious for treating opioid-exacerbated constipation (OEC).

INTRODUCTION: THE SPECTRUM OF OPIOID-RELATED CONSTIPATION

Chronic idiopathic constipation (CIC), a term that frequently overlaps with functional constipation (FC), has been reported in approximately 12% and 7% of the international and US populations. In the United States, constipation accounts for almost 1 million physician visits per annum.[1,2] Multiple pathogenic mechanisms are responsible for constipation, with opioids a common precipitant. Opioids are currently prescribed to more than 1 in 5 adults with chronic noncancer pain (CNCP), and opioid-induced constipation (OIC) is considered a secondary and direct consequence of their use.[3]

Although not considered a distinct functional gastrointestinal disorder, OIC shares the same symptom profile as FC, including both subjective and objective symptoms such as straining, incomplete evacuation, reduced defecatory frequency, and hard stools.[4,5] OIC is thought to affect more than 40% of individuals prescribed opioids for CNCP with a number needed to harm (number of individuals who must be treated with an opioid before developing constipation) of approximately 3.3.[6–8] Many patients are willing to reduce, skip, or completely discontinue opioids, which in most instances results in inadequate pain relief.[9] This limitation indicates that improved treatment algorithms, based on new terminology that reflects nuances in clinical progression and likelihood of response to specific therapies, are needed to combat OIC without minimizing analgesia (**Table 1**).

Department of Medicine, Division of Gastroenterology/Hepatology, Northwestern University, 676 N St Clair Street, Suite 1400, Chicago, IL 60611, USA
* Corresponding author.
E-mail address: darren.brenner@nm.org

Gastroenterol Clin N Am 51 (2022) 107–121
https://doi.org/10.1016/j.gtc.2021.10.007
0889-8553/22/© 2021 Elsevier Inc. All rights reserved.
gastro.theclinics.com

Table 1
Current definitions for OIC

Rome IV diagnostic criteria for OIC include new or worsening of 2 or more of the following after initiation of, changes, or increases in opioid therapy.[4] Loose stools rarely present without laxatives and:	Diagnostic criteria for OIC: Consensus Working Group Definition[5] "A change when initiating opioid therapy from baseline bowel habits that is, characterized by any of the following:"
<3 SBM per week	Reduction in BM frequency
Lumpy or hard stools (BSFS 1–2) >25% BM	Harder stool consistency (BSFS 1–2)
Straining >25% of BM	Worsening of straining
Sensation of incomplete evacuation >25% BM	Sensation of incomplete rectal evacuation
Sensation of blockage >25% BM	
Manual maneuvers (digital manipulation/ pelvic floor support) to assist >25% BM	

Abbreviations: BM, bowel movement; BSFS, bristol stool form scale; IBS, irritable bowel syndrome; SBM, spontaneous bowel movement.

Use of the term opioid-related constipation (ORC) provides the framework for a novel classification schema, which differentiates two subtypes of constipation associated with opioid use: OIC, constipation that specifically develops after the initiation of opioid therapy, and opioid-exacerbated constipation (OEC), worsening of pre-existing constipation symptoms due to opioids. In most instances, the two can be differentiated by an accurate history[6,7] (**Fig. 1**). This distinction may appear semantic but is important as up to 50% of patients taking opioids suffer from pre-existing constipation and may be more responsive to medications with proven efficacy against both the constipating effects of the opioids and other underlying pathogenic mechanisms.[10]

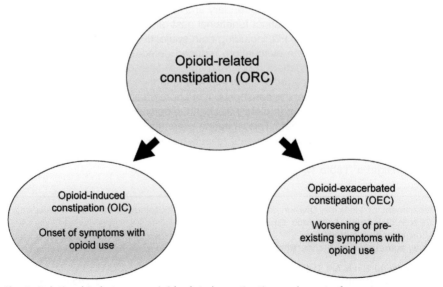

Fig. 1. Relationship between opioid-related constipation and onset of symptoms.

PATHOPHYSIOLOGY OF ORC

Opioids provide analgesia by binding to μ-opioid receptors in the central nervous system (CNS). However, these same receptors are also dispersed across the gastrointestinal mucosa with the highest concentrations identified in the stomach and colon. As opioids express no selective preference for μ-receptors in the CNS, they bind throughout the gastrointestinal tract, resulting in delayed gut transit, increased intestinal fluid reabsorption, and decreased fluid secretion.[11] Furthermore, in a retrospective study of 3452 laxative-refractory patients meeting Rome III criteria for FC undergoing pelvic floor physiologic testing at a tertiary center, patients receiving opioids had significantly higher resting anal sphincter tone, were more likely to have abnormal balloon expulsion tests (>1 minute), and met criteria for dyssynergic defecation more often than laxative-refractory individuals not consuming opioids. Rectal sensation was also significantly reduced in the cohort receiving opioids.[12] Opioids may mediate intestinal motility via alteration of the gut microbiome, although specific mechanisms have yet to be elucidated.[13] Thus, the pathogenesis of constipation in individuals consuming opioids is complex and likely multifactorial, and maximally effective treatment of ORC may require therapies directed at multiple targets.

TREATMENT OF ORC

ORC is frequently underidentified, leading to delays in treatment.[14] In a recent analysis of patient-opioid prescriber interactions, 64.4% of patients endorsed experiencing OIC, but 82.4% of prescribers failed to ask about symptoms and 33.8% did not receive a specific therapeutic recommendation.[15] In another survey of over 200 hospice agencies, 75% of agency primary contacts or hospice professionals reported that they had never used peripherally acting μ-opioid receptor antagonists (PAMORAs) to treat OIC.[16] Asking specifically about symptoms of constipation and previous laxative regimens may be revealing and indicate when treating OEC is more appropriate.[17]

First-line treatment of ORC is identical to FC. Based predominately upon anecdotal data, over-the-counter (OTC) fiber supplements, osmotic, and stimulant laxatives are safe, inexpensive, and effective in approximately 50% of cases. Should these initial interventions fail, 2 key questions must be answered: (1) when to switch to prescription therapy and (2) which therapeutic is most appropriate. Argoff and colleagues identified the Bowel Function Index (BFI) as the simplest and most accurate measure for identifying patients requiring treatment escalation, even when considering other patient-reported outcome measures such as the bowel function diary and the Patient Assessment of Constipation-Symptoms (PAC-SYM) questionnaire.[18] The BFI is a 3-item questionnaire validated to assess the severity of constipation-associated symptoms in individuals with OIC. The survey measures ease of defecation, sensation of incomplete evacuation, and an overall assessment of constipation-related symptoms over the course of the previous 7 days (**Fig. 2**). A BFI score of $\geq$ 30 has been recommended as the threshold for initiating prescription treatment in individuals with ORC nonresponsive to OTC agents. A score reduction of $\geq$ 12 points has been validated as clinically meaningful and shown to correlate patient preferences to individual therapies.[5,18,19]

In terms of choosing specific prescription therapy, the answer is predicated on the cause of the ORC. If the constipation is due to OIC, a PAMORA would be an appropriate next choice of therapy. However, if the symptoms are associated with OEC, a prescription laxative with evidence supporting its use across different constipation subtypes (ie, secretagogues, prokinetics) may prove more effective.

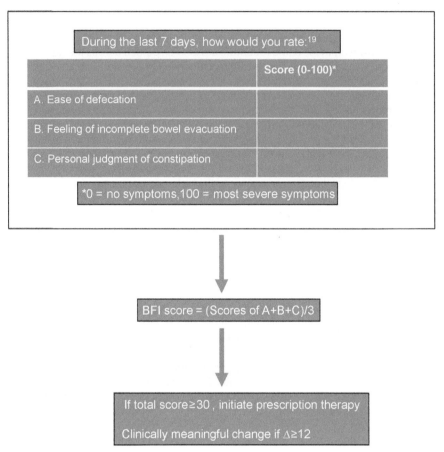

Fig. 2. The Bowel Function Index.

OTC TREATMENTS

Soluble fiber supplements (psyllium/ispaghula husk), osmotic (polyethylene glycol), and stimulant laxatives (senna, bisacodyl) are typically recommended as first-line treatments for ORC, but there is a paucity of high-quality studies supporting their use. Recently, the American Gastroenterological Association (AGA) published the first GI consensus guideline for the treatment of OIC, and strongly recommended OTC laxatives as first-line interventions, likely in part based on the fact that they are inexpensive and safe.[20–23] The most robust data supporting the use of OTCs stem from a randomized controlled crossover trial comparing the efficacy of polyethylene glycol (PEG 3350) to the PAMORA naloxegol.[24] In this study, equivalent numbers of patients endorsed subjective favorable preferences for one product over the other ($P = .92$) with most individuals noting a "strong" preference for their treatment of choice. This preference strongly correlated with a clinically meaningful response as identified via changes in BFI scores postintervention.

Unfortunately, for approximately 50% of individuals with OIC, OTC laxatives alone do not provide adequate relief.[25,26] For example, in a study of 322 patients taking daily opioids for cancer (4% of the study population) and non–cancer-related chronic pain, 81% reported continued constipation despite OTC laxative use and 58% reported persistent straining with bowel movements.[9] In a multinational survey of over 400 patients over a 24-week period, 94% of individuals using one laxative agent and 27% of those using 2 or more agents reported inadequate response (<3 BMs with at least one PAC-SYM score that was at least moderate).[27] For these patients, other strategies may be required.

PERIPHERALLY ACTING μ-OPIOID RECEPTORS ANTAGONISTS

PAMORAs are an FDA-approved class of therapies developed to reverse the constipating effects of opioids with minimal likelihood of compromising central analgesia or inducing opioid withdrawal.[28] These drugs, all derivatives of naloxone and naltrexone, have biochemical properties limiting their ability to cross the blood-brain barrier. Currently, 3 PAMORAs are approved in the United States for the treatment of OIC: methylnaltrexone, naloxegol, and naldemedine[6] (**Table 2**).

METHYLNALTREXONE

Methylnaltrexone (MNTX) was the first PAMORA to receive approval for the treatment of OIC, initially as a second-line agent for OIC in individuals with advanced illness receiving palliative care. It was subsequently approved for patients with CNCP and is the only PAMORA available in both subcutaneous (SC) and oral formulations. Its efficacy for treating OIC is supported by multiple randomized controlled trials (RCTs).

In a study enrolling 460 patients with nonmalignant pain-related OIC, individuals were randomized to receive SC injections of placebo or 12 mg of MNTX daily or every other day (alternating with placebo) for 4 weeks. Patients receiving daily and every other day injections of MNTX were significantly more likely to achieve a rescue-free bowel movement (RFBM) within 4 hours of receiving their initial injection compared with placebo (34.2% MNTX vs 9.9% placebo, P<.001). Furthermore, the percentage of injections resulting in RFBM in ≤4 hours was comparable between the MNTX groups (MNTX QOD 30.2%, MNTX QD 28.9%) but significantly greater than placebo (9%, P<.001 between groups).[29] A post-hoc analysis of 137 patients who initially received a 12 mg injection of MNTX daily revealed that patients who responded to at least 2 of the first 4 doses were more likely to experience a significant average increase in RFBMs (4.8 RFBM/wk) compared with those failing to achieve this endpoint (2.0 RFBM/wk; P<.001) Furthermore, the percentage of individuals achieving an average rate of ≥ 3 RFBMs was also significantly higher (81% vs 43%, P<.001). Thus, an initial response to treatment prognosticated better longer-term outcomes.[30]

In a later analysis, oral MTNX was also prospectively studied in 803 patients randomized to 150 mg, 300 mg, or 450 mg of MNTX QD or placebo.[31] An overall response was defined as ≥3 spontaneous bowel movements (SBMs) per week plus an increase of ≥1 SBM/wk from baseline for at least 3 of 4 weeks of the trial. A significantly higher percentage of individuals in the 300 and 450 mg cohorts achieved this endpoint compared with placebo (300 mg-49.3%, 450 mg-51.5%, placebo-38.3%; 300 mg vs placebo, P<.03; 450 mg vs placebo, P = .005). In addition, the proportion of dosing days resulting in an RFBM within 4 hours was significantly higher in patients receiving 300 mg (24.6%, P = .002) and 450 mg (27.4%, P<.0001) compared with placebo (18.2%).[31]

Both SC and oral MNTX were well-tolerated and serious adverse events were rare. In both studies, the most common treatment-emergent adverse events (TEAEs) occurring in individuals receiving MNTX included abdominal pain (19.3%), diarrhea (16.4%), and nausea (15.1%) in the SC and abdominal pain (8.0%), diarrhea (6.0%), and nausea

Table 2
FDA-approved treatments for OIC in patients with chronic noncancer pain with chemical structures

	Class (Biochemical Properties Preventing Transport Across Blood-Brain Barrier)	Class (Year of FDA Approval for OIC)	FDA-approved Dose and Route of Administration for OIC[a] CNCP	Primary Endpoint of Seminal Trials	Most Common TEAEs[c]	Clinical Considerations
Methylnaltrexone (MTNX)[54]	PAMORA (Quaternary compound (N-methylation) derived from naltrexone, positive charge and low lipid solubility)	2014 (s.c.) 2016 (p.o.)	12 mg daily s.c. 450 mg daily p.o.	s.c: % injections resulting in RFBM in ≤4 h p.o.: ≥ 3 SBMs/wk plus an increase of ≥1 SBM 3/4 wk	Abdominal pain, nausea, diarrhea	Only PAMORA available in s.c. form and also approved for patients with cancer. Consider in inpatient use given studies' outcome of RFBM within 4 h[51]
Naloxegol[56]	PAMORA (PEGylated derivative of naloxone, P-gp transporter substrate)	2014	25 mg daily p.o., on an empty stomach	12-wk response rate[b]	Diarrhea, abdominal pain, nausea	Can be crushed.[52] Weaker recommendation for patients using methadone.

Drug		Class/mechanism	Year	Dose	Endpoint	Side effects	Comments
Naldemedine[55]		PAMORA (Large steric side chain on naltrexone increasing polarity and molecular weight, P-gp transporter substrate)	2017	0.2 mg daily p.o.	12-wk response rate[b]	Abdominal pain, nausea, diarrhea	Has a "Strong" recommendation with high quality of evidence from the AGA based on trial data
Lubiprostone[53]		Chloride channel (ClC-2) agonist	2013	24 mcg twice daily p.o.	Δ Number of SBMs/wk from baseline at week 8[42] ≥3 SBM/wk for 9/12 wk + increase of 1 BM from baseline for all weeks[44]	Nausea, abdominal pain	Also approved for IBS and CIC, may be better for patients with worsening of pre-existing constipation. No risk of opioid withdrawal. Should not be given to patients using methadone.

[a] Dose adjustments recommended for hepatic and renal function, as well as patients taking CYP inhibitors.
[b] ≥ 3 SBMs/wk plus an increase of ≥ 1 SBM/wk from baseline for at least 9 of the 12 treatment weeks + 3 of last 4 weeks.
[c] No bowel perforations, serious cardiovascular events, or deaths in study drug groups.

(6.8%) in the oral MNTX cohorts, respectively.[32,33] There was no evidence of opioid withdrawal or major cardiovascular events.

NALOXEGOL

Naloxegol was the first oral PAMORA to receive FDA approval for treating OIC. This approval—for a daily dose of 25 mg—was based on 2 identical phase III studies (KODIAC-04 [N = 652], and KODIAC-05 [N = 700]) demonstrating sustained efficacy and safety over a 12-week period.[34] In these trials, durable responders were defined as having $\geq$3 SBMs/wk plus an increase of $\geq$1 SBM from baseline for $\geq$9 of 12 weeks inclusive of at least 3 of the final 4 weeks. Patients were randomized to receive 12.5 mg or 25 mg of naloxegol or placebo daily. In both studies, the response of patients receiving 25 mg daily was significant (KODIAC-04, 44.4% compared to 29.4% placebo [P = .001], KODIAC-05, 39.7% compared to 29.3% placebo [P = .02]). The response rates for the 12.5 mg cohorts were similar but not statistically significant for KODIAC-05. In an important subset analysis of individuals who had failed to respond to OTC laxatives before enrolling in KODIAC trials (KODIAC 04 N = 350, KODIAC 05 N = 370), data revealed that those receiving 25 mg daily in both trials were more likely to respond (48.7% vs 28.8% in placebo, P = .002, and 46.8% vs 31.4% in placebo, P = .01, respectively) and patients receiving 12.5 mg daily in KODIAC-04 had a statistically significant improvement (42.6% vs 28.8% in placebo, P = .03).[35]

The most common TEAEs in patients receiving naloxegol were diarrhea (5.4% in patients receiving 12.5 mg daily and 9.2% in patients receiving 25 mg daily) and abdominal pain (9.8% in the 12.5 group and 10.3% in the 25 mg group) and most were mild to moderate in severity. In KODIAC-04, 2 patients receiving naloxegol experienced myocardial infarctions, whereas in KODIAC-05, 2 events occurred in patients receiving placebo. Only one of these events was considered related to the study drug and occurred in an individual receiving placebo.[35] Eight patients reported symptoms consistent with opioid withdrawal including one in the placebo group and another in the treatment group who ran out of opioid medication. In a subsequent 52-week safety trial of 534 patients receiving 25 mg of naloxegol (KODIAC-08), TEAEs were similar with most mild to moderate in nature and occurring early in the course of therapy. Overall, naloxegol was well tolerated with only 11 patients discontinuing treatment because of diarrhea and 9 because of abdominal pain. In this long-term analysis, no cardiovascular events or episodes of opioid withdrawal were associated with naloxegol.[36]

NALDEMEDINE

Naldemedine is the most recent PAMORA approved for OIC in patients with CNCP and its efficacy is supported by 5 phase II/III trials.[37,38] Two identical 12-week phase III RCTs (COMPOSE-I and II) with a combined 1095 subjects evaluated with the same durable response endpoint utilized in the aforementioned naloxegol studies.[39] In COMPOSE-I, 47.6% of patients receiving 0.2 mg of naldemedine daily achieved this endpoint compared with 34.6% in the placebo group (P = .002). In COMPOSE-II, 52.5% of naldemedine-treated patients responded compared with 33.6% of those receiving placebo (P<.0001). COMPOSE-III, a 52-week trial, revealed that at 12, 24, 36, and 52 weeks, naldemedine-treated subjects (N = 621) experienced significantly increased rates of SBMs compared with placebo (P<.0001 at all timepoints).[40]

Diarrhea (8.0%) and abdominal pain (5.5%) were the two most common TEAEs reported in COMPOSE-I/II. There was no evidence of opioid withdrawal or cardiovascular events. In COMPOSE-III, TEAEs were similar between groups (68.4 vs 72.1%, respectively), with diarrhea (11%), and abdominal pain (8.2%) reported most frequently.

Notably, 11 cases of treatment-emergent opioid withdrawal were reported, with similar proportions occurring in the naldemedine (1.8%) and placebo (1.1%) cohorts.[40]

SECRETAGOGUES
Lubiprostone

Lubiprostone is a type-2 chloride channel activator that increases intestinal secretion and peristalsis.[41] Initially approved for the treatment of IBS-C in women (8 mcg twice daily) and CIC (24 mcg twice daily), it received subsequent FDA approval for OIC in individuals with nonmalignant pain syndromes in 2013. Presumably, lubiprostone reverses suppression of μ-receptor chloride secretion and improves intestinal transit time without affecting analgesia.[42] Because of its distinct mechanism of action, it has not been shown to reverse the central mediating effects of opioids.

Two identical phase III trials comparing lubiprostone to placebo yielded discordant results. In the first, patients with OIC were randomized to either lubiprostone 24 mcg twice daily (N = 209) or placebo (N = 204). The primary endpoint, the mean change from baseline in SBMs at week 8, was significantly higher in the lubiprostone cohort compared with placebo (3.3 vs 2.4, P = .005); however, this difference was not maintained at week 12.[42] In the second study, no significant differences in SBM frequency were detected between the cohorts at either 8 or 12 weeks.[43] Rates of adverse events were similar between groups with 63.5% of lubiprostone and 54.4% of placebo patients experiencing a TEAE. The most common TEAEs were nausea (15.4% in the lubiprostone group compared with 5.3% in the placebo group, P<.001), diarrhea, and abdominal distention.

In a third phase III trial, 431 patients with OIC were again randomized to either 24 mcg twice daily lubiprostone or placebo.[44] In the interim between the second trial and this subsequent study, new evidence emerged that methadone antagonizes the effects of lubiprostone at ClC-2 chloride channels, rendering it ineffective. As such, patients taking methadone were excluded.[45] Patients were considered primary responders if they experienced an increase of $\geq$1 SBM during all 12 weeks of the trial plus $\geq$3 SBM/wk for at least 9 of 12 weeks. A significantly greater percentage of lubiprostone-treated individuals (27.1%) met this endpoint compared with placebo (18.9%, P = .003). A greater mean change in SBM/wk frequency was also observed in the lubiprostone group (3.2 vs 2.4 placebo, P = .001) The most common TEAEs were diarrhea, nausea, vomiting, and abdominal pain (7.1% vs 0% in the placebo group). There was no evidence of opioid withdrawal in any of these 3 studies.[42–44]

Given the positive results of the third study, concerns emerged that the first two trial results were impacted by the enrollment of methadone patients. Subsequent post-hoc analyses excluding individuals consuming diphenylheptanes (methadone) were performed showing that patients taking nonmethadone opioids experienced significant increases in their numbers of SBMs.[46] Conversely, patients using methadone did not. Treatment ($\geq$1 SBM increase for 12 of 12 weeks) and full response ($\geq$3 SBMs/wk for at least 9 of 12 weeks) were also significantly greater in the nonmethadone cohorts. Given these outcomes, lubiprostone is not recommended for patients with OIC who use methadone.

Linaclotide

Linaclotide is a guanylate cyclase-C (GC-C) receptor agonist FDA-approved to treat both CIC (72, 145 mcg daily) and IBS-C (290 mcg daily). In a recently published phase II trial, adults with OIC associated with nonmalignant chronic pain were randomized to receive a once-daily dose of linaclotide 145 mcg (N = 87), linaclotide 290 mcg (N = 88), or placebo (N = 79) daily for 8 weeks. SBM frequency (SBMs/wk) and 6/8 week response (≥3 SBMs/wk plus an increase of ≥1 SBM/wk from baseline for 6 of 8 weeks) were measured; the response was "durable" if response was achieved for 3 of 4 weeks of treatment at the end of the trial.[47] Patients in both linaclotide cohorts experienced significantly greater mean changes in SBM rates compared with placebo (mean change 2.9 [145 mcg], 3.5 [290 mcg], 1.6 [placebo] at 8 weeks; P<.01 for both comparisons to placebo). Numerically, individuals receiving both doses of linaclotide had improvements in their 6/8-week responses (40.2% [145 mcg]; 47.1% [290 mcg]) compared with placebo (33.3%), with results approaching significance for the 290 mcg dose (P = .051). Diarrhea, the most common TEAE, occurred in 27.6%%, 36.8%, and 16.7% of patients in the linaclotide 145 mcg, linaclotide 290 mcg, and placebo groups, respectively.

Prokinetics

Prucalopride is a serotonergic $5-HT_4$ receptor agonist with prokinetic effects. It was recently approved by the FDA for treating CIC at a dose of 2 mg daily. A single phase-II trial in patients with OIC compared an average increase of ≥1 complete SBM per week over 4 weeks between prucalopride 2 mg (N = 66), 4 mg (N = 64), and placebo (N = 66).[48] In the prucalopride 2 mg and 4 mg groups, 60.7% and 69% met this endpoint, respectively, versus 43% of the placebo group (P = .01 for the 4 mg group). The most common TEAEs were abdominal pain (12.1% in the 2 mg group, 25% in the 4 mg group compared with 9.1% in the placebo group), nausea, and diarrhea. Headaches were infrequently reported (6.1% in the 2 mg prucalopride group and 7.8% in the 4 mg prucalopride group). A subsequent phase III trial was initiated but terminated early because of nonsafety, business-related reasons.

COMPARISONS OF THERAPIES AND UTILITY IN THE TREATMENT OF OIC VERSUS OEC

Several systematic reviews comparing the efficacy of treatments for OIC in individuals with CNCP have been published; all note differing levels of evidence, enrollment populations, primary outcome definitions, and the absence of direct head-to-head studies[21,49,50] (Table 3). In 2019, the American Gastroenterological Association (AGA) published guidelines for the treatment of OIC.[22] Naldemedine, naloxegol, and OTC laxatives received "strong" recommendations for use but only naldemedine was considered to have high-quality evidence. Methylnaltrexone received a "conditional" recommendation presumably due to the shorter duration and reduced rigor of the endpoints used in these studies. It is important to note, however, that there was no FDA guidance for defining an OIC population or trial outcomes available when the initial MNTX studies were completed. Lubiprostone and prucalopride did not receive formal recommendations because of evidence gaps. Data for linaclotide were published subsequent to the release of the AGA guideline. However, all 3 are medications with proven efficacy for treating alternative forms of constipation.

Where does this leave the practitioner when treating individuals across the spectrum of ORC? OTC laxatives should be used as first-line therapies: they are safe, inexpensive, and effective in approximately 50% of patients. If patients are laxative-refractory (subjectively or with a BFI score ≥ 30), and have OIC, PAMORAs are a natural next choice as they have proven efficacious, safe, and tolerable with limited potential to decrease central analgesia or induce withdrawal. For OEC, lubiprostone, linaclotide, and prucalopride may exhibit superior response as each has proven effective for treating nonopioid causes of constipation (Fig. 3). Ultimately, the most successful outcomes are likely to occur when individuals are appropriately categorized.

Table 3
Comparison of recent meta-analyses for treatments in OIC/ORC

	Nee, 2018	Hanson, 2019	Luthra 2019
	RR (95% CI) for Treatment Failure Compared to PBO	RR (95% CI) for Rate of Response Compared to PBO	RR (95% CI) for Failure to Achieve Average ≥3 BMs/wk or average ≥3 BMs/wk + ≥1 BM/wk Compared to PBO
Methylnaltrexone s.c.	0.75 (0.63–0.90) P = .006[a]	1.43 (1.21–1.68)[a]	0.74 (0.58–0.94), P = .61
Methylnaltrexone p.o.	NA	NA	0.91 (0.79–1.17), P = .23
Naldemedine	0.65, P<.001	1.51 (1.32–1.72)	0.67 (0.59–0.77), P = .80
Naloxegol	0.77 (0.61–0.97) P = .026	1.43 (1.19–1.71)	0.85 (0.71–1.01), P = .35
Lubiprostone	0.90 (0.83–0.97), P = .005	1.15 (0.97–1.37)	0.92 (0.79–1.07) P = .22
Linaclotide	NA	NA	NA
Prucalopride[b]	0.88 (0.68–0.98), P = .032	RR 1.57 (0.88–2.80)	NA

[a] Did not specify whether s.c. or p.o. or both; Hanson et al included patients with cancer.
[b] Where applicable, included incomplete trial data.

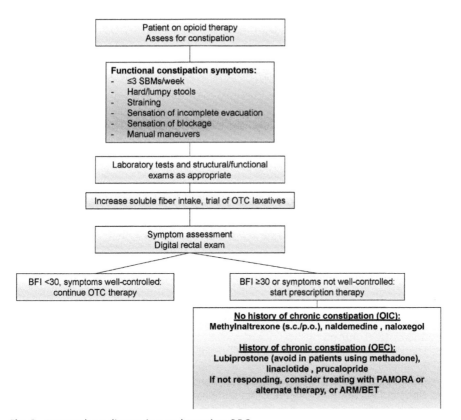

Fig. 3. Approach to diagnosing and treating ORC.

SUMMARY

Constipation is the most common adverse effect experienced by individuals taking opioids for CNCP, and it significantly impacts quality of life and optimization of analgesia. There are now multiple evidence-based therapies available to combat this disorder and which to choose is dependent upon the underlying causes of constipation. Differentiation may lead to better results, yet further studies are necessary assessing responses specifically in individuals with OEC. Future trials should also take into consideration whether outcomes are impacted by the specific opioid being consumed.

CLINICS CARE POINTS

- Opioid-induced constipation (OIC) develops in more than 40% of patients using opioids for chronic noncancer pain-related syndromes.
- Opioid-related constipation encompasses both opioid-induced and opioid-exacerbated constipation, which are differentiated by the relationship between the development of constipation and timing of opioid initiation.
- Over-the-counter laxatives are first-line treatments for opioid-induced and opioid-exacerbated constipation based on their clinical efficacy, ease of use, low cost, and safety profile.
- When over-the-counter laxatives fail, peripherally acting μ-opioid receptor antagonists (PAMORAs) are an appropriate next choice for individuals with opioid-induced constipation, whereas secretagogues or prokinetic agents may be more effective for patients with opioid-exacerbated constipation.

DISCLOSURE

J.J. Liu does not have any disclosures to report. D.M. Brenner has served as an advisor, consultant, or speaker for the following: Allergan (AbbVie), Ironwood, Laborie, Salix, Takeda, Alphasigma, Arena, Alynlam, Laborie, and Redhill Pharmaceuticals. He is also supported in research by an unrestricted gift from the Irene D. Pritzker Foundation.

REFERENCES

1. Ma C, Congly SE, Novak KL, et al. Epidemiologic burden and treatment of chronic symptomatic functional bowel disorders in the United States: a nationwide analysis. Gastroenterology 2021;160(1):88–98.e4.
2. Palsson OS, Whitehead W, Törnblom H, et al. Prevalence of Rome IV Functional Bowel Disorders Among Adults in the United States, Canada, and the United Kingdom. Gastroenterology 2020;158(5):1262–73.e3.
3. Dowell D, Haegerich TM, Chou R. CDC guideline for prescribing opioids for chronic pain–United States, 2016. JAMA 2016;315(15):1624–45.
4. Lacy BE, Mearin F, Chang L, et al. Bowel Disorders. Gastroenterology 2016; 150(6):1393–407.e5.
5. Camilleri M, Drossman DA, Becker G, et al. Emerging treatments in neurogastroenterology: a multidisciplinary working group consensus statement on opioid-induced constipation. Neurogastroenterol Motil 2014;26(10):1386–95.
6. Brenner DM, Stern E, Cash BD. Opioid-related constipation in patients with noncancer pain syndromes: a review of evidence-based therapies and justification for a change in nomenclature. Curr Gastroenterol Rep 2017;19(3):12.

7. Brenner DM, Barrett-Englert M, Cash BD. How to manage opioid-related constipation in individuals with chronic nonmalignant pain syndromes. Am J Gastroenterol 2020;115(3):307–10.

8. Brenner D, Chey W. An Evidence-Based Review of Novel and Emerging Therapies for Constipation in Patients Taking Opioid Analgesics. In: 2014. doi:10.1038/AJGSUP.2014.8.

9. Bell T, Panchal S, Miaskowski C, et al. The prevalence, severity, and impact of opioid-induced bowel dysfunction: Results of a US and European Patient Survey (PROBE 1). Pain Med 2009;10:35–42.

10. Ducrotté P, Milce J, Soufflet C, et al. Prevalence and clinical features of opioid-induced constipation in the general population: A French study of 15,000 individuals. United Eur Gastroenterol J 2017;5(4):588–600.

11. Sobczak M, Sałaga M, Storr MA, et al. Physiology, signaling, and pharmacology of opioid receptors and their ligands in the gastrointestinal tract: current concepts and future perspectives. J Gastroenterol 2014;49(1):24–45.

12. Nojkov B, Baker J, Menees S, et al. Is Dyssynergic Defecation an Unrecognized Cause of Chronic Constipation in Patients Using Opioids? Am J Gastroenterol 2019;114(11):1772–7.

13. Wang F, Meng J, Zhang L, et al. Morphine induces changes in the gut microbiome and metabolome in a morphine dependence model. Sci Rep 2018;8. https://doi.org/10.1038/s41598-018-21915-8.

14. Alvaro D, Caraceni AT, Coluzzi F, et al. What to do and what not to do in the management of opioid-induced constipation: a choosing wisely report. Pain Ther 2020;9(2):657–67.

15. Vallerand AH, Hendry S, Baldys E, et al. Analysis of Patient-Provider Interactions Regarding the Burden and Treatment of Opioid-Induced Constipation in Adults with Chronic Noncancer Pain. Pain Med Malden Mass 2019;20(5):889–96.

16. Sera L, McPherson ML. Management of Opioid-Induced Constipation in Hospice Patients. Am J Hosp Palliat Med 2017. https://doi.org/10.1177/1049909117705379.

17. Argoff CE. Opioid-induced constipation: a review of health-related quality of life, patient burden, practical clinical considerations, and the impact of peripherally acting μ-opioid receptor antagonists. Clin J Pain 2020;36(9):716–22.

18. Argoff CE, Brennan MJ, Camilleri M, et al. Consensus recommendations on initiating prescription therapies for opioid-induced constipation. Pain Med 2015;16(12):2324–37.

19. Rentz AM, Yu R, Müller-Lissner S, et al. Validation of the Bowel Function Index to detect clinically meaningful changes in opioid-induced constipation. J Med Econ 2009;12(4):371–83.

20. Ford AC, Moayyedi P, Chey WD, et al. American College of Gastroenterology monograph on management of irritable bowel syndrome. Am J Gastroenterol 2018;113(Suppl 2):1–18.

21. Hanson B, Siddique SM, Scarlett Y, et al. American Gastroenterological Association Institute Technical Review on the Medical Management of Opioid-Induced Constipation. Gastroenterology 2019;156(1):229–53.e5.

22. Crockett SD, Greer KB, Heidelbaugh JJ, et al. American Gastroenterological Association Institute guideline on the medical management of opioid-induced constipation. Gastroenterology 2019;156(1):218–26.

23. Paré P, Fedorak RN. Systematic review of stimulant and nonstimulant laxatives for the treatment of functional constipation. Can J Gastroenterol Hepatol 2014;28(10):549–57.

24. Brenner DM, Hu Y, Datto C, et al. A randomized, multicenter, prospective, crossover, open-label study of factors associated with patient preferences for naloxegol or PEG 3350 for opioid-induced constipation. Am J Gastroenterol 2019; 114(6):954–63.

25. Pappagallo M. Incidence, prevalence, and management of opioid bowel dysfunction. Am J Surg 2001;182(5A Suppl):11S–8S.

26. Christensen HN, Olsson U, From J, et al. Opioid-induced constipation, use of laxatives, and health-related quality of life. Scand J Pain 2016;11:104–10.

27. Coyne KS, LoCasale RJ, Datto CJ, et al. Opioid-induced constipation in patients with chronic noncancer pain in the USA, Canada, Germany, and the UK: descriptive analysis of baseline patient-reported outcomes and retrospective chart review. Clin Outcomes Res 2014;6:269–81.

28. Viscusi ER. Clinical Overview and Considerations for the Management of Opioid-induced Constipation in Patients With Chronic Noncancer Pain. Clin J Pain 2019; 35(2):174–88.

29. Michna E, Blonsky ER, Schulman S, et al. Subcutaneous methylnaltrexone for treatment of opioid-induced constipation in patients with chronic, nonmalignant pain: a randomized controlled study. J Pain 2011;12(5):554–62.

30. Michna E, Weil AJ, Duerden M, et al. Efficacy of Subcutaneous Methylnaltrexone in the Treatment of Opioid-Induced Constipation: A Responder Post Hoc Analysis. Pain Med 2011;12(8):1223–30.

31. Rauck R, Slatkin NE, Stambler N, et al. Randomized, Double-Blind Trial of Oral Methylnaltrexone for the Treatment of Opioid-Induced Constipation in Patients with Chronic Noncancer Pain. Pain Pract 2017;17(6):820–8.

32. Webster LR, Michna E, Khan A, et al. Long-term safety and efficacy of subcutaneous methylnaltrexone in patients with opioid-induced constipation and chronic noncancer pain: a phase 3, open-label trial. Pain Med 2017;18(8): 1496–504.

33. Rauck RL, Slatkin NE, Stambler N, et al. Safety of oral methylnaltrexone for opioid-induced constipation in patients with chronic noncancer pain. J Pain Res 2018; 12:139–50.

34. Movantik (naloxegol) Prescribing Information. Published online 2014. Available at: https://www.accessdata.fda.gov/drugsatfda_docs/label/2014/204760s000lbl. pdf.

35. Chey WD, Webster L, Sostek M, et al. Naloxegol for Opioid-Induced Constipation in Patients with Noncancer Pain. N Engl J Med 2014;370(25):2387–96.

36. Webster L, Chey WD, Tack J, et al. Randomised clinical trial: the long-term safety and tolerability of naloxegol in patients with pain and opioid-induced constipation. Aliment Pharmacol Ther 2014;40(7):771–9.

37. Stern EK, Brenner DM. Spotlight on naldemedine in the treatment of opioid-induced constipation in adult patients with chronic noncancer pain: design, development, and place in therapy. J Pain Res 2018;11:195–9.

38. Liu JJ, Quinton SE, Brenner DM. Naldemedine for the treatment of opioid-induced constipation in adults with chronic noncancer pain. Pain Manag 2020. https://doi. org/10.2217/pmt-2020-0019.

39. Hale M, Wild J, Reddy J, et al. Naldemedine versus placebo for opioid-induced constipation (COMPOSE-1 and COMPOSE-2): two multicentre, phase 3, double-blind, randomised, parallel-group trials. Lancet Gastroenterol Hepatol 2017;2(8): 555–64.

40. Webster LR, Nalamachu S, Morlion B, et al. Long-term use of naldemedine in the treatment of opioid-induced constipation in patients with chronic noncancer pain:

a randomized, double-blind, placebo-controlled phase 3 study. Pain 2018; 159(5):987–94.

41. Cuppoletti J, Malinowska DH, Tewari KP, et al. SPI-0211 activates T84 cell chloride transport and recombinant human ClC-2 chloride currents. Am J Physiol Cell Physiol 2004;287(5):C1173–83.

42. Cryer B, Katz S, Vallejo R, et al. A randomized study of lubiprostone for opioid-induced constipation in patients with chronic noncancer pain. Pain Med Malden Mass 2014;15(11):1825–34.

43. Spierings ELH, Drossman DA, Cryer B, et al. Efficacy and Safety of Lubiprostone in Patients with Opioid-Induced Constipation: Phase 3 Study Results and Pooled Analysis of the Effect of Concomitant Methadone Use on Clinical Outcomes. Pain Med Malden Mass 2018;19(6):1184–94.

44. Jamal MM, Adams AB, Jansen J-P, et al. A randomized, placebo-controlled trial of lubiprostone for opioid-induced constipation in chronic noncancer pain. Am J Gastroenterol 2015;110(5):725–32.

45. Cuppoletti J, Chakrabarti J, Tewari K, et al. Methadone but not morphine inhibits lubiprostone-stimulated Cl- currents in T84 intestinal cells and recombinant human ClC-2, but not CFTR Cl- currents. Cell Biochem Biophys 2013;66(1):53–63.

46. Webster LR, Brewer RP, Lichtlen P, et al. Efficacy of Lubiprostone for the Treatment of Opioid-Induced Constipation, Analyzed by Opioid Class. Pain Med Malden Mass 2018;19(6):1195–205.

47. Brenner DM, Argoff CE, Fox SM, et al. Efficacy and safety of linaclotide for opioid-induced constipation in patients with chronic noncancer pain syndromes from a phase 2 randomized study. Pain 2020;161(5):1027–36.

48. Sloots CEJ, Rykx A, Cools M, et al. Efficacy and Safety of Prucalopride in Patients with Chronic Noncancer Pain Suffering from Opioid-Induced Constipation. Dig Dis Sci 2010;55(10):2912–21.

49. Nee J, Zakari M, Sugarman MA, et al. Efficacy of Treatments for Opioid-Induced Constipation: Systematic Review and Meta-analysis. Clin Gastroenterol Hepatol 2018;16(10):1569–84.e2.

50. Luthra P, Burr NE, Brenner DM, et al. Efficacy of pharmacological therapies for the treatment of opioid-induced constipation: systematic review and network meta-analysis. Gut 2019;68(3):434–44.

51. Murphy JA, Sheridan EA. Evidence Based Review of Pharmacotherapy for Opioid-Induced Constipation in Noncancer Pain. Ann Pharmacother 2018;52(4):370–9.

52. Bui K, Birmingham B, Diva U, et al. An Open-Label, Randomized Bioavailability Study of Alternative Methods of Oral Administration of Naloxegol in Healthy Subjects. Clin Pharmacol Drug Dev 2017;6(4):420–7.

53. National Center for Biotechnology Information. PubChem Compound Summary for CID 157920, Lubiprostone. Available at: https://pubchem.ncbi.nlm.nih.gov/compound/Lubiprostone. February 17, 2021.

54. National Center for Biotechnology Information. PubChem Compound Summary for CID 5361917, Methylnaltrexone bromide. Available at: https://pubchem.ncbi.nlm.nih.gov/compound/Methylnaltrexone-bromide. February 17, 2021.

55. National Center for Biotechnology Information. PubChem Compound Summary for CID 54732242, Naldemedine. Available at: https://pubchem.ncbi.nlm.nih.gov/compound/Naldemedine. February 17, 2021.

56. PubChem. Naloxegol. Available at: https://pubchem.ncbi.nlm.nih.gov/compound/56959087. March 9, 2021.

A Pain in the Butt
Hemorrhoids, Fissures, Fistulas, and Other Anorectal Syndromes

Tisha N. Lunsford, MD[a], Mary A. Atia, MD[b],
Suaka Kagbo-Kue, MD[a], Lucinda A. Harris, MS, MD[a],*

KEYWORDS

- Anorectal pain • Anorectal itching • Anorectal disorders • Hemorrhoids • Proctalgia
- Biofeedback

KEY POINTS

- Causes for anorectal pain are classified as acute or chronic
- Most anorectal syndromes are benign, but inflammatory, infectious, and malignant causes must be ruled out
- Anorectal symptoms do not distinguish between underlying causes
- Coexisting disordered bowel habits must be addressed
- Coexisting defecatory dysfunction must be addressed

INTRODUCTION

About 25% of the population is affected by anorectal disorders.[1] This article provides an overview of these disorders and the approaches used to diagnose and treat them. Common structural anorectal disorders (hemorrhoids, fissures, fistulas, abscesses, solitary rectal ulcer syndrome [SRUS], rectal prolapse, anal cancers), rarer causes of anorectal pain (pruritis ani, sexually transmitted diseases, foreign bodies), and disorders of gut brain axis (proctalgia fugax and levator ani syndrome [LAS]) are addressed. Each of these disorders is clearly "a pain in the butt," and recognition is imperative because treatment significantly improves quality of life.

HEMORRHOIDS (PILES)

Hemorrhoids are present in all persons but are commonly underrecognized until they become symptomatic. The hemorrhoidal plexus plays pivotal roles in facilitating

[a] Division of Gastroenterology & Hepatology, Alix School of Medicine, Mayo Clinic, 13400 E. Shea Blvd, Scottsdale, AZ 85259, USA; [b] Arizona Digestive Health, 5823 W. Eugie Ave, Suite A, Glendale, AZ 85304, USA
* Corresponding author.
E-mail address: Harris.Lucinda@Mayo.edu

Gastroenterol Clin N Am 51 (2022) 123–144
https://doi.org/10.1016/j.gtc.2021.10.008
0889-8553/22/© 2021 Elsevier Inc. All rights reserved.

continence and protecting the anal sphincters from injury during defecation.[2] Historically, hemorrhoids have been referred to as piles from the Latin word *pila,* which translates roughly to "balls" and reflects a patient's sensation of the swollen hemorrhoid. Their exact prevalence is not known because most patients do not consult their physician regarding symptoms. The prevalence of symptomatic hemorrhoids increases with age with symptoms experienced by more than 50% of patients older than 50 years.[3] Although hemorrhoids do not impact mortality, they are distressing and negatively impact quality of life. Hemorrhoids develop when the venous drainage of the rectum is increased, resulting in dilation of the sinusoids supplied by the superior and middle hemorrhoidal arteries and the superior rectal artery. Factors that increase pressure in the pelvic floor contribute to the formation of hemorrhoids, and hemorrhoidal formation is a multifactorial process involving arteriovenous distension, downward protrusion of congested anal cushions, and progressive stretching and collapse of the support structure (mucosa, anoderm, supporting and anchoring connective tissue) over time.[4] These factors include constipation with straining, chronic frequent diarrhea, obesity, pregnancy and labor, anal intercourse, pelvic floor dysfunction, and decompensated cirrhosis complicated by ascites.[5]

Hemorrhoids are classified based on their location in relation to the dentate line, an anatomic landmark dividing the insensate rectal mucosa from the richly innervated anal skin.[4] Internal hemorrhoids develop proximal to the dentate line, whereas external hemorrhoids emerge distal. Internal hemorrhoids are painless because they have visceral innervation. External hemorrhoids are encased in squamous epithelium and therefore can become painful when swollen. The degree of internal hemorrhoid prolapse is graded from I to IV (**Fig. 1, Table 1**). This grading scale is relevant because it guides optimal treatment.

Symptomatic internal hemorrhoids classically present with painless hematochezia. The bleeding is described as streaks of bright red blood coating the stool, in the toilet bowl, or noted while wiping. Prolapse of internal hemorrhoidal tissue may also cause pruritus (due to mucous deposition) and fecal leakage.[6] External hemorrhoid symptoms include soiling or severe pain when thrombosed.

Although many patients attribute their perianal symptoms to hemorrhoids, there are several other pathologies to consider. Consequently, a perianal inspection and digital rectal examination (DRE) are crucial in the evaluation of all anorectal symptoms; this is best accomplished in the left lateral decubitus position with visual inspection of the perianal region performed both at rest and during Valsalva. A thrombosed external hemorrhoid is easily recognized as a tender blue bulge at the anal verge (**Fig. 2**); however, it is important to keep in mind that melanoma can mimic an external hemorrhoid. If not precluded by pain, anoscopy is an effective way to visualize the distal rectum and to detect internal hemorrhoids,[7] which develop along 3 anatomic planes: right anterior, right posterior, and left lateral.[8] Even when hemorrhoids are identified, further diagnostic testing via flexible sigmoidoscopy or colonoscopy is recommended to ensure that comorbid issues including polyps, malignancy, or colitis have been ruled out.

Initial treatment of hemorrhoids should include dietary and lifestyle changes. Conservative measures effective for the management of hemorrhoids include a high-fiber diet with adequate fluid intake (1.5– 2 L/d).[9] Recommended fiber intake is 20 to 25 g for females and 30 to 35 g for males.[10] Fiber supplementation is helpful because it can be used to treat both constipation and diarrhea—both known precipitants for the development of symptomatic hemorrhoids.[6] It is also advised to limit defecation time to 3 to 5 minutes. Warm water sitz baths alternating with cold compresses, use of stool softeners, and judicious use of nonsteroidal anti-inflammatory

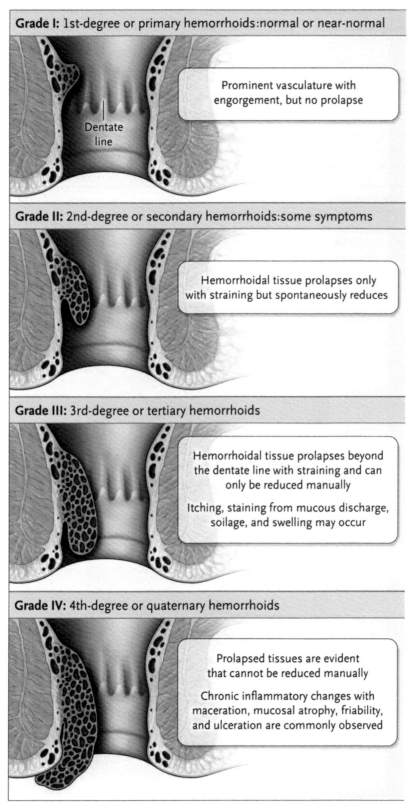

Fig. 1. Classification of internal hemorrhoids. (*Used with permission* of Mayo Foundation for Medical Education and Research, all rights reserved.)

Table 1
Classification of internal hemorrhoids

Grade	Description
I	Bulge internally with defecation
II	Prolapse with defecation, reduce spontaneously
III	Require digital reduction after prolapsing
IV	Incarcerated, cannot be reduced

Data from Qureshi WA. Office management of hemorrhoids. Am J Gastroenterol. 2018;113(6):795–98. https://doi.org/10.1038/s41395-018-0020-0.

drugs can also be helpful for mild intermittent symptoms. There are several over-the-counter remedies, such as Preparation H and Tucks pads that may also provide symptomatic relief. The active ingredients of these remedies, for example, hydrocortisone, witch hazel, phenylephrine, pramoxine, and various emollients, vary according to the

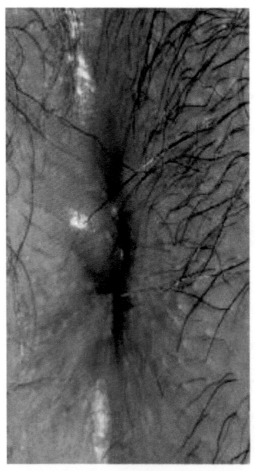

Fig. 2. Thrombosed external hemorrhoid. (*Used with permission* of Mayo Foundation for Medical Education and Research, all rights reserved.)

product and can vary from country to country. However, there is a paucity of quality clinical trial data demonstrating any long-term benefit[9] for these agents.

In most instances, conservative management is effective in treating the acute pain of external hemorrhoids because this usually resolves over 48 to 72 hours. Occasionally, the high pressure within the thrombus erodes the mucosa and bleeding ensues, often accompanied by relief of the pain. If the pain is severe, surgical evacuation of the thrombus may be warranted. In other circumstances, prolapsed internal hemorrhoids may become strangulated, thrombose, and induce pain or purulent foul-smelling discharge. Reduction may provide some temporary relief, but urgent surgical hemorrhoidectomy may be required. External and prolapsed internal hemorrhoids can be differentiated by the fact that external hemorrhoids are covered by anoderm with the clot lying beneath the skin, whereas internal hemorrhoids are covered by anal mucosa.

Office-based or surgical procedures can effectively treat internal hemorrhoids refractory to conservative therapy. The goal of the intervention is to decrease vascularity and redundant tissue with fixation of the tissue to the underlying structures to prevent further prolapse.[11] In general, the lower the grade, the more likely an office-based procedure, such as rubber band ligation, infrared photocoagulation, or sclerotherapy, will be successful. Rubber band ligation is the preferred office-based treatment due to increased efficacy[12] and low complication rate. This modality is used for 80% of patients.[6] Ligation completely encircles the redundant mucosa, vascular bundle, and connective tissue causing the entrapped tissue to necrose and slough; this results in refixation of the hemorrhoidal cushion and eliminates prolapse and associated hemorrhoid symptoms. A limitation of this intervention is that rubber band ligation does not treat external disease and is associated with variable recurrence rates requiring additional interventions.[13] Contraindications to this intervention include previous pelvic floor radiation therapy, anticoagulation, active inflammatory disease in the colon, pregnancy, and cirrhosis/portal hypertension. Surgery is indicated for those who cannot tolerate office-based procedures, who have failed nonsurgical treatment, or who have more severe disease. Surgical options include mucopexy, stapled hemorrhoidopexy, Doppler-guided hemorrhoidal artery ligation, and traditional hemorrhoidectomy. Compared with office-based procedures, surgery is more painful and associated with longer recovery times and higher complication rates, but recurrence rates are significantly lower.[14] After banding, 30% to 50% of individuals will have recurrence of hemorrhoids within 5 to 10 years compared with 2% to 5% after operative hemorrhoidectomy.[15]

ANAL FISSURE

The presence of an anal fissure should also be considered when patients present with anorectal pain. In many instances these are identified concurrently with hemorrhoids, and pain during defecation is one way to clinically differentiate them from hemorrhoids. Anal fissures are longitudinal tears of the squamous anoderm. As these lesions occur inferior to the dentate line, they are associated with significant pain with the quality of the pain usually described as similar to a "paper cut" or "passing shards of glass." Fissures can be classified as acute or chronic with acute fissures presenting as thin tears lasting less than 6 to 12 weeks and chronic fissures characterized by the presence of visible sphincter muscles fiber, indurated margins, and the formation of a sentinel pile (skin tag) distally and/or hypertrophied anal papillae proximally (**Fig. 3**).[16]

In a retrospective review, the average lifetime risk of developing an anal fissure was 7.8%[17] with nearly equal distribution among males and females. Fissures are most often seen in younger individuals with mean age of onset of 40 years[18]

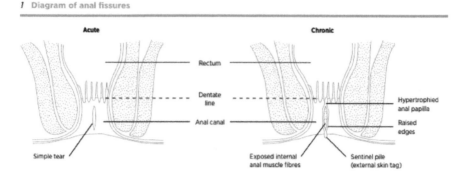

1 Diagram of anal fissures

Acute   Chronic

Rectum

Dentate
line

Anal canal

Hypertrophied
anal papilla

Raised
edges

Simple tear   Exposed internal   Sentinel pile
                               anal muscle fibres   (external skin tag)

Fig. 3. Diagram of anal fissures. (*From* Schlichtemeier S, Engel A. Anal fissure. Aust Prescr. 2016;39(1):14–7. https://doi.org/10.18773/austprescr.2016.007 with permission.)

Most acute idiopathic fissures (90%) develop in the posterior midline, owing to poor perfusion at this location. Ten percent of fissures occur anteriorly, and these are more common in women.[19] Fissures in the anterolateral position (<1% of fissures) are atypical and can be associated with other conditions such as Crohn's disease, granulomatous disease (ie, tuberculosis or sarcoidosis), infections (ie, syphilis, human immunodeficiency virus [HIV]/AIDS), or malignancy (ie, lymphoma or anal carcinoma).[13]

Classic teaching attributes the formation of anal fissures to constipation with the passage of large hard stools causing a tear in the anal mucosa. However, this association is not universally present in all patients. Fissures can also occur with diarrhea, anorectal surgery, or anoreceptive intercourse. Studies have found that patients with anal fissures have reduced vascularity and elevated pressures in the anal canal,[20] which contribute to localized ischemia. Ulceration with subsequent reactive spasm of the internal anal sphincter also reduces blood flow compounding the problem and delaying healing.

A DRE may not be feasible due to pain and associated anal sphincter spasm. Gentle effacement of the anus may allow visualization of the ulcer or tear. If a DRE is performed, a ridge may be palpated and suggests a fissure. Even if hemorrhoids are present, pain precipitated by DRE or a ridge appreciated during DRE are consistent with the presence of a coexistent fissure, and this should be treated as the primary source of symptoms. Features indicating a chronic fissure include a sentinel pile (skin tag) distally and/or hypertrophied anal papillae proximally (see **Fig. 3**)[16].

Nearly 50% of patients with acute anal fissures due to constipation will heal with conservative therapy: fluid and fiber supplementation and use of stool softeners as needed.[21] Warm sitz baths are also considered standard therapy for all anal fissures because benefits include improved cleanliness, decreased pain, and reduction of the hypertonicity of the anal sphincter potentiating healing.[18]

Pharmacologic therapy for chronic anal fissures includes topical nitrates or calcium channel blockers.[22] These medications often require a local compounding pharmacy. Physiologically, these medications are vasodilators that induce smooth muscle relaxation improving blood flow to the anoderm.[20] Topical nitroglycerin 0.2% ointment applied 2 to 3 times daily for 4 to 8 weeks is associated with healing of 50% chronic fissures. Headaches (reported in 20%–70% of individuals), orthostatic hypotension, and nausea limit its use. Topical calcium channel blockers (diltiazem 2% and nifedipine 0.3%–0.5%) applied 2 to 3 times daily for 4 to 8 weeks have similar mechanisms of action and rates of efficacy with lower incidences of side effects when compared with nitrates.[23] Counseling patients that headaches decrease as fissures heal may improve compliance.

Botulinum toxin injection is a secondary treatment option for chronic anal fissures. The mechanism of action of this botulinum toxin is blockade of acetylcholine release, producing temporary paralysis of the internal anal sphincter muscle with reduction in anal tone. There is lack of dose-dependent efficacy, and postintervention incontinence rates are unrelated to the dosage or formulation of botulinum neurotoxin used.[24] The most common side effects are temporary flatus and fecal incontinence occurring in approximately 18% and 5% of individuals, respectively.[18] Recurrence is common with documented rates as high as 42%; higher doses of Botox may improve healing.[13]

In a small study topical nitrates in combination with Botox versus Botox alone was found to significantly improve healing rates of chronic anal fissures at 6 weeks (66% versus 20%), but the statistical significance did not persist at 8 or 12 weeks (73% versus 60% and 66%, respectively).[25] A meta-analysis has also compared topical nitrates to the performance of Botox injection for the healing of chronic anal fissures and found that incomplete healing rates were comparable.[26] There was considerable heterogeneity in the nitrate studies, but recurrence rates of the fissures were similar in the 2 groups (Botox 19% versus nitrates 25%). There is also a meta-analysis comparing oral and topical calcium blockers in the treatment of anal fissures. When compared with oral therapy topical calcium channel blockers were associated with a significantly lower rate of unhealed fissures (21% versus 38%).[27] No head-to-head trials of both topical nitrates and calcium channel blockers versus botulinum toxin have been performed to date.

Patients who fail to respond to the aforementioned treatment strategies should consider internal anal sphincterotomy (IAS). IAS is superior to medical interventions with healing rates as high as 90% to 95%.[28] The small yet loathsome risk of fecal incontinence is the major drawback to operative intervention.

ANAL ABSCESSES AND FISTULAS

Anal abscesses and fistulas are manifestations of the same pathogenic process, with ~50% of abscesses evolving into fistulas. Anal abscesses usually originate from infected anal glands whose openings are located at the dentate line. These infections can spread into adjacent areas such as the posterior anal space, the perianal region, or the ischiorectal fossa but rarely into the supralevator space. Abscesses commonly present with throbbing anal pain worsened by Valsalva or sitting associated with a tender lump in the anal area with minimal fluctuance. Fever may or may not be present. If the abscess is in the suprasphincteric or intrasphincteric space, external inspection may appear normal but DRE reveals a palpable bulge. Diagnosis may require further investigation via rectal ultrasonography or pelvic computed tomography (CT) or MRI, which also provides additional information about the involved area and surrounding anatomic structure. The goal of management is adequate and dependent drainage, and the surgical approach depends on the location of the abscess.[29] Intravenous (IV) antibiotics should be given to immunocompromised individuals, patients with prosthetic heart valves, and individuals with extensive overlying cellulitis or concomitant systemic illness. After drainage, warm sitz baths, avoidance of constipation, and adequate pain control are recommended. About 30% of anal abscesses develop into fistulas after incision and drainage.

Diabetic and immunocompromised patients with incompletely treated abscesses are at increased risk for developing necrotizing fasciitis (Fournier gangrene).[29] These patients often present with high fevers, severe rectal pain, and fluctuance. Additional findings on physical examination include significant swelling of the buttock and perineum. Necrosis may be present. The infections are often polymicrobial and require surgical debridement along with broad-spectrum IV antibiotics. CT scans of the lower abdomen are helpful both in diagnosing and delineating the extent of the necrosis. Prompt recognition of this disorder is critical to survival.

Anal fistulas are abnormal connections between 2 epithelial lined spaces of the anus and rectum. Pain and bleeding during defecation is common. Anal fistulas are also associated with drainage, incontinence, anorectal swelling, and diarrhea. Most originate from infected anal glands; however, it is crucial to consider Crohn's disease in the differential. Transmural inflammation due to Crohn's disease disrupts the integrity of the mucosa of the anal canal causing fistula and/or abscess formation and in 45% of cases; perianal disease presents before or concurrent with the diagnosis of Crohn's disease.[30] The presence of perianal disease is a poor prognostic indicator for patients with Crohn's disease.[31]

Anal fistulas are associated with significant morbidity with several studies indicating a negative impact on quality of life.[32] Anal fistulas are classified as intersphincteric, transsphincteric, suprasphincteric, and extrasphincteric or fistula-in-ano (**Fig. 4**).[33] In addition to the physical examination, often performed under anesthesia, MRI and endoscopic ultrasonography of the pelvic floor can be used to further characterize anatomic abnormalities.

The management of fistulae not secondary to Crohn's disease is surgical[34] with the goal being removal of the fistula while maintaining continence of stool. Delayed or inadequate treatment can result in rare septicemia and/or tissue necrosis. Intersphincteric fistulas can be treated with a simple fistulotomy. High transsphincteric and suprasphincteric fistulas are more optimally managed with setons—tubular silastic structures placed through the fistula tract. The seton is progressively tightened at regular intervals until it eventually cuts through the sphincter.[35] Other surgical options include advancement flaps, tissue plugs, use of fibrin glue, or creation of a diverting colostomy or colectomy. The latter are considered last resorts for refractory disease that has not responded to medical therapy.

Anal fistulas related to Crohn's disease are far more challenging. Surgical treatment alone is associated with poor wound healing and a higher risk of incontinence. Furthermore, in a prospective randomized controlled trial, surgical placement of setons proved inferior to biologic therapy.[36] In this study, 126 patients with a single fistula were to be randomized to seton therapy alone, seton plus anti-tumor necrosis factor (TNF), or surgical closure after anti-TNF therapy. However, the study was closed at 44 patients by the safety monitoring board due to the failure of seton therapy alone to close fistulas. Consequently, combination medical and surgical management is preferred. Perianal abscesses should be adequately drained before starting immunosuppressive therapy, and biologic use under the care of a gastroenterologist with expertise in treatment of Crohn's disease is recommended with higher infliximab drug levels (>10.1–20.3 μm/mL) correlating with improved fistula healing.[37] Adjuvant use of antibiotics (ie, metronidazole or ciprofloxacin) and/or immunomodulators to prevent immunogenicity is often routinely used. Steroids are not effective in healing perianal fistulas, may increase sepsis risk, and should not be used for this indication.[31] Despite combination therapy, only one-third of patients with Crohn's disease achieve remission (defined as closure of external openings with resolution of drainage),[38] and relapse rates remain high with current therapies.

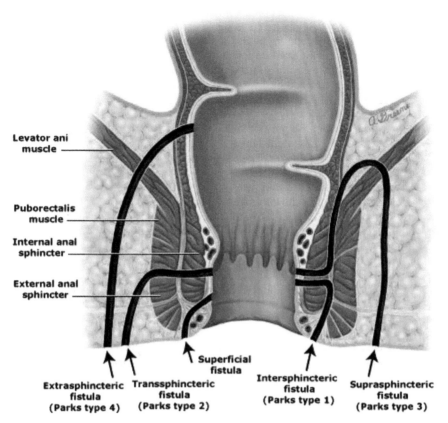

Levator ani muscle

Puborectalis muscle

Internal anal sphincter

External anal sphincter

Superficial fistula

Extrasphincteric fistula (Parks type 4)

Transsphincteric fistula (Parks type 2)

Intersphincteric fistula (Parks type 1)

Suprasphincteric fistula (Parks type 3)

Fig. 4. Parks classification of anal fistula. (*From* Parks AG. Pathogenesis and treatment of fistuila-in-ano. Br Med J. 1961;1(5224):463–9. https://doi.org/10.1136/bmj.1.5224.463 with permission.)

SQUAMOUS CELL CARCINOMA OF THE ANUS

Anal cancer is a rare malignancy with an incidence rate of less than 1% annually. Most are squamous cell carcinomas (SCC) with less frequent types including adenocarcinoma, neuroendocrine tumors, melanoma, gastrointestinal stromal tumors, Paget disease (intraepithelial adenocarcinoma), and lymphoma.[39] Based on the most recent Surveillance, Epidemiology and End Results program data, the median age at diagnosis is 62 years with women diagnosed slightly more often than men.[40] The rates of anal cancers in the United States are increasing by 2% each year over the past decade.[41]

Human papillomavirus (HPV) is the predominant risk factor for anal SCC because 88% of anal SCCs contain HPV DNA, most commonly subtypes 16 and 18.[42] Integration of HPV DNA into the host genome is the mechanism driving carcinogenesis. As HPV is the most common sexually transmitted disease in the United States, HPV vaccines have the potential to prevent anal and other HPV-associated cancers in the future.[43] Less common risk factors include HIV, anal condyloma accuminata, immunosuppression, organ transplant, anoreceptive intercourse, and smoking.

SCC of the anus arises from a precursor lesion, anal intraepithelial neoplasia (AIN). AIN is dysplastic tissue histologically classified as low or high grade,[41] and progression of AIN to anal cancer occurs in 10% of cases annually.[44]

Symptoms of anal cancer are nonspecific; therefore, the diagnosis of anal cancer is often delayed because symptoms are attributed to other benign anorectal conditions.[45] In addition, reluctance of the patient to discuss symptoms and the provider to perform a thorough anorectal examination may further prolong time to diagnosis. Rectal bleeding is the most common presenting symptom (45%) followed by anorectal pain, identification of palpable growths, and fecal incontinence. About 20% to 33% of individuals are asymptomatic at the time of diagnosis.[43] DRE, anoscopy, and/or endoscopic evaluation will identify irregularities ranging from subtle thickening of the anal canal to ulcerations to exophytic masses. As lymphatic drainage distal to the dentate line is directed to the inguinal nodes, physical examination for inguinal lymphadenopathy should also be pursued. Locoregional disease is best identified via transanal ultrasonography or rectal MRI. A PET scan or conventional CT of the chest, abdomen, and pelvis is also recommended to assess for metastatic disease (**Table 2**).

Given the efficacy of screening for cervical dysplasia, current goals of care extend beyond treatment to screening and prevention. However, owing to the low incidence of anal SCC, guidelines for universal screening do not exist. Certain high-risk groups may benefit from screening with anal Papanicolaou test every 1 to 2 years including the following: patients with HIV, men having sex with men, and women with histories of cervical or vulvar dysplasia. If abnormal cytology is detected, follow-up with high-resolution anoscopy with biopsy should be pursued. The limitation of anal Papanicolaou test is its low sensitivity with false-negative rates ranging from 23% to 45%.[41]

Management of SCCs of the anal canal continues to evolve. Before the 1980s abdominoperineal resection (APR) of the anorectum was considered first-line therapy for anal cancer. However, owing to its morbidity and detrimental impact on quality of life, it has been replaced by chemoradiation as the first-line intervention. Per National Comprehensive Cancer Network guidelines, variations of the Nigro protocol with 5-fluorouracil (5-FU) and mitomycin-C are the gold standard for stage I to III disease.[43] These protocols have increased sphincter preservation and improved survival. Adverse effects are common, are primarily related to radiation, and include dermatitis, tenesmus, diarrhea, nausea, and weakness. Owing to these radiation-induced complications, which often require pauses in therapy, there is increasing interest in radiotherapy dose adaptation using escalation or deescalation strategies.[46] Stage I disease may be treated with local excision if the anal sphincter is not involved. Stage IV disease requires systemic chemotherapy (5-FU with cisplatin) and radiation with surgery reserved for palliative purposes. The development of immune checkpoint

Table 2	
Staging of anal squamous cell carcinoma	
Stage	**Description**
I	Tumor < 2 cm, node negative, no distant disease
II	Tumor > 2 cm but not invading nearby organs, node negative
III	Tumor invading nearby organs and/or positive regional lymph nodes
IV	Distant disease present

Data from Szmulowicz UM, Wu JS. Squamous cell carcinoma of the anal canal: a review of the aetiology, presentation, staging, prognosis and methods available for treatment [published correction appears in Sex Health. 2018 Nov;15(5):480]. Sex Health. 2012;9(6):593–609. https://doi.org/10.1071/SH12010.

inhibitors provides potential new therapies, which may improve disease-free survival and quality of life.[46]

SOLITARY RECTAL ULCER SYNDROME

SRUS is a chronic, rare, and benign finding commonly associated with functional defecation disorders. SRUS has an estimated prevalence of 1 in 100,000, with a slight female preponderance. This condition occurs predominately in young adults in the third to fourth decades of life but has also been described in children and the elderly.[47,48] The true prevalence of SRUS may be underestimated because of its misclassification as rectal polyps or inflammatory bowel disease (IBD). The pathophysiologic mechanism of SRUS is poorly understood and may involve multiple factors. The most common hypothesis implicates chronic direct mucosal trauma and hypoperfusion leading to local ischemia and ulceration. Chronic trauma is thought to be due to constipation-associated straining and rectal digitation of impacted stool.[49,50] Paradoxic contraction of the puborectalis muscle, commonly identified in individuals with functional defecation disorders, rectal prolapse, and rectal intussusception may also reduce local blood flow resulting in ischemic changes. About one-quarter of cases may occur in patients with previous rectal surgery.[51]

Typical clinical features include rectal pain, rectal bleeding that may be copious, mucoid discharge, severe constipation, tenesmus, prolonged straining, incomplete evacuation, and abdominal and pelvic pain.[52] Up to 25% of patients may be asymptomatic with SRUS identified during routine colonoscopy.

Diagnosis is based on clinical presentation, endoscopic findings, and histology. Endoscopic findings vary ranging from patchy erythema to mucosal ulceration or the formation of polypoid lesions (**Fig. 5**). Solitary ulcers are found in approximately 20% of cases, making the name of the disorder a misnomer. Ulcers vary in size and are most frequently located on the anterior rectal wall. Biopsy of the ulcer is diagnostic with characteristic histologic findings inclusive of fibromuscular obliteration of the lamina propria with collagen deposition and displacement of the muscularis mucosa. Inflammation is absent in most cases, but the presence of this nonspecific finding can make the diagnosis challenging. SRUS may coexist with IBD and malignancy, hence multiple biopsies should be obtained, and reexamination may be warranted when the diagnosis remains in doubt.

The role of supportive studies such as barium enema, endoanal ultrasonography, defecography, anorectal manometry, and MRI, although not providing a definitive diagnosis, can increase the index of suspicion and provide information on contributing risk factors such as rectocele, rectal prolapse, and intussusception. However, these studies are not routinely necessary.

The treatment of SRUS is challenging because of the lack of validated therapies and high rates of treatment failure. Treatment depends on disease severity and the presence of other underlying pathologic condition (**Fig. 6**). The condition may resolve with conservative therapy aimed at treating coexistent constipation. When constipation is due to a functional defecation disorder, pelvic floor physical therapy and biofeedback may be beneficial. Topical therapy with mesalamine, sucralfate, or corticosteroid enemas may facilitate mucosal healing.[50] Severe and/or refractory cases may require endoscopic or surgical intervention. More recently, local endoscopic therapy with argon plasma coagulation (APC) has been described.[53] Limited studies have reported effective bleeding control and ulcer healing with APC in refractory cases not responding to conservative measures.[53] Surgery requires careful patient selection because it may result in nerve damage and exacerbate baseline constipation. A variety of surgeries

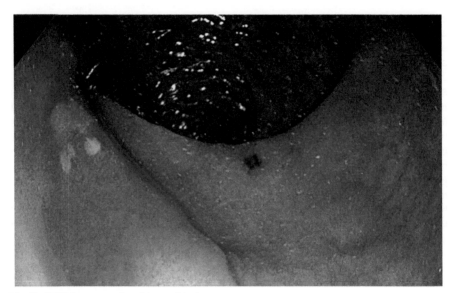

Fig. 5. SRUS image: polypoid rectal lesion.

have been described based on disease phenotype[54] including rectopexy and the Delorme procedure, but success rates only approach 50%. About 30% of patients with coexistent rectal prolapse will require surgical intervention.[54] Rarely, colostomy or coloanal anastomosis is performed in patients who have failed other surgical measures.[55]

PROCTALGIA FUGAX

Proctalgia fugax is defined by Rome IV criteria as sudden, infrequent episodes of severe, localized pain in the rectum most commonly lasting seconds to no more than 30 minutes with complete resolution between attacks.[56] It has an estimated prevalence ranging between 3% and 14% with a slight female predominance.[57,58] Persistent symptoms are incongruent with a diagnosis of proctalgia fugax, and a

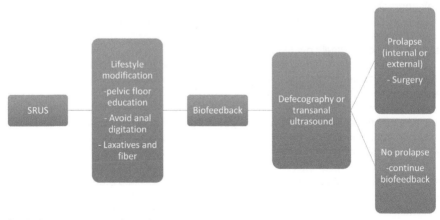

Fig. 6. SRUS treatment algorithm.

diagnosis of chronic proctalgia should be considered (**Fig. 7**). The cause of this disorder is unknown, but hypotheses range from a spastic disorder of colonic and anal smooth muscle to a rare hereditary hypertrophic myopathy of the internal anal sphincter.[59,60] Patients are usually asymptomatic during clinical consultation, and diagnosis relies on a careful clinical history and negative physical and endoscopic examination. Most patients cannot identify inciting triggers, and although proctalgia fugax has traditionally been thought to be more of a nocturnal disorder, this may be due to recall with awakening rather than reality.[61] Proctalgia fugax tends to follow a relapsing-remitting course, with fleeting symptoms that limit the yield of physiologic testing such as anorectal manometry and render prophylactic treatment impractical. Radiographic evaluation is infrequently warranted but may be considered when symptoms persist despite reassurance. Pelvic floor MRI can be used to rule out masses, and endoanal ultrasonography can identify the presence of internal anal sphincter hypertrophy. As intermittent spasm is a suggested cause, treatments aimed at relaxation of the internal anal sphincter have all been proposed, including warm sitz baths, tap water enemas, biofeedback, digital dilation and massage, sublingual (0.3 mg) or topical nitroglycerin (0.3%), topical (2%) or oral (diltiazem 80 mg twice a day) calcium channel blockers, clonidine 150 µg twice a day, inhaled β-agonist salbutamol, intrarectal or intravaginal benzodiazepines (diazepam 5–10 mg suppository), smooth muscle relaxants (such as dicyclomine), intersphincteric injection of botulinum A toxin, and even myotomy.[62,63] Unfortunately, well-controlled studies to support these interventions are lacking and utility of pharmacotherapy is often limited by side effects.

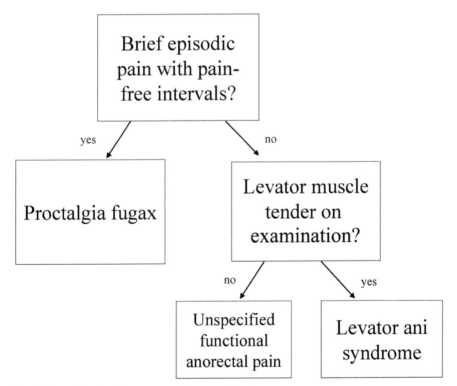

Fig. 7. Rome IV: chronic or recurrent anorectal pain.

Botulinum injections increase the risk of fecal incontinence, and there is lack of data supporting surgical interventions. In a recent systematic review, Jeyarajah and colleagues[63] recommend the following therapeutic progression for patients with frequent, debilitating episodes of proctalgia fugax: (1) reassurance and warm baths, (2) topical glyceryl trinitrate 0.2% p.r.n., (3) salbutamol inhalation 200 g p.r.n., (4) warm water enemas, (5) clonidine 150 μg twice a day, (6) local anesthetic block, and (7) botulinum toxin injection into the anal sphincters. Current guidelines do not endorse these interventions.[56]

LEVATOR ANI SYNDROME AND UNSPECIFIED FUNCTIONAL ANORECTAL PAIN

LAS and unspecified functional anorectal pain (UFAP) are functional anorectal pain disorders characterized by recurrent or persistent pain in the region of the rectum lasting greater than 30 minutes in the absence of organic pathology. LAS is differentiated from UFAP by the presence of tenderness on palpation of the levator ani muscle during DRE.[64] LAS and UFAP have a reported prevalence of 6% with a female preponderance. Most affected patients range in age from 30 to 60 years, with the condition peaking at age 45 years. Only 30% of affected individuals seek medical care despite their negative impact on quality of life.[65] The exact cause and pathophysiology of these disorders is poorly understood. It has been proposed that chronic levator muscle spasm exacerbated by stress, anxiety, trauma, prolonged sitting, childbirth, defecation, sexual intercourse, and pelvic and spinal surgeries may play a role. Patients present with dull or pressurelike pain in the rectum, which may be constant or recurrent, and often report radiation to the thighs or perineal or gluteal regions. The pain usually worsens with sitting and has been described as the feeling of a "lump" in the rectum.[1] Diagnosis is based on Rome IV criteria (see **Fig. 6**). Appropriate testing to exclude alternative diagnoses and underlying organic disease is necessary even with typical history and examination findings. One should bear in mind that extraintestinal disorders like interstitial cystitis and endometriosis, which can cause pelvic floor myalgia, may also produce rectal pain.[66] Depending on patient age, risk factors, and symptom severity, diagnostic workup may include pelvic ultrasonography, MRI, defecography, and endoscopic evaluation.[67]

LAS is thought to be associated with defecatory dysfunction[68] because biofeedback therapy improves evacuation in more than 90% in the short term. In addition to biofeedback, conservative treatment includes lifestyle measures to relax the pelvic floor including sitz baths, levator ani internal massage, and medical therapy with muscle relaxants and antispasmodics such as gabapentin, cyclobenzaprine, and tricyclic antidepressants.[58] Minimally invasive therapies have included local injection therapy and electrogalvanic stimulation. Local injection therapy with anesthetics (such as lidocaine and bupivacaine) and botulinum toxin and have provided variable outcomes.[69] Direct electrogalvanic stimulation of the levator ani muscle via an intraanal probe initially showed significant efficacy, but more recent studies have revealed minimal to no response and electrogalvanic stimulation.[70,71] Sacral nerve stimulation and surgery have been proved to be ineffective.[72,73]

PRURITUS ANI

Pruritus ani is a common and underreported condition thought to impact up to 5% of the population and is used to classify conditions resulting in itching, irritation, and consequences of scratching in the perianal skin such as burning and excoriation.[74] This condition is most often idiopathic in cause, has a male predominance, and is thought to be related to sensitization and a pathologic cycle of "itch-scratch-more uncontrollable itch" further resulting in stimulation and irritation of C-fibers in the peri-anal skin.[75] Rarely is a unifying cause or singular targeted treatment successful, and symptoms often recur. Given the broad differential diagnoses to consider with this complaint, in addition to a detailed medical, sexual, and travel history, a simplified algorithmic approach as denoted by the ITCH acronym for initial evaluation is extremely informative because it provides categorical context to potential causes.[76] (**Table 3**).

After the history is obtained, careful anorectal examination is crucial to not only iden-tify possible causes but also assess the degree of insult from scratching. Associated excoriation, lichenification, and superinfection often result from repeated attempts to achieve relief with overzealous cleansing or use of wet wipes that contain offending chemicals that propagate symptoms. In addition to physical and endoscopic exami-nations such as anoscopy, flexible sigmoidoscopy, or colonoscopy, referral to derma-tology for culture or biopsy of suspicious areas is recommended in those who fail empirical treatment or whose history suggests an atypical or unrelenting presenta-tion.[35] Initial treatment of pruritus ani is most often empirical and based on expert opinion over evidence. Patients should be counseled to have realistic expectations because improvement in symptoms often takes time and depends on adherence to lifestyle and behavioral changes. Patient education needs to prioritize the patient's un-derstanding of the role that scratching plays in exacerbating symptoms and is critical to improving outcomes.[20] Gentle rectal hygiene and perianal care along with advice, when appropriate, to bulk stool, use sitz baths, shower with a detachable nozzle after defecation, and keep the perianal area dry by pat drying or using a blow dryer on the cool cycle may be beneficial. Tight clothing should be avoided, and cotton undergar-ments are preferred over nylon. In addition to education and lifestyle modifications, medical therapy may be necessary, even if just to temporarily provide relief to allow for behavioral modification. Topical or oral antihistamines may be helpful especially when used at night. The use of topical witch hazel pads is controversial. Various forms of barrier creams are available for use after drying is performed, and an example of a trusted product is Balneol.[76] Topical hydrocortisone has been studied and found to provide temporary relief; however, its use should be limited in duration because of the risk of epidermal atrophy.[77] Some patients may also respond to oral low-dose tri-cyclic antidepressants.[20] Topical capsaicin (0.006%) cream applied 3 times daily for 14 days[78] or topical tacrolimus ointment (0.3%) for 4 weeks may decrease itch inten-sity and frequency.[79] For refractory cases, intradermal and subcutaneous injection

Table 3	
ITCH: Acronym for evaluation of pruritus ani	
Acronym	**Examples**
I: Infection	*Candida albicans*, herpes simplex virus, condyloma acuminatum, HIV, *Treponema pallidum* (syphilis), Gonorrhea, *Enterobius vermicularis* (pinworm), bacterial infection
T: Topical irritants	Soaps, detergents, tight clothing, nylon undergarments, scents
C: Cutaneous and cancer	Cutaneous: lichen planus, psoriasis, contact dermatitis, seborrhea Cancer: Paget, skin cancers, mycosis fungoides
H: Hypersensitivity	Foods ("C's": cola, coffee, citrus, chocolate, and calcium) Medications: chemotherapy, colchicine, quinidine.

From Henderson PK, Cash BD. Common anorectal conditions: evaluation and treatment. Curr Gas-troenterol Rep. 2014; 16:408; with permission.

("tattooing") of the perianal region with methylene blue dye, which is thought to destroy sensory nerve endings, has been described with some impressive results. However, potential drawbacks include need for saddle block anesthesia, hypoesthesia of the perianal region, blue perianal discoloration, fecal seepage, and skin necrosis. Methylene blue intradermal injection therapy consists of a total of 20 mL (5 mL 1% methylene blue and 15 mL 1% lidocaine) infiltrated using a small-gauge needle to cover the affected perianal skin up to the dentate line.[80]

SEXUALLY TRANSMITTED DISEASES INDUCING ANAL PAIN

It is important in certain instances when patients present with severe pain and mucopurulent discharge with or without blood to obtain a sexual history[29]; these are usually caused by unprotected anal receptive sexual practices and can present with anal/rectal pain, urgency, mucopurulent discharge, diarrhea, and/or bleeding. Patients with underlying HIV may be more severely affected and may be coinfected with several organisms. Syphilis, herpes simplex virus (HSV), gonorrhea, chlamydia, and lymphogranuloma venereum (LGV) can all cause severe proctitis.[29] These organisms can vary in how invasive they are in the rectal mucosa. For instance, *Neisseria gonorrhea* and certain serotypes of chlamydia (D to K) only invade the columnar epithelium, whereas serotypes L1, L2, and L3 of *Chlamydia trachomatis* that cause LGV,

Table 4
Sexually transmitted proctitis: diagnosis and treatment

Causative Organism	Diagnostic Investigations	Suggested Treatment of Initial Infection
Chlamydia *Chlamydia trachomatis*, serotypes D–K)	NAAT from rectal, endocervical, or urethral swabs	Azithromycin 1 g po, single dose OR Doxycycline 100 mg po bid for 7 d
Lymphogranuloma venereum (*Chlamydia trachomatis* serotypes L1, L2, and L3)	Culture, direct immunofluorescence, or nucleic acid detection from a rectal lesion and lymph node specimen	Doxycycline 100 mg PO bid for 21 d OR Erythromycin base 500 mg qid for 21 d
Gonorrhea (*Neisseria gonorrhea*)	Gram stain (gram-negative diplococci) and bacterial cultures from anogenital and pharyngeal swab	Ceftriaxone 250 mg IM in a single dose AND Azithromycin 1 g orally in a single dose
Herpes simplex virus	Viral culture or PCR from vesicular lesions	Acyclovir 400 mg PO tid for 7–10 d OR Acyclovir 200 mg po 5 times a day for 7–10 d
Syphilis (*Treponema pallidum*)	Darkfield examination and test to detect *T pallidum* from lesion exudate or tissue	Benzathine penicillin G 2.4 million units IM in a single dose OR Ceftriaxone 1–2 g IV/IM for 10–14 d OR Doxycycline 100 mg bid for 14 d

Abbreviations: bid, twice daily; IM, intramuscular; NAAT, nucleic acid amplification test; po, per os (by mouth), PCR, polymerase chain reaction; qid, 4 times a day; tid, 3 times a day.

Adapted from Lohsiriwat V. Anorectal emergencies. World J Gastroenterol. 2016;22(26):5867–78. https://doi.org/10.3748/wjg.v22.i26.5867 with permission.

Treponema pallidum (syphilis), and HSV are known to pass through the columnar and stratified epithelium.[29] As a result, LGV can cause inguinal adenopathy, deep rectal ulcers, and severe proctitis. **Table 4** summarizes the treatment and diagnostic laboratory tests for these various infections. Flexible sigmoidoscopy with adequate anesthesia is generally required to obtain the necessary samples for diagnosis.

FOREIGN BODIES

Foreign bodies in the rectum present the clinician with a challenge in diagnosis. The patient may be reluctant to disclose an accurate history. Foreign bodies occur rarely but usually are related to trying to obtain sexual pleasure. A calm, accepting, and reassuring demeanor may be particularly important, and a history of sexual practices and preferences can be pertinent.[29] The patient may have tried to unsuccessfully remove the foreign body so a gentle discussion of rectal manipulation may be revealing. An even smaller percentage of cases may be found to be related to criminal assault, illegal trafficking of drugs, or even an embarrassing accident. There is also a concern in some instances for perforation particularly when the patient presents with abdominal or pelvic pain, fever, tachycardia or peritoneal signs. A plain abdominal film or CT may reveal the diagnosis. Depending on the object, endoscopic removal may be possible. In some instances, surgical removal is necessary.

SUMMARY

This article summarizes a broad spectrum of painful anorectal disorders. It is imperative that health care providers understand the different causes of the various anorectal syndromes that produce pain to diagnose these conditions and manage patient expectations. All these conditions underscore the *importance of a comprehensive anorectal examination*. An appropriate workup that is both cost effective and in line with the suspected underlying cause has been outlined, and it is important to be cognizant of coexisting conditions, psychosocial concerns, and possible complications. In addition to understanding the differential diagnosis, providers need to understand the risk factors for the spectrum of conditions and prioritize timely treatment considering the potential for adverse impacts on quality of life.

CLINICAL PEARLS

- There is no substitute for physical examination of the perianal area, and when appropriate a digital rectal examination or anoscopy should be performed to aid in the diagnosis of hemorrhoids, fissures, fistulas, and other anorectal disorders.

- The dentate line defines hemorrhoidal disease: internal hemorrhoids develop proximally (area of decreased sensation) and hence present with painless bleeding or itching, whereas external hemorrhoids emerge distally (area rich in innervation) and present with soiling and pain when thrombosed.

- Anal fissures can be acute or chronic and form distal to the dentate line. These fissures usually present with severe pain because of ischemia. Initial treatment starts with local care (warm soaks, attention to bowel function), but refractory fissures may require topical nitrates/calcium channel blockers, botulinum injection therapy, or surgery.

- Anal abscesses and fistulas are manifestations of the same pathogenic process, with ~50% of abscesses evolving into fistulas. Although antibiotics are a primary treatment, immunocompromised individuals may develop necrotizing fasciitis and require surgical debridement, and patients with Crohn's disease may require multimodality therapy with setons, biologics, antibiotics, and possibly surgery.

- Proctalgia fugax, levator ani, and unspecified functional anorectal pain syndrome may all involve defecatory dysfunction. Appropriate diagnostic workup includes imaging and evaluation of pelvic floor function. Treatment should be geared toward improving defecation, possibly topical therapies and addressing biopsychosocial concerns.

- A careful sexual history may alert the clinician to risk factors for rarer anorectal disorders like condyloma acuminatum, sexually transmitted proctitis, squamous cell cancer of the anus, and foreign bodies.

DISCLOSURES

Tisha Lunsford: Biomerica InFoods IBS technology; Lucinda A Harris has done consulting for Allergan, Alnylam, Ironwood, Salix Pharmaceuticals, Takeda (Formerly Shire), Commonwealth Laboratories and the Rome Foundation and has research funding with Alakos.

REFERENCES

1. Patcharatrakul T, Rao SSC. Update on the pathophysiology and management of anorectal disorders. Gut Liver 2018;12:375–84.
2. Jacobs DO. Hemorrhoids: what are the options in 2018? Curr Opin Gastroenterol 2018;34:46–9.
3. Riss S, Weiser FA, Schwameis K, et al. The prevalence of hemorrhoids in adults. Int J Colorectal Dis 2012;27:215–20.
4. Qureshi W. Office management of hemorrhoids. Am J Gastroenterol 2018;113: 795–8.
5. Mott T, Lattimer K, Edwards C. Hemorrhoids: diagnosis and treatment options. Am Fam Physician 2018;97:172–8.
6. Guttenplan M. The evaluation and office management of hemorrhoids for the gastroenterologist. Curr Gastroenterol Rep 2017;19:30.
7. Kelly SM, Sanowski RA, Foutch PG, et al. A prospective comparison of anoscopy and fiber endoscopy in detecting anal lesions. J Clin Gastroenterol 1986;8: 658–60.
8. Jacobs D. Clinical practice. Hemorrhoids N Engl J Med 2014;371:944–51.
9. Altomare DF, Giannini I. Pharmacological treatment of hemorrhoids: a narrative review. Expert Opin Pharmacother 2013;14:2343–9.
10. Veronese N, Solmi M, Caruso MG, et al. Dietary fiber and health outcomes: An umbrella review of systematic reviews and meta-analyses. Amer J Clin Nutr 2018;107:436–44.
11. Sun Z, Migaly J. Review of hemorrhoid disease: prevention and management. Clin Colon Rect Surg 2016;29:22–9.
12. Johanson JF, Rimm A. Optimal nonsurgical treatment of hemorrhoids: a comparative analysis of infrared coagulation, rubber band ligation, and injection sclerotherapy. Am J Gastroenterol 1992;87:1600–6.
13. Wald A, Bharucha AE, Cosman BC, et al. ACG clinical guideline: management of benign anorectal disorders. Am J Gastroenterol 2014;109:1141–57.
14. MacRae HM, McLeod RS. Comparison of hemorrhoidal treatment modalities: a meta-analysis. Dis Colon Rectum 1995;38:687–94.
15. Chen HL, Woo XB, Cui J, et al. Ligature versus stapled hemorrhoidectomy in the treatment of hemorrhoids: a meta-analysis of randomized controlled trials. Surg Laproscopc Endosc Percutan Tech 2014;24:285–9.
16. Schlichtemeier S, Engel A. Anal Fissure Aust Prescr 2016;39:14–7.

17. Mapel DW, Schum M, Von Worley A. The epidemiology and treatment of anal fissures in a population-based cohort. BMC Gastroenterol 2014;14:129.
18. Beaty JS, Shashidharan M. Anal fissure. Clin Colon Rectal Surg 2016;29:30–7.
19. Zaghiyan KN, Fleshner P. Anal fissure. Clin Colon Rectal Surg 2011;24:22–30.
20. Lacy BE, Weiser K. Common anorectal disorders: diagnosis and treatment. Curr Gastroenterol Rep 2009;11:413–9.
21. Perry WB, Dykes SL, Buie WD, et al. Standards Practice Task for of the American Society of Colon and Rectal Surgeons. Practice parameters for the management of anal fissures. Dis Colon Rectum 2010;53:1110–5.
22. Nelson RL, Thomas K, Morgan J, et al. Non surgical therapy for anal fissure. Cochrane Database Syst Rev 2012;(2):CD003431.
23. Sajid MS, Whitehouse PA, Sains P, et al. Systematic review of the use of topical diltiazem compared with glycerltrinitrate for the nonoperative management of chronic anal fissure. Colorectal Dis 2013;15:19–26.
24. Bobkiewicz A, Francuzik W, Krokowicz L, et al. Botulinum toxin injection for treatment of chronic anal fissure: Is there any dose-dependent efficiency? A meta-analysis. World J Surg 2016;40:3064–72.
25. Lysy J, Israelit-Yatzkan Y, Sestiery-Ittah M, et al. Topical nitrates potentiate the effect of botulinum toxin in the treatment of patients with refractory anal fissure. Gut 2001;48:221–4.
26. Sahebally SM, Meshkat B, Walsh SR, et al. Botulinum toxin injection vs topical nitrates for chronic anal fissure: an updated systematic review and meta-analysis of randomized controlled trials. Colorectal Dis 2018;20:6–15.
27. Sahebally SM, Ahmed K, Cerneveciute, et al. Oral versus topical calcium channel blockers for chronic anal fissure – a systematic review and meta-analysis of randomized controlled trials. Int J Surg 2017;44:87–93.
28. Richard CS, Gregoire R, Piewes EA, et al. Internal sphincterotomy is superior to topical nitroglycerin in the treatment of chronic anal fissure: results of a randomized, controlled trial by the Canadian colorectal surgical trials group. Dis Colon Rectum 2000;43:1048–58.
29. Lohsiriwat V. Anorectal Emergencies. World J Gastroenterol 2016;22:5867–78.
30. Pogacnik JS, Salgado G. Perianal Crohn's disease. Clin Colon Rectal Surg 2019;32:377–85.
31. Lopez N, Ramamoorthy S, Sandborn WJ. Recent advances in the management of perianal fistulizing Crohn's disease: lessons for the clinic. Expert Rev Gastroenterol Hepatol 2019;13:563–77.
32. de Groof EJ, Sahami S, Lucas C, et al. Treatment of perianal fistula in Crohn's disease: a systematic review and meta-analysis comparing seton drainage and anti-tumor necrosis factor treatment. Colorectal Dis 2016;18:667–75.
33. Parks AG, Gordon PH, Hardcastle JD. A classification of fistula-in-ano. Br J Surg 1976;63:1–12.
34. Amato A, Bottini C, De Nardi P, et al. Evaluation and management of perianal abscess and anal fistula: SICCR position statement. Tech Coloproctol 2020;24:127–43.
35. Schubert MC, Sridhar S, Schade RR, et al. What every gastroenterologist needs to know about common anorectal disorders. World J Gastroenterol 2009;15:3201–9.
36. Wasmann KA, de Groof EJ, Stellingwerf ME, et al. Treatment of perianal fistulas in Crohn's Disease, seton versus anti-TNF versus surgical closure following anti-TNF [PISA]: A randomised controlled trial. J Crohns Colitis 2020;14:1049–56.

37. Yarur AJ, Kanagala K, Stein DJ, et al. Higher infliximab trough levels are associated with perianal fistula healing in patients with Crohn's disease. Aliment Pharmacol Ther 2017;45:933–40.

38. Panes J, Reinisch W, Rupniewska E, et al. Burden and outcomes for complex perianal fistulas in Crohn's disease: Systematic review. World J Gastroenterol 2018;24:4821–34.

39. Szmulowicz UM, Wu JS. Squamous cell carcinoma of the anal canal: a review of the aetiology, presentation, staging, prognosis and methods available for treatment. Sex Health 2012;9:593–609.

40. SEER data base. Available at: https://seer.cancer.gov/statfacts/html/anus.html. March 27, 2021.

41. Osborne MC, Maykel J, Johnson EK, et al. Anal squamous cell carcinoma: An evolution in disease and management. World J Gastroenterol 2014;20:13052–9.

42. Daling JR, Madeleine MM, Johnson LG, et al. Human papillomavirus, smoking, and sexual practices in the etiology of anal cancer. Cancer 2004;101:270–80.

43. Morton M, Meinitchouk N, Bleday R. Squamous cell carcinoma of the anal canal. Curr Probl Cancer 2018;42:486–92.

44. Devaraj B, Cosman BC. Expectant management of anal squamous dysplasia in patients with HIV. Dis Colon Rectum 2006;49:36–40.

45. Lohsiriwat V. Treatment of hemorrhoids: A coloproctologist's view. World J Gastroenterol 2015;21:9245–52.

46. Martin D, Balermpas P, Winkelmann R, et al. Anal squamous cell carcinoma - State of the art management and future perspectives. Cancer Treat Rev 2018; 65:11–21.

47. Poddar U, Yachha SK, Krishnani N, et al. Solitary rectal ulcer syndrome in children: A report of 140 Cases. J Pediatr Gastroenterol Nutr 2020;71:29–33.

48. Zhu QC, Shen RR, Qin HL, et al. Solitary rectal ulcer syndrome: clinical features, pathophysiology, diagnosis and treatment strategies. World J Gastroenterol 2014;20:738–44.

49. Abid S, Khawaja A, Bhimani SA, et al. The clinical, endoscopic and histological spectrum of the solitary rectal ulcer syndrome: a single-center experience of 116 cases. BMC Gastroenterol 2012;12:72.

50. Forootan M, Darvishi M. Solitary rectal ulcer syndrome: A systematic review Medicine. Baltimore) 2019;98:e14662.

51. Felt-Bersma RJF. Solitary rectal ulcer syndrome. Curr Opin Gastroenterol 2021; 37:59–65.

52. Sadeghi A, Biglari M, Forootan M, et al. Solitary Rectal Ulcer Syndrome: A Narrative Review. Middle East J Dig Dis 2019;11:129–34.

53. Shah A, Bohra S, Desai S. Argon plasma coagulation-an effective treatment for solitary rectal ulcer syndrome: A single-center experience from western India. Indian J Gastroenterol 2021;40:35–40. https://doi.org/10.1007/s12664-020-01089-w.

54. Gouriou C, Siproudhis L, Chambaz M, et al. Solitary rectal ulcer syndrome in 102 patients: Do different phenotypes make sense? Dig Liver Dis 2021;53:190–5.

55. Gouriou C, Chambaz M, Ropert A, et al. A systematic literature review on solitary rectal ulcer syndrome: is there a therapeutic consensus in 2018? Int J Colorectal Dis 2018;33:1647–55.

56. Carrington EV, Popa SL, Chiarioni G. Proctalgia Syndromes: Update in diagnosis and management. Curr Gastroenterol Rep 2020;22:35.

57. Drossman DA, Li Z, Andruzzi E, et al. US householder survey of functional gastro-intestinal disorders. Prevalence, sociodemography, and health impact. Dig Dis Sci 1993;38:1569–80.

58. Thompson WG. Proctalgia fugax. Dig Dis Sci 1981;26:1121–4.

59. Bharucha AE, Lee TH. Anorectal and pelvic pain. Mayo Clin Proc 2016;91:1471–86.

60. König P, Ambrose NS, Scott N. Hereditary internal anal sphincter myopathy causing proctalgia fugax and constipation: further clinical and histological char-acterization in a patient. Eur J Gastroenterol Hepatol 2000;12:127–8.

61. de Parades V, Etienney I, Bauer P, et al. Proctalgia fugax: demographic and clin-ical characteristics. What every doctor should know from a prospective study of 54 patients. Dis Colon Rectum 2007;50:893–8.

62. Boquet J, Moore N, Lhuintre JP, et al. Diltiazem for proctalgia fugax. Lancet 1986;1(8496):1493.

63. Jeyarajah S, Chow A, Ziprin P, et al. Proctalgia fugax, an evidence-based man-agement pathway. Int J Colorectal Dis 2010;25:1037–46.

64. Rao SS, Bharucha AE, Chiarioni G, et al. Functional anorectal disorders. Gastro-enterology 2016;S0016-5085(16):00175.

65. Ng CL. Levator ani syndrome - a case study and literature review. Aust Fam Physician 2007;36:449–52.

66. Faubion SS, Shuster LT, Bharucha AE. Recognition and management of nonrelax-ing pelvic floor dysfunction. Mayo Clin Proc 2012;87(2):187–93.

67. Bharucha AE, Trabuco E. Functional and chronic anorectal and pelvic pain disor-ders. Gastroenterol Clin North Am 2008;37:685–ix.

68. Rao SS, Benninga MA, Bharucha AE, et al. ANMS-ESNM position paper and consensus guidelines on biofeedback therapy for anorectal disorders. Neurogas-troenterol Motil 2015;27:594–609.

69. Nugent E, Beal M, Sun G, et al. Botulinum toxin A versus electrogalvanic stimu-lation for levator ani syndrome: is one a more effective therapy? Tech Coloproctol 2020;24:545–51.

70. Hull TL, Milsom JW, Church J, et al. Electrogalvanic stimulation for levator syn-drome: how effective is it in the long-term? Dis Colon Rectum 1993;36:731–3.

71. Chiarioni G, Nardo A, Vantini I, et al. Biofeedback is superior to electrogalvanic stimulation and massage therapy for the treatment of levator ani syndrome. Gastroenterology 2010;138:1321–9.

72. Dudding TC, Thomas GP, Hollingshead JR, et al. Sacral nerve stimulation: an effective treatment for chronic functional anal pain? Colorectal Dis 2013;15:1140–4.

73. Atkin GK, Suliman A, Vaizey CJ. Patient characteristics and treatment outcome in functional anorectal pain. Dis Colon Rectum 2011;54:870–5.

74. Nasseri YF, Osborne M. Pruritis ani: diagnosis and treatment. Gastroenterol Clin N Amer 2013;42:801–13.

75. Ansari P. Pruritus Ani. Clin Colon Rectal Surg 2016;29:38–42.

76. Henderson PK, Cash BD. Common anorectal conditions: evaluation and treat-ment. Curr Gastroenterol Rep 2014;16:408.

77. Al-Ghnaniem R), Short K, Pullen A, et al. 1% hydrocortisone ointment is an effec-tive treatment of pruritus ani: a pilot randomized controlled crossover trial. Int J Colorectal Dis 2007;22(12):1463.

78. Lysy J, Sistiery-Ittah M, Israelit Y, et al. Topical capsaicin—a novel and effective treatment for idiopathic intractable pruritus ani: a randomised, placebo controlled, crossover study. Gut 2003;52:1323–6.

79. Suys E. Randomized study of topical tacrolimus ointment as possible treatment for resistant idiopathic pruritus ani. J Am Acad Dermatol 2012;66(2):327–8.

80. Kim JH, Kim DH, Lee YP. Long-term follow-up of intradermal injection of methylene blue for intractable, idiopathic pruritus ani. Tech Coloproctol 2019;23:143–9.

Psychological and Nutritional Factors in Pelvic Floor Disorders

Sarah Quinton, PsyD[a], Bethany Doerfler, MS, RDN[b],*

KEYWORDS

- Pelvic floor disorders • Dyssynergic defecation • Multidisciplinary care
- Psychogastroenterology • Dietary fiber • Malnutrition • Obesity • Dietary pattern

KEY POINTS

- Psychological and nutritional factors can play a profound role in the development and maintenance of gastrointestinal (GI)-related pelvic floor dysfunction.
- Adherence to treatment and ability to benefit from treatment may be impacted by these factors and should be addressed in this patient population.
- This is an understudied area and multidisciplinary options may provide a pathway towards care.

PSYCHOLOGICAL AND NUTRITIONAL FACTORS IN PELVIC FLOOR DISORDERS

Introduction

Gastrointestinal (GI) pelvic floor disorders (PFDs) are complex, multifactorial, and not as well understood or studied as urogynecological PFDs. While gut–brain interactions of multiple functional bowel disorders have been fairly well described, there is less research examining psychosocial factors contributing to the development and maintenance of GI related-pelvic floor dysfunction (GI-PFD). Psychological and nutritional factors impact GI-PFDs and have important implications in a patient's ability to benefit from and adhere to treatment. By nature, GI-PFDs are multifactorial in both their development and maintenance. As such, interdisciplinary interventions are recommended[1–3] but have seen limited implementation.

Psychological Factors in Pelvic Floor Disorders

Psychological distress

GI pelvic floor dysfunction including constipation, fecal incontinence, and pelvic pain are all associated with increased psychological distress. Comorbid psychological

[a] Q Wellness; [b] Division of Gastroenterology and Hepatology, Northwestern University Feinberg School of Medicine, 676 N. Saint Clair Street, Suite 1400, Chicago, IL 60611, USA
* Corresponding author. Division of Gastroenterology and Hepatology, Northwestern University Feinberg School of Medicine, 676 N. Saint Clair Street, Suite 1400, Chicago, IL 60611, USA
E-mail address: bethany-doerfler@northwestern.edu
Twitter: @DrSQuinton (S.Q.); @DoerflerBethany (B.D.)

Gastroenterol Clin N Am 51 (2022) 145–156
https://doi.org/10.1016/j.gtc.2021.10.009
0889-8553/22/© 2021 Elsevier Inc. All rights reserved.
gastro.theclinics.com

disorders such as depression, anxiety, adjustment disorder, obsessive-compulsive disorder, posttraumatic stress disorder, and somatization have been well described in individuals with disorders of gut–brain interaction (DGBI) including PFDs, but much of this research has focused primarily on women with urogynecological conditions.[4–8] Less well known is the role of comorbid psychological factors in defecatory dysfunction.

Psychological distress is seen as both a consequence of GI symptoms and a risk factor for the development of DGBI.[4] While both anxiety and depression are common, anxiety disorders are most prevalent, with estimates of up to 50% of patients having a comorbid anxiety disorder.[4,9] Depression has been identified in 30% to 40% of patients with a DGBI.[9–12] Comorbid psychiatric disorders occur in 50% to 90% of patients with IBS,[13–15] and somatic disorders having been found in 40% to 60% of patients with DGBI.[12]

Quality of life (QoL) and daily functioning are also negatively impacted. Significant impairment in QoL has been documented in patients with IBS, constipation, fecal incontinence, and other DGBI[12,16–21] including pelvic floor dysfunction compared with healthy controls.[22–24] QoL was found to be more negatively impacted in those with dyssynergic defecation than slow transit constipation,[10] and those with constipation complicated by fecal incontinence (often described as overflow incontinence) demonstrated worse QoL than individuals with isolated fecal incontinence.[25,26]

Trauma, Abuse, and Stressful Life Events

Traumatic experiences, sexual, physical, and emotional abuse, and medical traumas are not uncommon in individuals with pelvic floor dysfunction. Stressful life events (SLEs) other than abuse have also been found to be risk factors for subsequent development of a DGBI and/or increased symptom severity.[4,27] The role of trauma and SLE's has implications on physiologic, psychological, and behavioral functioning and can impact treatment adherence.

Rates of sexual abuse in individuals with PFD range from 17% to 48%, with the overwhelming majority identifying as female.[22–24,28] A history of sexual abuse has been associated with an increased prevalence of chronic pelvic pain, dyspareunia, and urinary dysfunction.[29–31] Sexually abused women are more likely to present with multiple GI and genitourinary PFDs [32] with greater rates of pelvic floor dyssynergia documented in this population.[33]

Nonsexual traumas including physical abuse, SLEs, and medical trauma are also identified more frequently in patients with PFDs. Physical abuse has been reported in 31% to 74% of subjects with constipation.[22,24,34] Fecal incontinence is associated with sexual and physical abuse, as well as medical trauma (pelvic surgery, childbirth). The most robust research linking trauma to defecatory disorders has been in children and adolescents. Several studies have indicated that children with functional defecation disorders have a significantly higher prevalence of SLEs[27] and there is a significant association between sexual, physical, and verbal abuse and fecal incontinence in these populations.[35–39]

Impact on Pelvic Floor Functioning

Medical injuries are known risk factors for anal sphincter dysfunction,[40] but less well understood is the connection between psychological distress, trauma, abuse, and the pathophysiology of pelvic floor dysfunction. In general, psychological distress, trauma, and SLEs are significant risk factors for the later development of functional bowel disorders.[41] Trauma exposure is associated with pelvic floor hyperactivity, with more severe trauma and PTSD associated with more severe pelvic dysfunction.[42]

Avoidance of painful defecation and withholding despite recurrent defecatory urges are seen as common behaviors in childhood and can perpetuate a maladaptive cycle leading to dyschezia.[43] Women with PFD have been shown to demonstrate higher pelvic tone and it has been hypothesized that hypertonus is a natural trauma-related defense mechanism.[44]

Impact on Treatment Adherence

Treatment effectiveness is often directly associated with a patient's ability or willingness to engage in therapeutic recommendations. Many environmental, financial, cultural, and psychological factors influence compliance. For example, patients anxious about potential adverse events associated with recommended treatments are less likely to engage in these interventions. Patients with abuse histories may forego treatments they find to be invasive, embarrassing, or painful—especially if these treatments reactivate or replicate the original trauma. Finally, a lack of trust or feelings of dismissal by medical personnel is associated with reduced medical compliance.[45] Nonadherence is most problematic in chronic conditions requiring continuous intervention.

Clinical Care Points

- Psychological distress, trauma, and adverse life events are prevalent in individuals with PFDs.
- These factors should be routinely assessed in this patient population.
- Psychological factors can negatively impact engagement in treatment recommendations.

PSYCHOLOGICAL INTERVENTIONS AND THEIR ROLE IN PELVIC FLOOR DYSFUNCTION
Psychogastroenterology

Psychological therapies have historically been used to treat complex medical conditions, and there is a growing understanding of the value of these interventions in gastroenterology practice.[45–49] Environmental triggers, psychological disorders, trauma, and SLEs all play a role in the development, pathophysiology, and maintenance of GI disorders. These factors are associated with poorer outcomes, higher medical costs, increased surgical rates, and reduced adherence to treatment recommendations.[4,50,51] Psychogastroenterology is a specialized field that integrates an understanding of GI functioning and psychological science to develop patient-centric, nonmedicinal treatment protocols.

The largest collection of evidence validating the effectiveness of gut-brain psychotherapies arises from the treatment of irritable bowel syndrome. Cognitive-behavioral therapy (CBT), gut-directed hypnotherapy (GDH), and mindfulness are the most well-developed and studied interventions for GI illness and offer promise for those with pelvic floor dysfunction. Less well studied are trauma-focused interventions. As a higher prevalence of trauma is identified in individuals with pelvic floor dysfunction, further development of treatment protocols inclusive of trauma therapy represents a fertile area for research.

Gut–brain Psychotherapies in Pelvic Floor Disorders

Cognitive-behavioral therapy
CBT was first developed by Aaron Beck to treat mood disorders[52] but has since been adapted for use in a number of medical conditions. It is widely studied in the treatment

of GI illness, especially IBS. Recent systematic reviews and meta-analyses have shown CBT to be highly effective for treating IBS symptoms in both the short- and long-term.[6,7,53] CBT protocols have also been developed for other GI conditions including inflammatory bowel disease and esophageal dysfunction with preliminary data indicating benefits.[5]

CBT emphasizes how the relationship between an individual's physical experiences, thoughts, feelings, and behaviors can be maladaptive or adaptive to their situation. In gut-focused CBT, patients and therapists identify areas, such as maladaptive thoughts, contributing to increased symptoms, and difficulty coping. Most frequently, GI-CBT targets altered central nervous system (CNS) processing, motility, pain perception, and visceral hypersensitivity through the identification of maladaptive cognitive, psychological, and behavioral processes. For example, a patient experiencing abdominal discomfort (physical sensation) may become anxious (feeling) about an upcoming dinner event which they think may include foods likely to worsen their symptoms (thought). This appraisal of increased threat can contribute to activation in the CNS leading to worsening symptoms and can also impact behaviors (such that the patient may avoid dining out or eating certain foods) leading to reduced social interaction, QoL, and the increased potential health consequences such as weight loss and malnutrition.

In GI-PFD, the potential benefits of CBT have yet to be tested. However, given the symptom overlap between PFD and other functional disorders such as IBS, it is reasonable to assume that improvements may occur. For example, patients with dyssynergic defecation may believe evacuation requires straining or prolonged toileting time, and these thoughts and behaviors can perpetuate and worsen the functioning of the muscles, nerves, and ligaments of the pelvic floor. While the physical toileting behaviors are frequently addressed in pelvic floor physical therapy, the aberrant cognitions driving them often remain unopposed. CBT can be used to identify rigid or mistaken beliefs and help patients reframe thoughts to be more productive, or in line with therapeutic goals. In patients with traumatic experiences, particularly sexual abuse, pelvic floor physical therapy may not only be anxiety-provoking but also has the potential to reactivate symptoms of PTSD. CBT can increase ones' awareness of bodily signals, such as increased tension, and provide opportunities for patients to use relaxation strategies and adaptive cognitions (i.e., I am safe and trust my therapist) to reduce symptom burden.

Gut-directed hypnotherapy

GDH has been studied as a treatment of GI illness since the 1980s, and similar to CBT, most of the research has focused on functional disorders such as IBS.[54,55] GDH has been shown to be effective, and in many instances as equally effective as CBT for treating GI illnesses with similar short and long-term benefits.[53] Multiple IBS hypnotherapy protocols exist, the most well studied being the Manchester and North Carolina Protocols. These protocols have also been adapted for use in other GI conditions such as IBD and esophageal disorders.[56–59]

The focus in GDH is on teaching patients to achieve physically relaxed yet cognitively focused states whereby they are receptive to suggestions regarding healthy functioning of the GI tract. Although not fully understood, GDH targets altered CNS processing, motility, pain perception, and visceral hypersensitivity through techniques that normalize pain perception in the brain and modulate motor and colonic sensory functioning.[54] Hypnotherapy has also been found to reduce gut inflammation and improve coping and resilience by providing useful personalized relaxation skills.[5] As the pain associated with pelvic floor dysfunction is hypothesized to be related to dysregulation of the CNS with hyporesponsiveness of the hypothalamic–pituitary–adrenal axis,[60] GDH may represent a beneficial adjunctive therapy to address this issue in patients undergoing pelvic floor physical therapy.

Mindfulness and Mindfulness-Based Stress Reduction

Mindfulness is the cultivation of awareness and acceptance of present moment circumstances. Mindfulness-based treatments (MBTs) use relaxation training and meditation practices, often in a structured way, to enhance coping. Mindfulness protocols have been developed for use in health care[61] and successfully used for conditions including IBS.[62,63] Many MBTs are based on the work of John Kabat-Zinn, who first adapted the use of these principles for mindfulness-based stress reduction (MBSR). Developed in the 1970s as an 8-week course to help individual's cope with chronic illness, MBSR is predicated on a combination of meditation, awareness, and nonjudgment of present experience (including thoughts, feelings, behaviors, and bodily sensations), and yoga.[64] Reduced levels of mindfulness have been associated with pain catastrophizing and hypervigilance to pain[60] which are known to impact those with PFDs.

Although the data are less robust than for CBT and GDH, MBTs have also been found to be effective for treating GI conditions.[6,7,62,63] MBSR, in particular, has proven highly effective in reducing symptoms of, and improving QoL in individuals with IBS.[63] There are no RCTs evaluating MBTs for treating GI-PFD. Research has been limited to case studies of women with urogynecological pelvic floor dysfunction whereby a combination of mindfulness-based and CBT has shown utility in reducing symptoms of pain. Mindfulness may benefit patients with GI-PFD by bringing awareness of the roles stress, emotions, and behaviors play in their symptoms. A key aspect of mindfulness it to bring awareness to the present moment, including awareness of bodily sensations. Some patients with GI-PFD report being unaware of tension in their pelvic floor, or having histories of ignoring the urge to defecate, eventually losing awareness of their bodies' own natural signals. Patients with trauma may even disassociate from sensations within their pelvic floors or associate their pelvic regions with uncomfortable thoughts and feelings. Mindfulness-based therapies may prove to be a beneficial adjunctive approach.

CLINIC CARE POINTS

- A large body of evidence supports the use of psychotherapies for treating disorders of gut–brain interaction.
- Brain–gut psychotherapies seem efficacious in reducing visceral hypersensitivity, catastrophic cognitions, and disruptive illness behaviors.
- More research is needed assessing the benefits of psycho and trauma-specific therapies in GI-PFDs

NUTRITIONAL FACTORS IN PELVIC FLOOR DISORDERS
Role of Nutritional Status in Pelvic Floor Dysfunction

Eating behaviors and nutritional status can contribute to the development and maintenance of global GI symptoms commonly experienced in PFD. Both underweight and overweight status impact PFD via different mechanisms. PFD contributes to both upper and lower GI symptoms including abdominal pain, bloating, and altered bowel patterns. Patients often have a natural drive to control abdominal symptoms and stool consistency with dietary alterations. While dietary modification improves GI symptoms in DGBI[65], the role of diet modification has not been studied specifically in the context of PFD. However, nutritional intake and status have important implications in the treatment of pelvic floor dysfunction.

Obesity and Pelvic Floor Dysfunction

Obesity contributes to PFD by increasing intraabdominal pressure. In a large cross-sectional analysis of 3440 women selected from National Health and Nutrition Examination Survey (NHANES) data collected between 2005 and 2010, overweight and obese women reported higher rates of more than 1 PFD than women of normal weight (30.4% [95% confidence interval (CI): 25.8–35.0] vs 15.1% [95% CI: 11.6–18.7]). Specifically, urinary incontinence (30.4%, (95% CI: 25.8–35.0]), fecal incontinence (15.1%, [95% CI: 11.6–18.7]) and multiorgan prolapse [3.6 (95% CI: 2.0–5.2] vs 1.7 [95% CI: .6–2.9], $P < .001$) were more commonly identified. This relationship did not differ by racial or ethnic group.[66] Weight loss improves PFD by reducing intra-abdominal pressure, but this improvement seems to benefit urinary incontinence more so than other forms of PFD based on recent studies[67] Effective weight loss strategies such as reducing food volume, increasing fruits, vegetables, and fiber may also improve treatment response in PFD in obese individuals but rigorous studies are lacking.

Undernutrition and Comorbidity with Restrictive Eating Disorders

Eating disorders (EDs) can complicate the diagnosis and treatment of DBGI and PFD as suboptimal nutritional status directly contributes to altered GI motility, pelvic floor muscular dyscoordination, and increased symptom burden. A recent systematic review of 195 publications examined GI symptoms and objective GI work up in patients with EDs. For those with anorexia nervosa (AN), a high prevalence of subjectively reported abdominal pain (45%), distention (28.4%), constipation (10%), and diarrhea (7%) were reported in the pooled studies. Equally elevated prevalence rates were observed in bulimia nervosa (BN) for abdominal pain (39%) abdominal distention (32%), nausea (17.9%), constipation (7%), and diarrhea.[68] Objectively, across studies, gastroparesis was confirmed via gastric emptying scan in 24.5% of those with AN and 15.2% of those with BN.[68]

Low body weight and chronic food restriction can contribute to subjective GI symptoms and may impair treatment outcomes in PFD although research on this relationship is lacking. While abdominal fullness can drive oral restriction, it also matches objectively measured delayed gastric emptying.[68] Pelvic floor anatomic variants are also commonly observed in individuals with delayed gastric and intestinal emptying. In a study of 206 patients with gastroparesis assessed at an academic medical center, 88.9% were found to have rectoceles compared with 60% of nongastroparesis GI controls ($P = .008$). There were, however, no differences in rates of dyssynergic defecation between the 2 cohorts ($P = .88$).

Gastric emptying can improve after long-term disordered earing rehabilitation, however, symptoms can persist potentially complicating adherence to treatment.[68–71]

Overall, disordered eating behaviors such as food avoidance, meal skipping, and self-directed elimination diets are highly prevalent in DGBI but have not been systematically described in PFD.[71–73] Often these disordered eating patterns are motivated by mitigation of symptoms as opposed to a drive for thinness.[71] Disordered eating should be assessed as it is associated with higher risks of developing avoidant/restrictive food intake disorder (ARFID) or orthorexia nervosa (ON). Estimates of these disorders in patients with DGBI can be as high as 44% but have not been measured in PFD.[71]

Estimating Nutritional Needs and Screening for Nutritional Risk

Best practices for nutritional interventions in PFD need to be established but should begin with both nutrition assessments and implementation of specific diet recommendations. Consultation with a registered dietician nutritionist (RDN) trained in GI disorders should be considered for patients with PFD—especially those with overlapping DGBI. A comprehensive nutrition assessment may reveal inadequate or inappropriate intake of calories, protein, or other nutrients leading to weight and muscle loss. Adults should be weighed and measured and have their BMI calculated and weight history assessed for any unplanned weight loss or gain.[74,75] Nutrition assessments can also help identify maladaptive eating, or attitudes and beliefs associated with disordered eating.[76] A total body weight loss of 5% or more within 1 month, as well as a body mass index less than 18.5 kg/m2, are indicators of nutritional risk. Eating behaviors increasing the nutritional risk that should be addressed by both a GI RDN as well as a GI health psychologist include exclusion of specific food groups, avoidance of eating resulting in severely restricted calories, and reluctance to expand consumed foods in the absence of symptoms.[76]

Role of Fiber to Promote Laxation

Individuals with PFD are often advised to avoid straining during a bowel movement. The consumption of adequate dietary fiber (>25 g/d) along with additional fluid intake can improve laxation through increasing stool weight and bulk. Wheat bran is the most widely studied source of added fiber but should be increased cautiously in individuals with PFD and DGBI as it can exacerbate symptoms of bloating and pain due to its high fructan content.[77]

Soluble fiber from psyllium and fruits such as kiwi, prunes, and mango improve weekly defecatory frequency, stool texture, and decrease laxative use.[78,79] Kiwi may provide the best outcome/side-effect ratio as a recent study revealed that kiwi increases spontaneous bowel movement rates without inducing the abdominal pain or bloating reported with consumption of wheat bran or psyllium.[80] Presumably, the difference relates to kiwi's polysaccharide complex which increases water retention properties in stool.

While increased fiber from healthy foods such as fruits, vegetables, and whole grains is advised for overall nutrition, data are lacking to suggest formal targets for patients with GI pelvic floor dysfunction. Due to the minimal potential for negative side effects, clinicians should recommend increased consumption of fruit-based fibers—especially kiwi fruits—in patients with chronic constipation.

The limitation of short-chain carbohydrates including fermentable oligosaccharides, disaccharides, monosaccharides, and polyols (low FODMAP) is often recommended by health care providers for patients with IBS,[65] and recent meta-analyses confirm the efficacy of the low FODMAP diet for controlling bloating and abdominal pain[81]. This diet has 3 phases: the elimination phase, reintroduction phase, and personalization phase. It is recommended that a trained GI RDN be involved in the implementation and management of the diet due to its complexities and the need to prevent excessive restriction[65,81] Concurrent IBS is common in patients with GI PFD, and a low FODMAP diet may be used to treat symptoms. However, patients should be made aware that the dietary changes are meant to control IBS symptoms and are not expected to impact transit time or PFD. Importantly, restrictive diets such as the low FODMAP diet should be avoided in individuals with concurrent disordered eating.

CLINICS CARE POINTS

- Function of the pelvic floor is negatively impacted by being over or underweight.
- Optimizing soluble fibers and fluid intake are helpful for simple constipation but have not directly been studied as a treatment of pelvic floor dysfunction.
- Assessment of nutritional status and muscle mass should be part of a multi-disciplinary plan of care.
- An overall healthy diet offering diverse food choices and adequate protein and calories should be encouraged.

SUMMARY

Current methods for treating GI-PFD tend to focus on the physical symptoms and retraining of the pelvic floor musculature (primarily through biofeedback) but do not necessarily address psychological, nutritional, and behavioral factors contributing to and arising from PFD. An interdisciplinary approach, including providers trained in psychogastroenterology and GI nutrition, is well suited to address the complexity of these disorders. Although further research assessing the impact of specific behavioral and nutritional approaches is needed, interdisciplinary therapy has proven highly effective for other DGBI.

DISCLOSURE

The authors have nothing to disclose.

REFERENCES

1. Vrijens D, Berghmans B, Nieman F, et al. Prevalence of anxiety and depressive symptoms and their association with pelvic floor dysfunctions-A cross sections cohort study at a Pelvic Care Centre. Neurologu and Urodynamics 2017;36:1816–23.
2. Davis KJ, Kumar D, Wake MC. Pelvic floor dysfunction: a scoping study exploring current service provision in the IK, interprofesional collaboration and future management priorities. Int J Clin Pract 2010;64:1661–70.
3. Chatoor D, Soligo M, Emmanuel A. Organising a clinical service for patients with pelvic floor disorders. Best Pract Res Clin Gastroenterol 2009;23:611–20.
4. Van Oudenhove L, Levy RL, Crowell MD, et al. Biopsychosocial aspects of functional gastrointestinal disorders: how central and environmental processes contribute to the development and expression of functional gastrointestinal disorders. Gastroenterology 2016;150:1355–67.
5. Ballou S, Keefer L. Psychological interventions for irritable Bowel Syndrome and Inflammatory Bowel Disease. Clin Transl Gastroenterol 2017;8(1):e214.
6. Ford AC, Lacey BE, Harris LA, et al. Effects of Antidepressants and psychological therapies in Irritable Bowel Syndrome: An updated systematic review and meta-analysis. Am J Gastroenterol 2019;114:21–39.
7. Black CJ, Thakur ER, Houghtan LA, et al. Efficacy of psychological therapies for irritable bowel syndrome: systematic review and network meta-analysis. Gut 2020;69:1441–51.
8. Taft TH, Bedell A, Craven MR, et al. Initial assessment of post-traumatic stress in a US cohort of Inflammatory bowel disease patients. Inflamm Bowel Dis 2019; 25(9):1577–85.

9. Bouchoucha M, Hejnar M, Devroede G, et al. Anxiety and depression as markers of multiplicity of sites of functional gastrointestinal disorders: a gender issue? Clin Res Hepatol Gastroenterol 2013;37:422–30.

10. Whitehead WE, Palsson OS, Levy RR, et al. Comorbidity in irritable bowel syndrome. Am J Gastroenterol 2007;102:2767–76.

11. Addolorato G, Mirijell A, D'Angelo C, et al. State and trait anxiety and depression in patients affected by gastrointestinal disease: psychometric evaluation of 1641 patients referred to an internal medicine outpatients setting. Int J Clin Pract 2008; 62:1063–9.

12. Vu J, Kushnir V, Cassell B, et al. The impact of psychiatric and extraintestinal comorbidity on quality of life and bowel symptom burden in functional GI disorders. J. Neurogastroenterol Motil 2014;26:1323–32.

13. Whitehead WE, Palsson O, Jones KR. Systematic review of the comorbidity of irritable bowel syndrome with other disorders: what are the causes and implications? Gastroenterology 2002;122:1140–56.

14. Palsson OS, Whitehead WE. Psychological treatment in functional gastrointestinal disorders: A primer for the Gastroenterologist. J Clin Gastroenterol Hepatol 2013; 11:208–16.

15. Harley Sobin W, Heinrich TW, Drossman DA. Central neuromodulators for treating functional GI disorders: A primer. Am J Gastroenterol 2017;112:693–702.

16. Drossman DA, Chang L, Bellamy N, et al. Severity in irritable bowel syndrome: a Rome Foundation working team report. Am J Gastroenterol 2011;106-:1749.

17. Lea R, Whorwell PJ. Qaulity of life in irritable bowel syndrome. Pharmacoeconomics 2001;19(6):643–53.

18. Koloski NA, Tally NJ, Boyce PM. The impact of functional gastrointestinal disorders on quality of life. Am J Gastroenterol 2000;95:67–71.

19. Ballou S, Keefer L. The impact of irritable bowel syndrome on daily functioning: characterizing and understanding daily consequences of IBS. J Neurogastroenterol Motil 2017;29e12982.

20. Bordeianou L, Rockwood T, Baxter N, et al. Does incontinence severity correlate with quality of life? Prospective analysis of 502 consecutive pateints. Colorectal Dis 2008;10:273–9.

21. Malmstrom TK, Andresen EM, Wolinsky FD, et al. Urinary and fecal incontinence and quality of life in African Americs. J Am Geriatr Soc 2010;58:1941–5.

22. Rao SS, Patcharatrakul T. Diagnosis and treatment of dyssynergic defecation. J Neurogastroenterol Motil 2016;22(3):423–35.

23. Rao SS, Seaton K, Miller MJ, et al. Psychological profiles and quality of life differ between patients with dyssynergia and those with slow transit constipation. J Psychosom Res 2007;63(4):441–9.

24. Rao SS, Tuteja AK, Vellema T, et al. Dyssynergic defecation: demographics, symptoms, stool patterns, and quality of life. J Clin Gastroenterol 2004;38(8): 680–5.

25. Cauley CE, Savitt LR, Weinstein M, et al. A quality of life comparison of two fecal incontinent phenotypes: isolated fecal incontinence versus concurrent fecal incontinence with constipation. Dis Colon Rectum 2019;62:63–70.

26. Bordeianou L, Hicks CW, Olariu A, et al. Effect of coexisting pelvic floor disorders on Fecal Incontinence Quality of Life scores: a prospective survey-based study. Dis Colon Rectum 2015;58:1091–7.

27. Philips EM, Peeters B, Teeuw AH, et al. Stressful life events in children with functional defecation disorders. J Pediat Gastroenterol Nutr 2015;61(4):384–92.

28. Cichowski SB, Dunivan GC, Komesu YM, et al. Sexual abuse history and pelvic floor disorders in women. South Med J 2013;106(12):675–8.

29. Davila GW, Bernier F, Franco J, et al. Bladder dysfunction in sexual abuse survivors. J Urol 2003;170(2):476–9.

30. Jundt K, Scheer I, Schiessl B, et al. Physical and sexual abuse in patients with overactive bladder: is there an association? Int Urogynecol J Pelvic Floor Dysfunct 2007;18:449Y453.

31. Peters KM, Carrico DJ, Ibrahim IA, et al. Characterization of clinical cohort of 87 women with interstitial cystitis/painful bladder syndrome. Urology 2008;71(4): 634–64.

32. Beck JJ, Elzevier HW, Pelger RC, et al. Multiple pelvic floor complaints are correlated with sexual abuse history. J Sex Med 2009;6:193–8.

33. Leroi AM, Berkelmans I, Denis P, et al. Anismus as a marker of sexual abuse: consequences of abuse on anorectal motility. Dig Dis Sci 1995;40(7):1411–6.

34. Noelting J, Eaton JE, Choung RS, et al. The incidence rate and characteristics of clinically diagnosed defecatory disorders in the community. J Neurogastroenterol Motil 2016;28:1690–7.

35. van der Wal MF, Benninga MA, Hirasing RA. The prevalence of encopresis in a multicultural population. J Pediat Gastroent Nutr 2005;40:345–8.

36. Foreman DM, Thambirajah M. Encopresis was associated with child sexual abuse. Child Abuse Negl 1998;22(5):337.

37. Feehan CJ. Encopresis [corrected] secondary to sexual assault. J Am Acad Child Adolesc Psychiatry 1995;34(11):1404.

38. Boon F. Encopresis and sexual assault. J Am Acad Child Adolesc Psychiatry 1991;30:509–10.

39. Rajindrajith S, Devanarayana NM, Benninga MA. Fecal Incontinence in adolescents Is associated with child abuse, somatization, and poor health-related quality of life. J Pediatr Gastroenterol Nutr 2016;62(5):698–703.

40. Rao SS, Tetangco EP. Anorectal Disoders: An update. J Clin Gastroenterol 2020; 54(7):606–14.

41. Chitkara DK, van Tilburg MA, Blois-Martin N, et al. Early life riskfactors that contribute to irritable bowel syndrome in adults: a systematic review. Am J Gastroenterol 2008;103:765–74.

42. Karsten MDA, Wekker V, Bakker A, et al. Sexual function and pelvic floor activity in women: the role of traumatic events and PTSD symptoms. Eur J Psychotraumatol 2020;11. https://doi.org/10.1080/20008198.2020.1764246.

43. Whitehead WE, Lorenzo CD, Leroi AM, et al. Conservative and behavioral management of constipation. Neurogastroenterol Motil 2009;21(Suppl 2):55–61.

44. Laan E, van Lunsen R. The overactive pelvic floor: Female sexual functioning. In: Padoa A, Rosenbaum TY, editors. The overactive pelvic floor. Switzerland: Springer International Publishing; 2016. p. 17–29.

45. Youssef A, Wiljer D, Mylopoulos M, et al. "Caring about me": a pilot framework to understand patient-centered care experience in integrated care-a qualitative study. BMJ 2020;10(7):e034970.

46. Kinsinger SW, Ballou S, Keefer L. Snapshot of an integrated psychosocial gastroenterology service. World J Gastroenterol 2015;21:1893–9.

47. Riehl ME, Kinsinger S, Kahrilas PJ, et al. Role of a health psychologist in the management of functional esophageal complaints. Dis Esophagus 2015;28:428–36.

48. Keefer L. Behavioral medicine and gastrointestinal disorders: the promise of positive psychology. Nat Rev Gastroenterol Heaptology 2018;15:378–86.

49. Keefer L, Palsson OS, Pandolfino JE. Best practice update: incorporating psycho-gastroenterology into management of digestive disorders. Gastroenterology 2018;154:1249–57.
50. Szigethy EM, Allen JI, Reiss M, et al. White paper AGA: the impact of mental and psychosocial factors on the care of patients with inflammatory bowel disease. Clin Gastroenterol Hepatol 2017;15:986–97.
51. Keefer L, Kane SV. Considering the bidirectional pathways between depression and IBD: recommendations for comprehensive IBD care. Gastroenterol Hepatol 2017;13:164–9.
52. Beck AT. The past and future of cognitive therapy. J Psychother Pract Res 1997;6: 276–84.
53. Laird KT, Tanner-Smith EE, Russell AC, et al. Short-term and long-term efficacy of psychological therapies for irritable bowel syndrome: a systematic review and meta-analysis. Clin Gastroenterol Hepatol 2016;14:937–47.
54. Vasant DH, Whorwell PJ. Gut-focused hypnotherapy for functional gastrointestinal disorders: Evidence-base, practical aspects, and the Manchester Protocol. J Neurogastroenterol Motil 2019;31:e13573.
55. Flik CE, Laan W, Zuithoff NPA, et al. Efficacy of individual and group hypnotherapy in irritable bowel syndrome (IMAGINE): a multicenter randomised controlled trial. Lancet Gastroenterol Hepatol 2019;4:20–31.
56. Mawdsley JE, Jenkins DG, Macey MG, et al. The effect of hypnosis on systemic and rectal mucosal measures of inflammation in ulcerative colitis. Am J Gastroenterol 2008;103:1460–9.
57. Keefer L, Taft TH, Kiebles JL, et al. Gut-directed hypnotherapy significantly augments clinical remission in quiescent ulcerative colitis. Aliment Pharmacol Ther 2013;38:761–71.
58. Miller V, Whorwell PJ. Treatment of inflammatory bowel disease: a role for hypnotherapy? Int J Clin Exp Hypn 2008;56:306–17.
59. Riehl ME, Pandolfino JE, Palsson OS, et al. Feasibility and acceptability of esophageal-directed hypnotherapy for functional heartburn. Dis Esophagus 2016;29:490–6.
60. Dunkley CR, Brotto LA. Psychological treatment for provokes vestibulodynia: Integration of mindfulness-based and cognitive behavioral therapies. J Clin Psychol 2016;72(7):637–65.
61. Gotink RA, Chu P, Busschbach JJ, et al. Standardised mindfulness-based interventions in healthcare: an overview of systematic reviews and meta-analyses of RCTs. PLoS ONE ONE 2015;10:e0124344.
62. Zernicke KA, Campbell TS, Blustein PK, et al. Mindfulness-based stress reduction for the treatment of irritable bowel syndrome symptoms: a randomized wait-list controlled trial. Int J Behav Med 2013;20:385–96.
63. Naliboff BD, Smith SR, Serpa JG, et al. Mindfulness-based stress reduction improves irritable bowel syndrome (IBS) symptoms via specific aspects of mindfulness. J Neurogastroenterol Motil 2020;32:e13828.
64. Kabat-Zinn J. Full catastrophe living: using the wisdom of your body and mind to face stress, pain, and illness. New York: Doubleday Dell Publishing; 1990.
65. Chey WD, Keefer L, Whelan K, et al. Behavioral and Diet Therapies in Integrated Care for Patients With Irritable Bowel Syndrome. Gastroenterology 2021;160(1): 47–62.
66. Nygaard I, Barber MD, Burgio KL, et al. Prevalence of symptomatic pelvic floor disorders in US women. JAMA 2008;300(11):1311–6.

67. Zikos TA, Kamal AN, Neshatian L, et al. High Prevalence of Slow Transit Constipation in Patients With Gastroparesis. J Neurogastroenterol Motil 2019;25(2): 267–75.

68. Riedlinger C, Schmidt G, Weiland A, et al. Which Symptoms, Complaints and Complications of the Gastrointestinal Tract Occur in Patients With Eating Disorders? A Systematic Review and Quantitative Analysis. Front Psychiatry 2020; 11:195.

69. Benini L, Todesco T, Grave RD, et al. Gastric emptying in patients with restricting and binge/purging subtypes of anorexia nervosa. Am J Gastroenterol 2004;99: 1448–54.

70. Rigaud D, Bedig G, Merrouche M, et al. Delayed gastric emptying in anorexia nervosa is improved by completion of a renutrition program. Dig Dis Sci 1988; 33:919–25.

71. Simons M, Taft TJ, Doerfler B, et al. Narrative review: risk of eating disorders and nutritional deficiencies with dietary therapies for irritable bowel syndrome. NGM in press.

72. Reed-Knight B, Squires M, Chitkara DK, et al. Adolescents with irritable bowel syndrome report increased eating-associated symptoms, changes in dietary composition, and altered eating behaviors: a pilot comparison study to healthy adolescents. Neurogastroenterol Motil 2016;28(12):1915–20.

73. White JV, Guenter P, Jensen G, et al, The Academy Malnutrition Work Group, the A.S.P.E.N. Malnutrition Task Force, A.S.P.E.N. Board of Directors. Consensus statement of the academy of nutrition and dietetics/american society for parenteral and enteral nutrition: characteristics recommended for the identification and documentation of adult malnutrition (Undernutrition). J Acad Nutr Diet 2012;112:730–8.

74. Groetch M, et al. Dietary therapy and nutrition management of eosinophilic esophagitis: a work group report of the american academy of allergy, asthma, and immunology. J Allergy Clin Immunol Pract 2017;5(2):312–24.

75. Scarlata K, Catsos P, Smith J. From a dietitian's perspective, diets for irritable bowel syndrome are not one size fits all. Clin Gastroenterol Hepatol 2020;18(3): 543–5.

76. Skodje GI, Sarna VK, Minelle IH, et al. Fructan, rather than gluten, induces symptoms in patients with self-reported non-celiac gluten sensitivity. Gastroenterology 2018;154(3):529–39.

77. Rush EC, Patel M, Plank LD, et al. Kiwifruit promotes laxation in the elderly. Asia Pac J Clin Nutr 2002;11(2):164–8.

78. Chan AO, Leung G, Tong T, et al. Increasing dietary fiber intake in terms of kiwifruit improves constipation in Chinese patients. World J Gastroenterol 2007; 13(35):4771–5.

79. Chey SW, Chey WD, Jackson K, et al. Exploratory comparative effectiveness trial of green kiwifruit, psyllium, or prunes in US patients with chronic constipation. Am J Gastroenterol 2021;116(6):1304–12.

80. Varjú P, Farkas N, Hegyi P, et al. Low fermentable oligosaccharides, disaccharides, monosaccharides and polyols (FODMAP) diet improves symptoms in adults suffering from irritable bowel syndrome (IBS) compared to standard IBS diet: A meta-analysis of clinical studies. PLoS One 2017;12(8):e0182942.

81.. Zhan Y-L, Zhan Y-A, Dai S-X. Is a low FODMAP diet beneficial for patients with inflammatory bowel disease? A meta-analysis and systematic review. Clin Nutr 2018;37(1):123–9.

Evaluation and Treatment of Urinary Incontinence in Women

Elisa R. Trowbridge, MD[a],*, Elizabeth F. Hoover, DO[b]

KEYWORDS

- Urinary incontinence • Pelvic floor disorder • Evaluation • Treatment

KEY POINTS

- Urinary incontinence (UI) is a common disorder that disproportionately affects women.
- Careful history taking and physical examination are often sufficient for correct diagnosis, and invasive testing is generally not needed in cases of uncomplicated UI.
- A cough stress test is critical to the correct diagnosis of stress urinary incontinence.
- Treatment options are broad and include lifestyle changes, pelvic floor exercises, medications, office-based minor procedures, and surgery.

INTRODUCTION

Epidemiology, Economic Impact, and Quality of Life

Urinary incontinence (UI) is a common diagnosis, broadly defined as the involuntary loss of urine. The prevalence of UI in men and women varies widely, ranging from 15% to 75%, but disproportionately affects women more than men.[1] Notably, the prevalence of UI has increased over the last decade in both, with suspected attribution to increasing rates of both obesity and diabetes.[2] The economic impact of UI has seen steady growth since the 1990s, with annual direct costs estimated more than $16 billion.[3] The indirect costs of UI are also notable as one study has pointed out that, of all workers treated for UI, 23% of women missed work (compared to 8% of men) and had an average total annual work absence of 28.7 hours (between inpatient and outpatient treatment services).[4]

UI has significant social, physical, and psychological implications on patients' general wellbeing.[2,5] Women with UI are three times more likely to have concurrent major depression.[5] Patients reporting UI have noted increased stress levels associated with

[a] Department of Obstetrics & Gynecology/Urology, University of Virginia, Division Director, Female Pelvic Medicine and Reconstructive Surgery, PO BOX 801305, Charlottesville, VA 22908-1305, USA; [b] Department of Obstetrics & Gynecology, University of Virginia, PO BOX 800712, Charlottesville, VA 22908, USA
* Corresponding author.
E-mail address: etrowbridge@virginia.edu

Gastroenterol Clin N Am 51 (2022) 157–175
https://doi.org/10.1016/j.gtc.2021.10.010
0889-8553/22/© 2021 Elsevier Inc. All rights reserved.

their symptoms, significant discomfort in normal social situations, and interference with their daily activities.[6] Patients express concerns about having accidents outside of the home and even disruption of work meetings due to frequent bathroom trips. UI can predispose patients to skin irritation, pressure ulcers, and falls (particularly in geriatric populations and those with nocturnal incontinence).[7] These risks have been indicated as one of the factors that lead families to seek nursing home care for those affected.[7]

NORMAL PHYSIOLOGY AND PATHOGENESIS
Physiology

The lower urinary tract is comprised of the bladder, an organ composed of mucosa and layers of smooth muscle (detrusor muscle), and the urethra (**Fig. 1**).[8] The urethra contains two sphincters: the internal urethral sphincter (IUS) and the external urethral sphincter (EUS). The IUS is primarily composed of smooth muscle and α-adrenergic receptors and receives sympathetic innervation, while the EUS is primarily composed of striated muscle which allows for voluntary contraction via somatic innervation. The detrusor muscle of the bladder is innervated by both the sympathetic (β-adrenergic receptors) and parasympathetic (cholinergic receptors) nervous system. Sympathetic stimulation results in bladder filling via detrusor relaxation and sphincter contraction while parasympathetic stimulation causes bladder emptying through detrusor contraction and sphincter relaxation (**Fig. 2**).

Most individuals remain continent throughout their lifetimes, so complaints of UI should be thorough evaluated.[9] Normal age-related changes in the urinary tract, however, can contribute to the development of incontinence in otherwise healthy individuals. These include the following:

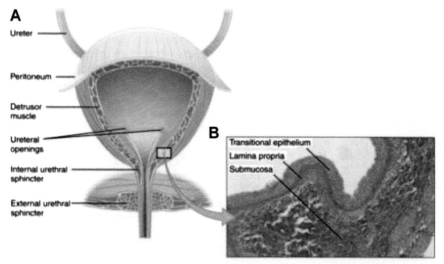

Fig. 1. The lower urinary tract. Anatomy of the lower urinary tract: (*A*) bladder and urethra and (*B*) cross-section of the bladder wall. (*From* Betts JG, Young KA, Wise JA, Johnson E, Poe B, Kruse OK, Johnson JE, Womble M, DeSaix P. (eds). Anatomy and Physiology: Gross anatomy of urine transport. Houston, Texas. OpenStax. 2013; with permission. Accessed 3/17/21: https://openstax.org/books/anatomy-and-physiology/pages/25-2-gross-anatomy-of-urine-transport.)

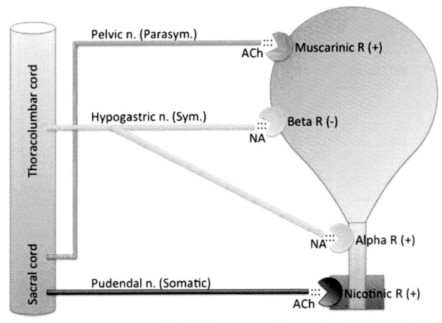

Fig. 2. Autonomic innervation of the bladder. Autonomic innervation of the bladder: Sympathetic stimulation at Beta (β3) receptors in the detrusor muscle and alpha (α1) receptors in the urethra results in bladder filling via detrusor relaxation and sphincter contraction. Parasympathetic stimulation at muscarinic (M3) receptors in the detrusor muscle causes bladder emptying through detrusor contraction and sphincter relaxation. (*From* Hu HZ, Granger N, Jeffery ND. Pathophysiology, Clinical Importance, and Management of Neurogenic Lower Urinary Tract Dysfunction Caused by Suprasacral Spinal Cord Injury. J Vet Intern Med. 2016;30(5):1575-1588. https://doi.org/10.1111/jvim.14557 with permission.)

- Detrusor hyperactivity
- Decreased bladder capacity and contractility
- Hypoestrogenic state in postmenopausal women
- Urethral hypermobility

Women who have recently given birth, particularly via vaginal delivery, commonly experience transient incontinence secondary to normal physiologic changes in pregnancy. Some women will experience persistent UI even after the postpartum recovery period which ranges from 6 to 12 months.[10] In the elderly, sources of UI outside of the urogenital tract should also be ruled out before more invasive evaluations.[9] These can include delirium, infections, depression, stool impaction, decreased mobility, drug effects, and syndromes associated with increased urinary output (hyperglycemia, hypercalcemia, congestive heart failure).[7]

Types of Incontinence

The most encountered types of incontinence include stress, urgency, overflow, and mixed UI (**Box 1**). *Stress urinary incontinence* (SUI) is defined as the involuntary leakage of urine with physical exertion, coughing, laughing, or sneezing.[11] Urine leakage occurs due to increased intraabdominal pressure and an inability to maintain the normal pressure gradient between the bladder and urethra.[12] SUI is more common

---

Box 1
Differential Diagnosis of Urinary Incontinence in Women

Stress urinary incontinence

Urgency urinary incontinence

Overflow urinary incontinence

Mixed urinary incontinence

Anatomic causes

Genitourinary fistulas

Urethral diverticulum

Congenital urethral anomalies

Functional/Transient causes

Infection

Drug effects

Restricted mobility

Dementia/delirium

Excessive urine production secondary to medical comorbidities (DM, CHF, etc.)

---

among women and is often associated with a history of pelvic floor weakness secondary to vaginal delivery, trauma, or surgery.[9,12,13]

Urgency urinary incontinence (UUI) is the complaint of involuntary leakage of urine accompanied by or immediately preceded by urgency.[11] The underlying mechanism associated with UUI is detrusor overactivity and most commonly does not have an identifiable cause, but can result from neurogenic or myopathic bladder dysfunction.[12,13] *Overactive bladder* (OAB) is a term commonly used to describe the symptoms associated with urinary urgency incontinence and has recently become the preferred term to describe the spectrum of urgency urinary disorders. It should be noted that a diagnosis of OAB does not require the presence of UI and must be made in the absence of a urinary tract infection (UTI).[12] Patients who report voiding greater than eight times in 24 hours meet the accepted frequency threshold for OAB and their symptoms are often also accompanied by nocturia, which occurs in the absence of a UTI or other urinary pathology.[11,12,14] OAB can be further subdivided to "wet" and "dry" to describe those with or without associated UI.

Overflow urinary incontinence is the involuntary loss of urine associated with bladder overdistention.[11] The underlying cause of overflow incontinence is usually related to bladder outlet obstruction or inadequate detrusor contraction.[13] This type of incontinence is more common among men and is often the result of urinary retention due to outlet obstruction associated with prostatic hypertrophy.[12] When overflow incontinence does occur in women, it is most associated with outlet obstruction secondary to severe pelvic organ prolapse (POP), excessive tension after a UI surgical procedure, or detrusor underactivity of unknown etiology.[12,15]

Patients can also present with combined symptoms of both stress and UUI, defined as *mixed urinary incontinence*. In patients who report equally bothersome symptoms of SUI and UUI, urodynamic testing can be helpful in determining the best treatment method[13] (further described below). Though less common, anatomic and functional causes of UI should also be considered when evaluating patients with complaints of urinary leakage (see **Box 1**).

Subjective Evaluation and Diagnostic Testing

A thorough history and physical examination are critical to the appropriate diagnosis of patients with complaints of UI. A careful assessment of reported symptoms is important in determining the type of incontinence as the type dictates further clinical testing. Additionally, it is essential to determine the impact of patients' symptoms on their lifestyles, as this will help guide management strategies. A study evaluating patient-centered treatment goals among women with pelvic floor disorders (of which UI is included) reported that these conditions are associated with decreased quality of life and increased cost expenditures more so than substantial morbidity or mortality.[16] Setting patient-centered goals is a simple, quick task that physicians can discuss during visits to help guide treatment and prioritize outcomes most important to patients.

History

The evaluation of incontinence should begin with a thorough discussion of symptoms. **Table 1** reviews common complaints reported by patients. The provider should also evaluate the duration, frequency, and severity of these symptoms, as well as their impact on emotional well-being and daily function. It can be difficult for patients to quantify the amount of urinary leakage they are experiencing; asking if they require the use of mini liners, pads, or adult diapers, and how many times per day they are changing these protective garments can help provide an initial measure of incontinence severity.

While some complaints are subjective, several simple questionnaires exist to help determine symptom severity. Short forms of the Incontinence Impact Questionnaire (IIQ-7) and the Urogenital Distress Inventory (UDI-6) have been developed and validated to aid in quickly assessing the life impact and distress that incontinence has on a patient.[17] These can be helpful in both the initial assessment of patients and as tools to measure symptom improvement at subsequent visits.

Other factors to consider include past surgeries, injuries, obstetric history, number of vaginal versus cesarean deliveries, use of forceps or vacuum during vaginal delivery, weight of largest child at birth, menopausal status, history of UTIs, night-time awakenings to urinate or wetting the bed, type of fluid intake, and current medication use. Reviewing a patient's intake of alcohol or caffeine and use of over-the-counter medications such as antihistamines or nasal decongestants is also important, as these agents can also contribute to UI symptoms.[9]

In women, the presence of POP should be assessed as this can be associated with or the primary source of incontinence.[12,18] Women with pelvic prolapse may complain of vaginal pressure and may report the need to "splint" (replace the prolapsed tissue or put pressure inside the vagina) to urinate or pass bowel movements.

Urinalysis

A urinalysis (dipstick) should be performed in all patients with urinary complaints of frequency, urgency, or incontinence to rule out infection as the source of symptoms.[19] A urine dipstick positive for leukocyte esterase and nitrites suggests the presence of a UTI and in this situation, urine should be sent for culture and appropriate antibiosis initiated.[20] If incontinence symptoms are not improved after treatment, further workup is indicated.

It is worthwhile to note that among the elderly population the presence of asymptomatic bacteriuria increases with age and can make the concurrent evaluation of incontinence more complicated.[21] Asymptomatic bacteriuria in female patients is defined as two (2) consecutive clean-catch urine samples growing at least 10^5 CFU/mL of no more than 2 species of microorganisms. This must occur in the absence

Table 1 Common complaints associated with types of incontinence		
Stress Incontinence	Urgency Incontinence	Overflow Incontinence
1. Leakage with coughing, laughing, sneezing	1. Strong sensation of needing to void that can't be ignored	1. Constant leakage or dribbling
2. Leakage with high impact exercise	2. Inability to reach the toilet before leakage occurs	2. Unknowingly leaking urine
3. Coital incontinence	3. Leaking large amounts of urine	

of an indwelling urinary catheter with the second positive specimen collected within 7 days of the first culture. This process is benign and, in most cases, does not result in a UTI; thus, antibiotic treatment is not indicated[22] and further evaluation for another source of incontinence is warranted.

While the presence of red blood cells on a urine dipstick in the setting of a UTI can be normal, if infection is not present, follow-up urine microscopy is indicated.[23] Guidelines vary for cut-off values of the number of red blood cells per high-power field (RBCs/HPF) and range from 2 to 25 RBC/HPF.[24] A 2019 systematic review noted that only a small proportion of women with microscopic hematuria will be diagnosed with a urologic malignancy and thus, routine cystoscopy to evaluate for bladder cancers in the setting of microscopic hematuria is not currently recommended for most women.[24]

Voiding diary, pad test
A voiding diary is a helpful, noninvasive tool to objectively quantify patients' voiding, and incontinence patterns (**Fig. 3**). Voiding diaries can range from 24 hours to a week. Patients are instructed to document the amount of urine output with each void, episodes of urine leakage, amount of urine leakage, circumstances under which urine leakage occurred (stress, urge, both), whether changing of pads was necessary, and the amount/type of fluid consumed during the day. The data obtained from these diaries have been validated as accurate for evaluating incontinence.[12] While patients who record 24 hours of data can provide a reliable picture of their symptoms, those who provide more data (48–72 hours) may provide a more complete assessment of their incontinence and be able to avoid more invasive testing.[25]

Some patients find it difficult to differentiate between excessive vaginal discharge and UI. In these cases, a pad test can be helpful in distinguishing between the 2. The patient is given pyridium (phenazopyridine), which will stain the urine orange, and instructed to wear a pad. If the pad is saturated with orange color, the presence of urine leakage is confirmed.

Physical examination
The physical examination can aid in the exclusion of certain contributing factors to UI and should include both a pelvic examination and neurologic evaluation. Patients should be instructed to avoid urinating just before their examination and present with a full bladder. With the patient in lithotomy position, the examination should start with the vulva to evaluate for signs of postmenopausal atrophy (thinning of vaginal tissues, loss of architecture, labial fusion). Atrophy of the urogenital tissues occurs due to the loss of estrogen production and can result in stress urinary incontinence (SUI) secondary to decreased urethral support. Visual inspection of the urethra in combination

Date:	Column 1	Column 2	Column 3	Column 4	Column 5	Column 6
Time	Urinate in toilet Amount	Had urine loss beyond control	Amount of urine loss 1, 2, 3 or 4	Description of Urine Loss, enter S, U or B	Pad Change	Fluid Intake amount and type of fluid
12 AM						
1 AM						
2 AM						
3 AM						
4 AM						
5 AM						
6 AM						
7 AM	8 oz					8oz coffee
8 AM		✓	2	U	✓	
9 AM						
10 AM	6 oz					
11 AM						
NOON						12oz Coke
1 PM	4 oz					
2 PM						
3 PM						4oz Tea
4 PM						
5 PM						
6 PM						8oz Water
7 PM		✓	3	S	✓	
8 PM	8 oz					
9 PM						
10 PM						
11 PM						

Time out of bed: _____ AM   Time to bed: _____ PM

Fig. 3. 3-day voiding diary. University of Virginia Female Pelvic Medicine and Reconstructive Surgery Clinic, Three-day voiding diary. Column 3: 1= < ½ teaspoon or slight moisture, 2 = ½ teaspoon −1 tablespoon or wetted underwear, 3 = 1 tablespoon - less than 1/3 cup or wetted outerwear, 4 = ¼ cup or more, soaked outerwear. Column 4: S = stress, U = urge, B = both.

with palpation of the bladder neck through the anterior wall of the vagina is helpful in evaluating the presence of urethral masses or diverticula. Vaginal support should be evaluated for the presence of cystocele, rectocele, or uterine prolapse/enterocele.[26] If present, an attempt should be made to reduce the prolapsed tissue to determine if the severity of the presence of incontinence symptoms is being masked[20.] Leakage of urine that occurs only after the reduction of pelvic prolapse is considered occult SUI.[27] The vaginal walls should also be inspected for the presence of fistulae. If a fistula is suspected, it is important to differentiate whether the connection is between the ureter and the vagina or the bladder and the vagina; this can easily be accomplished with a double dye test.[12] Pelvic floor muscle strength should be evaluated during the pelvic examination, as well.

Performing a rectal examination is also helpful in the evaluation of UI. Assessment of rectal tone, presence of fecal impaction, or rectovaginal fistulas can all aid in the appropriate diagnosis of UI. Fecal impaction and constipation may lead to UI secondary to increased pressure from the stool on the bladder. This pressure can lead to decreased bladder filling and SUI, or inappropriate bladder contraction and urinary urgency. Finally, evaluation of the motor and sensory function of the lower extremities and perineum can help determine if incontinence is due to neurologic pathology. Sacral dermatomes 2 through 4 contain the parasympathetic neurons responsible for controlling micturition and their motor and sensory function can be easily evaluated via the assessment of the bulbocavernosus reflex.[20,28] Lightly brushing the labia majora with a soft Q-tip should elicit contraction of the external anal sphincter muscles if this neural pathway is intact. Loss of this reflex may indicate the presence of a lower motor neuron lesion and should prompt the examiner to inquire about the presence of fecal incontinence or defecatory dysfunction symptoms.

Cough stress test

A cough stress test should be performed in all patients with complaints of UI. In a lithotomy/supine position, the patient is instructed to Valsalva or forcefully cough, and visualization of urine leakage from the urethra is indicative of a positive test. Immediate urine loss with cough suggests SUI, while delayed leakage is more likely to be associated with UUI.[9] If the test is negative, it should be repeated with the patient in a standing position or after retrograde-filling the bladder. If the standing cough stress test is also negative and the pretest probability for SUI remains high, further evaluation via multi-channel urodynamics is indicated. This is particularly important to evaluate occult incontinence, leakage of urine that occurs only after the reduction of pelvic prolapse, to assure that surgical intervention corrects both the POP and the concomitant UI.[29]

Postvoid residual urine volume

A postvoid residual (PVR) is the volume of urine remaining in the bladder after spontaneous urination. Once a patient has voided, a PVR can be obtained by performing an in and out catheterization of the bladder or by ultrasound. A PVR can be helpful in the evaluation of patients who describe urinary retention, symptoms suggestive of bladder outlet obstruction, or overflow incontinence. A PVR of less than 50 mL is considered normal, while greater than 200 mL suggests insufficient bladder emptying.[9] An elevated PVR in the absence of POP is abnormal in women and an evaluation of bladder emptying with a pressure-flow urodynamic study is indicated.[19]

Multi-channel urodynamic studies and cystoscopy

A multichannel urodynamic study gathers data during both the filling and voiding phases of urination and assesses urethral function (**Fig. 4**A).[30] The study measures intravesical pressure (Pves), intra-abdominal pressure (Pabd), detrusor pressure (Pdet), urethral pressure (Pura), urinary flow rate (Q), and sphincter electromyography (EMG). When used together they can diagnose dysfunction of the bladder, urethra, and pelvic floor. The urodynamic study, such as anorectal manometry, attempts to

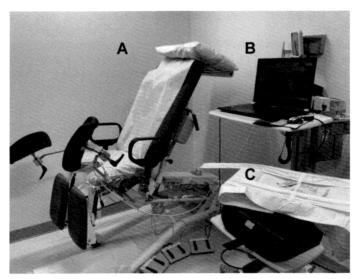

Fig. 4. Multi-Channel Urodynamic Study Equipment. University of Virginia, Multi-Channel Urodynamics procedure room: (*A*) examination chair with urine collection system, (*B*) software to collect data, (*C*) catheters for bladder filling and pressure monitoring.

reenact voiding patterns to better understand the etiology of the patient's complaints. There are 5 components of a urodynamic evaluation:

- *Complex uroflowmetry* is the test first performed. The patient is asked to come in with a full bladder and empties into a funnel connected to a calibrated scale that calculates the urinary flow rate over time to assess possible obstructive or functional voiding abnormalities.
- *Complex cystometry* is completed by placing catheters in the bladder and vagina (see **Fig. 4**B). The patient's bladder is slowly filled with water to assess bladder capacity and compliance. In addition, the testing determines abnormalities of detrusor activity and sensation which are consistent with urge incontinence.
- *Urethral pressure profilometry* evaluates the intraluminal urethral pressure along its length by slowly pulling a pressure catheter through the urethra. Though not diagnostic, very low closure pressures are associated with severe forms of SUI.
- *Pressure–flow study* is the last test performed in the urodynamic evaluation for which the patient is asked to empty the bladder with pressure catheters in place to assess the bladder pressure required to void. This study evaluates the relationship of the bladder pressure against the flow rate to help establish causes of voiding dysfunction.
- *EMG* is performed by placing bilateral EMG pads in the perianal region to evaluate the contractile activity and innervation of the perineal muscles involved with voiding. Muscular overactivity may indicate a possible cause of voiding difficulty.

It is not currently recommended that urodynamic testing be used in the initial evaluation of uncomplicated UI, as it does not provide superior data over an in-office physical examination.[31,32] Women should be referred for urodynamic studies if their physical examination does not support their symptoms (negative cough stress test with a complaint of SUI), if they have a past medical history of multiple incontinence surgeries, or if their incontinence symptoms do not improve with treatment or surgery.[20]

Cystoscopy directly visualizes the urethra and bladder and can be easily performed in the office setting. Cystoscopy can be helpful in the evaluation of patients with microscopic hematuria, concern for bladder outlet obstruction, or concern for fistula.[12]

Associations with Gastrointestinal Disorders

Constipation and fecal incontinence have been associated with UI.[33] As space in the pelvis is limited, when stool volume increases, distention of the bowels can result in increased pressure on the bladder and UI symptoms may develop. Increased pressure on the bladder may inhibit complete bladder filling and patients may experience stress or overflow incontinence. Patients may also experience urge incontinence symptoms secondary to inappropriate bladder contraction as a result of increased pressure on the bladder. These are conditions that affect 50% of nursing home residents and even with appropriate treatment, are persistent problems due to dementia and immobility.[34] In patients who report constipation or fecal incontinence, inquiry of concurrent UI is worthwhile.

Treatment

Lifestyle modifications: weight loss, timed voids, fluid restriction, and pelvic floor exercises

For women with stress, urge, or mixed incontinence, weight loss, timed voiding, and fluid restriction have been proven as effective treatments.[20] In a randomized controlled trial, behavioral therapy (education, bladder training with scheduled voids, and pelvic floor exercises) resulted in a 50% decrease in the number of incontinence episodes as recorded in a voiding diary.[35] Timed voiding can be used to help prevent excessive bladder fullness, particularly in cases of SUI, or to increase the time between voids by establishing a voiding schedule in those patients with urgency incontinence.

Obesity is a well-established risk factor for SUI.[33] Studies have shown that even moderate weight loss (an 8% reduction in body weight) is associated with a 47% decrease in weekly incontinence episodes.[36,37] Patients should also be counseled on limiting their daily fluid intake to 48 to 64 fluid ounces per day and decreasing or eliminating caffeine from their diet as both have been associated with all types of UI.[20,38–40] If patients with incontinence are waking up to void during sleeping hours (nocturia), counseling regarding decreasing, or eliminating fluid intake before bed can be a helpful strategy.

Pelvic floor exercises, or Kegel exercises, aim to strengthen the levator ani muscles of the pelvic floor and voluntary periurethral muscles.[12,20] In women with mild to moderate stress, urge, or mixed incontinence, this approach to symptom management can be an effective first-line treatment.[41] Pelvic floor exercises can be performed alone or in combination with biofeedback (pressure catheter and myographic monitoring that provides visual or auditory cues to the patient that they are performing exercises correctly) or electrical stimulation (intravaginal electrodes which activate muscles), though studies have shown that these modalities may not provide additional benefit over pelvic floor exercises alone.[42,43]

Pessaries

Pessaries have been used for centuries to treat POP; more recently, pessaries have been developed specifically for the treatment of SUI (**Fig. 5**).[44] Incontinence pessaries are placed inside the vagina and provide mechanical support to the bladder neck and

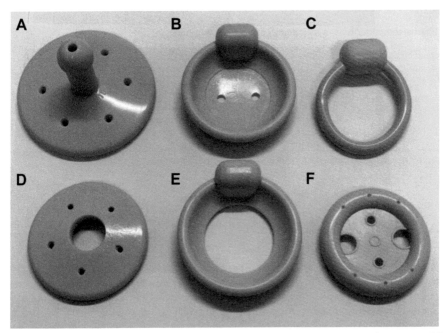

Fig. 5. Pessaries. Variety of pessaries: (A) Gellhorn, (B) incontinence dish with support, (C) incontinence ring, (D) Shaatz, (E) incontinence dish without support, (F) ring with support.

urethra conferring continence through elevation of the bladder neck and/or obstruction.[12,45] Pessaries are a reasonable treatment option for patients who are not ideal surgical candidates or for use as a temporizing option until surgery is scheduled. Studies have shown that in women who have been successfully fit for incontinence pessaries, over 50% were satisfied with the results and continued use greater than 6 months.[46] With appropriate use and fitting, complications associated with pessary use (vaginal erosions, bleeding, infection, urinary retention, etc.) are negligible. Patients who are able to perform their own pessary maintenance should remove the device, wash it with mild soap and water, and reinsert it at least every 3 months. These patients should also be seen in the clinic once a year to assure proper fit. Alternatively, patients who do not want to manage and care for their pessaries are followed up in the clinic every 3 to 5 months for a pessary check. At this visit, the pessary is removed, and a speculum examination is performed to check for vaginal erosion caused by vaginal atrophy. If vaginal erosion is identified, the pessary is not replaced, and the patient is prescribed topical estrogen cream for 3 to 4 weeks to heal the erosions. Subsequently, the pessary can be reinserted.

Pharmacotherapy
Based on current recommendations, pharmacologic therapies should be reserved for the treatment of OAB or UUI, as no effective options exist for treating stress or overflow incontinence.[20] The primary drug categories used for the treatment of UI are antimuscarinic and beta-agonist agents (**Table 2**). Antimuscarinic agents work by blocking parasympathetic signaling and inhibit involuntary detrusor contraction. Beta-agonist agents relax the detrusor muscle, allowing for increased bladder capacity via the activation of Beta-3 receptors in the detrusor. A systematic review of

Table 2
Pharmacotherapy for the treatment of urinary incontinence

Drug Category	Drug Name	Mechanism of Action	Side Effects
Antimuscarinics	Oxybutynin (Ditropan), Tolterodine (Detrol), Trospium (Santura), Solifenacin (Vesicare), Darifenacin (Enablex), Fesoterodine (Toviaz)	Blocks parasympathetic muscarinic receptor signaling (bladder M2, M3 receptors), inhibiting involuntary detrusor contractions	Dry mouth, blurry vision, dizziness, palpitations, constipation, headache, fatigue, cognitive changes
Beta-agonists	Mirabegron (Myrbetriq)	Activation of beta-3 receptors relaxes the detrusor muscle of the bladder and results in increased storage capacity	Hypertension, tachycardia, headache, diarrhea

antimuscarinics for the treatment of urgency incontinence has shown moderate improvements compared with placebo,[47] and long-term compliance with these medications is low due to side effects. Additionally, there is concern that long term use of antimuscarinic medications may increase the risk for dementia.[9,20,48] The beta-agonist agent, Mirabegron, is a newer medication (released in 2012) that has shown similar efficacy to antimuscarinic medications for the relief of urgency incontinence.[9,49] Given the drug's milder side effect profile, this may be a good option for patients who do not tolerate antimuscarinic agents.

Antidepressant medications such as Duloxetine and Imipramine have been used to treat UI, but efficacy and compliance among patients is minimal.[20,48] Genitourinary syndrome of menopause (GSM), the normal thinning of the vulva, vagina, urethra, and bladder that occurs among postmenopausal women, is due to a lack of estrogen, and results in loss of normal architecture and support. Vaginal estrogen has shown benefit in decreasing UI among postmenopausal women with this syndrome. It is safe and can be an effective stand-alone or adjunctive therapy option (**Fig. 6**).[20,50]

Botox and neuromodulation

Third-line treatments for UI include intradetrusor injection of onabotulinumtoxin-A (Botox), sacral neuromodulation (SNM), and percutaneous tibial nerve stimulation. Botox acts by blocking the presynaptic release of acetylcholine from motor neurons, thus reducing the strength of muscle contractions. Botox is FDA approved for patients suffering from OAB or urgency incontinence who have failed conservative management. In a study comparing the use of antimuscarinic therapy to Botox injections, patients in both treatment groups were found to have similar reductions in incontinence episodes per day, but more patients in the Botox group reported complete resolution of incontinence.[51] Botox injections can be completed in the office setting or the operating room, and effects typically last 6 months; patients should be counseled about possible postprocedure side effects including UTI, urinary retention, and the possible need for temporary self-catheterization (**Fig. 7**).[20]

SNM is an additional third-line treatment of refractory urge incontinence, nonobstructive urinary retention, and fecal incontinence (**Fig. 8**). The two-stage procedure involves placement of a lead through the S3 foramen which stimulates sacral nerves that inhibit parasympathetic motor neurons, there-by reducing bladder contractions.[20] Similarly, percutaneous tibial nerve stimulation involves afferent nerve stimulation that

High-estrogen environment   Low-estrogen environment

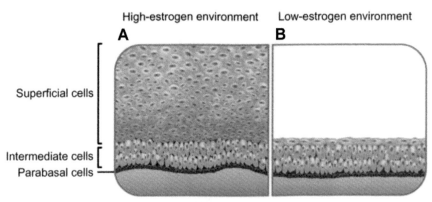

Fig. 6. Effect of the loss of estrogen on vaginal and urethral tissues. Estrogen effect on tissues: (A) Appearance of mucosal tissues under high estrogen environment (pre-menopausal state of use of topical estrogen) – superficial cell layer is plump and well supported. (B). Appearance of musical tissues under low estrogen environment. (*From* Reiter S. Barriers to effective treatment of vaginal atrophy with local estrogen therapy. Int J Gen Med. 2013;6:153–158. https://doi.org/10.2147/IJGM.S43192 with permission.)

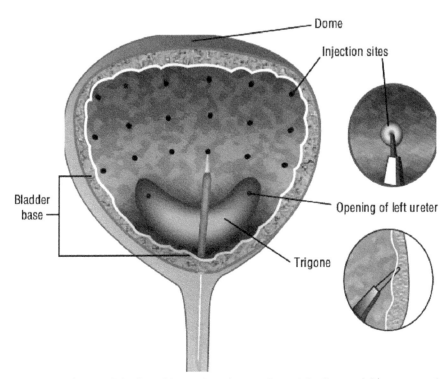

Fig. 7. Intra-detrusor injection of Botox. Intradetrusor Botox injections: a rigid cystoscope is placed into the bladder and the bladder is partially distended with saline. A catheter with an injection needle tip is then inserted through the cystoscope to inject Botox into the detrusor muscle of the bladder. Care is taken to avoid the trigone of the bladder. (*From* Allergan FDA Botox Highlights of Prescribing Information (2018). https://www.accessdata.fda.gov/drugsatfda_docs/label/2018/103000s5307lbl.pdf.)

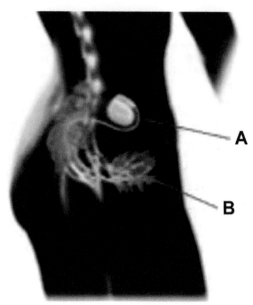

A

B

Fig. 8. Sacral Neuromodulation Device. Sacral neuromodulation device placement: The procedure is completed in 2 stages; a permanent electrode (*B*) is placed in the lower back and leads are placed through S3 foramen so that appropriate stimulation of the sacral nerves is obtained. After a test period, the second stage is completed to connect a permanent indwelling battery (*A*) to the electrode. (*Courtesy of Medtronic, Fridley, MN.*)

reduces parasympathetic motor output but is an office-based treatment that requires weekly treatment of 12 weeks followed by maintenance treatments every 3 to 4 months.[20]

In a randomized controlled trial comparing the effectiveness of intradetrusor Botox injection and SNM among women with refractory UUI, Botox resulted in slightly reduced rates of daily incontinence episodes, but with high risk of UTI and need for temporary self-catheterization.[52] While SNM may provide less efficacious results, for women who are not willing to self-catheterize, it may be a reasonable alternative treatment option.

Surgery

Sling procedures

UI is most often initially managed with the conservative treatments described above, but for women with stress or mixed UI who do not achieve adequate symptom relief with these interventions, or for those who decline conservative management, surgical intervention is indicated. The goal of surgical management is to restore appropriate bladder neck support and is most commonly achieved with placement of a synthetic mid-urethral mesh sling (**Fig. 9**).[12,20,53] In a study comparing cure rates of mid-urethral slings to pelvic floor physical therapy, patients in the surgery group reported 90% improvement compared with 64% in the physical therapy group.[54] Mid-urethral slings are most placed via the retropubic or transobturator technique, with both shown to be equally effective and with similar patient satisfaction rates.[55] The retropubic technique is associated with greater morbidity (bladder perforation, greater intraoperative blood loss, and voiding dysfunction) while the transobturator technique is associated with more groin pain.[20]

A   **B**

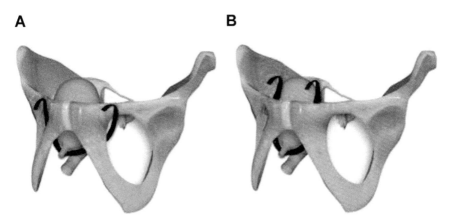

Fig. 9. Mid-urethral Slings: (*A*) Transobturator placement, (*B*) Suprapubic placement. (*From* Alila Medical Media. Available at https://www.alilamedicalmedia.com/media/412e5516-b6d3-4ae4-9242-4f40d94e641f-mid-urethral-sling-transobturator-versus-retropubic?hit_num=2&hits=4&page=1&per_page=100&prev=b6446b48-4ce1-4a87-b604-f8eeec067ecd&search=%22mid-urethral%22+sling; with permission)

Among patients who are not candidates for mesh slings or decline this option, the autologous fascial sling (usually created from the rectus sheath or fascia lata of the quadriceps muscle) and Burch colposuspension procedures represent effective alternative surgical options. A 2007 study comparing these 2 procedures showed the superiority of the autologous fascial sling.[56] However, the autologous fascial sling is associated with greater morbidity including higher rates of UTIs, urge incontinence, voiding dysfunction, and need for surgical revision. Due to these complications, the procedure is not among the more common surgeries used for the treatment of UI.[56]

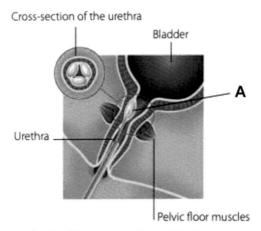

Fig. 10. Injection of Urethral Bulking Agents. Urethral bulking agents: (*A*) a cystoscope is used to visualize the mucosa of the urethra and inject bulking agents circumferentially into the urethra to rebuild normal urethral closure. (*From* Bulkamid Urethral Bulking System, A Minimally Invasive Treatment For Stress Urinary Incontinence. Available at https://www.accessdata.fda.gov/cdrh_docs/pdf17/P170023C.pdf).

Urethral bulking agents

In women with refractory stress incontinence after surgery or those who cannot undergo surgery, agents can be injected into the tissues surrounding the bladder neck and proximal to the urethra to increase urethral resistance and thus decrease urinary leakage (**Fig. 10**). Meta-analysis of several studies has demonstrated that urethral bulking agents are significantly less effective than surgery in the treatment of SUI.[57]

SUMMARY

Given the prevalence and quality of life impact of UI, it is important to query and discuss even minor symptoms with patients. With appropriate evaluation and diagnosis, UI can be well-managed. There are a variety of treatment options available. Should conservative interventions fail, more invasive therapies may be effective.

CLINICS CARE POINTS

- UI is a common diagnosis with prevalence rates as high as 75% in the general population.

- Initial evaluation of uncomplicated UI should include a pelvic examination, urinalysis, cough stress test, and postvoid residual. Voiding diaries are helpful for the objective quantification of UI patterns.

- It is important to evaluate for concurrent symptoms of constipation or fecal incontinence during the evaluation of UI. Patients with chronic constipation or fecal impaction are at higher risk of UI secondary to increased pressure of stool on the bladder. Those with both urinary and fecal incontinence should be evaluated for loss of sacral innervation.

- Consideration of urodynamic testing is warranted in cases of complicated UI or negative cough stress test with symptoms suggestive of stress incontinence.

- In overweight or obese patients, moderate weight loss can improve continence.

- Conservative interventions such as timed voiding, pelvic floor strengthening exercises, and fluid restriction can improve incontinence symptoms. In postmenopausal women, the use of topical estrogen can often provide symptom relief.

- Antimuscarinic and beta-agonist medications used to treat UI are effective but poorly tolerated.

- Midurethral slings are both safe and effective for the management of refractory SUI.

DISCLOSURES

The authors have nothing to disclose.

REFERENCES

1. Nygaard I, Barber MD, Burgio KL, et al. Prevalence of symptomatic pelvic floor disorders in US women. JAMA 2008;300(11):1311–6.
2. Markland AD, Richter HE, Fwu CW, et al. Prevalence and trends of urinary incontinence in adults in the United States, 2001 to 2008. J Urol 2011;186(2):589–93.
3. Wilson L, Brown JS, Shin GP, et al. Annual direct cost of urinary incontinence. Obstet Gynecol 2001;98(3):398–406.
4. Thom DH, Nygaard IE, Calhoun EA. Urologic diseases in America project: urinary incontinence in women-national trends in hospitalizations, office visits, treatment and economic impact. J Urol 2005;173(4):1295–301.
5. Melville JL, Delaney K, Newton K, et al. Incontinence severity and major depression in incontinent women. Obstet Gynecol 2005;106(3):585–92.

6. Irwin DE, Milsom I, Kopp Z, et al. Impact of overactive bladder symptoms on employment, social interactions and emotional well-being in six European countries. BJU Int 2006;979(1):96–100.

7. Ouslander JG, Reyes B. Clinical problems associated with the aging process. In: Jameson J, Fauci AS, Kasper DL, et al, editors. Harrison's Principles of Internal Medicine, 20e. New York: McGraw-Hill; 2018.

8. Perucchini D, DeLancey JOL. Functional anatomy of the pelvic floor and lower urinary tract. In: Baessler K, Burgio KL, Norton PA, et al, editors. Pelvic floor Re-education. London: Springer; 2008.

9. Carr R. Urinary Incontinence. In: South-Paul JE, Matheny SC, Lewis EL, editors. Current Diagnosis & Treatment: Family Medicine, 5e. New York: McGraw-Hill; 2020.

10. Giugale LE, Moalli PA, Canavan TP, et al. Prevalence and predictors of urinary incontinence at 1 year postpartum. Female Pelvic Med Reconstr Surg 2021;27(2): e436–41.

11. Haylen BT, de Ridder D, Freeman RM, et al. An International Urogynecological Association (IUGA)/International Continence Society (ICS) joint report on the terminology for female pelvic floor dysfunction. Int Urogynecol J 2010;21(1):5–26.

12. Tarnay CM, Medendorp AR, Cohen SA, et al. Urinary Incontinence & Pelvic Floor Disorders. In: DeCherney AH, Nathan L, Laufer N, et al, editors. Current Diagnosis & Treatment: Obstetrics & Gynecology, 12e. New York: McGraw-Hill; 2019.

13. Lue TF, Tanagho EA. Urinary Incontinence. In: McAninch JW, Lue TF, editors. Simth & Tanagho's General Urology, 19e. New York: McGraw-Hill; 2020.

14. Nygaard I. Clinical practice: Idiopathic urgency urinary incontinence. N Engl J Med 2010;363(12):1156–62.

15. Miyazato M, Yoshimura N, Chancellor MB. The other bladder syndrome: underactive bladder. Rev Urol 2013;15(1):11–22.

16. Hullfish KL, Bovbjerg VE, Gibson J, et al. Patient-centered goals for pelvic floor dysfunction surgery: what is success, and is it achieved? Am J Obstet Gynecol 2002;187(1):88–92.

17. Uebersax JS, Wyman JF, Shumaker SA, et al. Short forms to assess life quality and symptom distress for urinary incontinence in women: The incontinence impact questionnaire and the urogenital distress inventory. Neurourol Urodyn 1995;14:131–9.

18. Burrows LJ, Meyn LA, Walters MD, et al. Pelvic symptoms in women with pelvic organ prolapse. Obstet Gynecol 2004;104(5 Pt 1):982–8.

19. Evaluation of uncomplicated stress urinary incontinence in women before surgical treatment. Committee Opinion No. 603. Obstet Gynecol 2014;123(6):1403–7.

20. Urinary incontinence in women. Practice Bulletin No. 155. American College of Obstetricians and Gynecologists. Obstet Gynecol 2015;126:c66–81.

21. Monane M, Gurwitz JH, Lipsitz LA, et al. Epidemiologic and diagnostic aspects of bacteriuria: a longitudinal study in older women. J Am Geriatr Soc 1995;43(6): 618–22.

22. Mody L, Juthani-Mehta M. Urinary tract infections in older women: a clinical review. JAMA 2014;311(8):844–54.

23. Davis R, Jones JS, Barocas DA, et al. Diagnosis, evaluation and follow up of asymptomatic microhematuria (AMH) in adults. AUA Guideline. J Urol 2012; 188(6 suppl):2473–81.

24. Jeppson PC, Jakus-Waldman S, Yazdany T, et al. Developed by the American Urogynecologic Society Systematic Review Committee. Microscopic Hematuria as

a Screening Tool for Urologic Malignancies in Women. Female Pelvic Med Reconstr Surg 2021;27(1):9–15.

25. Groutz A, Blaivas JG, Chaikin DC, et al. Noninvasive outcome measures of urinary incontinence and lower urinary tract symptoms: a multicenter study of micturition diary and pad tests. J Urol 2000;164(3 Pt 1):698–701.

26. Bump RC, Mattiasson A, Bo K, et al. The standardization of terminology of female pelvic organ prolapse and pelvic floor dysfunction. Am J Obstet Gynecol 1996; 175:10–7.

27. Jundt K, Wagner S, von Bodungen V, et al. Occult incontinence in women with pelvic organ prolapse - Does it matter? Eur J Med Res 2010;15(3):112–6.

28. Previnaire JG. The importance of the bulbocavernosus reflex. Spinal Cord Ser Cases 2018;4(2).

29. Nager CW. The urethra is a reliable witness: simplifying the diagnosis of stress urinary incontinence. Int Urogynecol J 2012;23:1649–51.

30. Blaivas J. Multichannel urodynamic studies. Urology 1984;23(5):421–38.

31. Rosier PF, Gajewski JB, Sand PK, et al. Executive summary: The International Consultation on Incontinence 2008 – Committee on: "Dynamic Testing"; for urinary incontinence and for fecal incontinence. Part 1: Innovations in urodynamic techniques and urodynamic testing for signs and symptoms of urinary incontinence in female patients. International Consultation on Incontinence 2008 Committee on Dynamic Testing. Nuerourol Urodyn 2010;29:140–5.

32. Nager CW, Brubaker L, Litman HJ, et al. A randomized trial of urodynamic testing before stress-incontinence surgery. N Engl J Med 2012;366:1987–97.

33. Holroyd-Leduc JM, Straus SE. Management of urinary incontinence in women: scientific review. JAMA 2004;291(8):986–95.

34. Leung FW, Schnelle JF. Urinary and fecal incontinence in nursing home residents. Gastroenterol Clin North Am 2008;37(3):697–707.

35. Subak LL, Quesenberry CP, Posner SF, et al. The effect of behaviors therapy on urinary incontinence: a randomized controlled trial. Obstet Gynecol 2002; 100:72–8.

36. Subak LL, Wing R, West DS, et al. Weight loss to treat urinary incontinence in overweight and obese women. PRIDE Investigators. N Engl J Med 2009;360: 481–90.

37. Phelan S, Kanaya AM, Subak LL, et al. Weight loss prevents urinary incontinence in women with type 2 diabetes: results from the Look AHEAD trial. Look AHEAD Research Group. J Urol 2012;187:939–44.

38. Gleason JL, Richter HE, Redden DT, et al. Caffiene and urinary incontinence in US women. Int Urogynecol J 2013;24:295–302.

39. Bradley CS, Erickson BA, Messersmith EE, et al. Symptoms of Lower Urinary Tract Dysfunction Research Network (LURN). Evidence of the impact of diet, fluid intake, caffeine, alcohol and tobacco on lower urinary tract symptoms: a systematic review. J Urol 2017;198(5):1010–20.

40. How much water should you drink when you have incontinence? In: National Association for Continence. 2020. Available at: https://www.nafc.org/bhealth-blog/how-much-water-should-you-drink-when-you-have-incontinence. March 15, 2021.

41. Dumoulin C, Hay-Smith EJ, Habée-Séguin GM. Pelvic floor muscle training versus no treatment, or inactive control treatments, for urinary incontinence in women. Cochrane Database Syst Rev 2014;5:CD005654.

42. Mørkved S, Bø K, Fjørtoft T. Effect of adding biofeedback to pelvic floor muscle training to treat urodynamic stress incontinence. Obstet Gynecol 2002;100(4): 730–9.

43. Goode PS, Burgio KL, Locher JL, et al. Effect of behavioral training with or without pelvic floor electrical stimulation on stress incontinence in women: a randomized controlled trial. JAMA 2003;290(3):345–52.

44. Shah SM, Sultan AH, Thakar R. The history and evolution of pessaries for pelvic organ prolapse. Int Urogynecol J Pelvic Floor Dysfunct 2006;17(2):170–5.

45. Magali R, Ross S. Clinical practice guideline No. 186 – Conservative management of urinary incontinence. J Obstet Gynaecol Can 2018;40(2):e119–25.

46. Donnelly MJ, Powell-Morgan S, Olsen AL, et al. Vaginal pessaries for the management of stress and mixed urinary incontinence. Int Urogynecol J 2004;15: 302–7.

47. Reynolds WS, McPheeters M, Blume J, et al. Comparative effectiveness of anticholinergic therapy for overactive bladder in women: a systematic review and meta-analysis. Obstet Gynecol 2015;125:1423–32.

48. Nambiar AK, Bosch R, Cruz F, et al. EUA guidelines on assessment and nonsurgical management of urinary incontinence. Eur Urol 2018;73:596–609.

49. Maman K, Aballea S, Nazir J, et al. Comparative efficacy and safety of medical treatments for the management of overactive bladder: as systematic literature review and mixed treatment comparison. Eur Urol 2014;65:755–65.

50. Dessole S, Rubattu G, Ambrosini G, et al. Efficacy of low-dose intravaginal estriol on urogenital aging in postmenopausal women. Menopause 2004;11(1):49–56.

51. Visco AG, Brubaker L, Richter HE, et al. Anticholinergic therapy vs onabotulinumtoxinA for urgency urinary incontinence. Pelvic Floor Disorders Network. N Engl J Med 2012;376:1803–13.

52. Amundsen CL, Richter HE, Menefee SA, et al. OnabotulinumtoxinA vs sacral neuromodulation on refractory urgency urinary incontinence in women: a randomized clinical trial. JAMA 2016;316(13):1366–74.

53. Anger JT, Weinburg AE, Albo ME, et al. Trends in surgical management of stress urinary incontinence among female Medicare beneficiaries. Urology 2009;74: 283–7.

54. Labrie J, Berghmans BL, Fischer K, et al. Surgery versus physiotherapy for stress urinary incontinence. N Engl J Med 2013;369:1124–33.

55. Ford AA, Rogerson L, Cody JD, et al. Mid-urethral sling operations for stress urinary incontinence in women. Cochran Database Syst Rev 2015;7:CD006375.

56. Albo ME, Richter HE, Brubaker L, et al. Burch colposuspension versus fascial sling to reduce urinary stress incontinence. N Engl J Med 2007;635:2143–55.

57. Kirchin V, Page T, Keegan PE, et al. Urethral injection therapy for urinary incontinence in women. Cochrane Database Syst Rev 2012;Issue 2:CD003881.

Pelvic Organ Prolapse

Sarah Collins, MD, Christina Lewicky-Gaupp, MD*

KEYWORDS

- Pelvic organ prolapse • Uterovaginal prolapse • Vaginal bulge • Enterocele
- Uterine procidentia • Anterior compartment prolapse
- Posterior compartment prolapse

KEY POINTS

- The diagnosis of anatomic pelvic organ prolapse (POP) requires only a pelvic examination, but a medical history is key to determining if the patient is symptomatic.
- Management of POP is driven by the degree of bother and impact on a patient's quality of life and can include expectant management, use of a pessary, or surgical treatment.
- Surgical management of POP can be accomplished through various routes of entry and techniques. The risks and benefits of each and the individual patient's values and goals should be considered during treatment counseling, which can be facilitated with shared decision-making instruments.

INTRODUCTION

The most common presenting symptom of pelvic organ prolapse (POP) is a sensation of a vaginal "bulge" that is protruding to the opening or outside of the vagina.[1] In a study of more than 1900 women, the reported complaint of a vaginal bulge was highly (>77%) correlated with stage II and higher prolapse.[2] However, prolapse can also be associated with other symptoms, including urinary incontinence, a sensation of incomplete bladder emptying, difficulty with defecation, and needing to splint or apply pressure to the vaginal bulge to facilitate emptying of the bladder or rectum.[3] Vaginal bulge symptoms can be associated with significantly decreased quality of life and diminished ability to perform daily activities, exercise, and sexual activity.[4]

Prolapse can affect the anterior vaginal wall, and the resulting defect formally is called "anterior vaginal wall prolapse," but "cystocele" is a commonly used term. Prolapse can also affect the posterior compartment ("posterior vaginal wall prolapse," commonly called a "rectocele") or the vaginal apex ("uterine"/"cervical"/"vaginal vault

Department of Obstetrics and Gynecology, Division of Female Pelvic Medicine and reconstructive Surgery Northwestern University, Feinberg School of Medicine Chicago, 250 E. Superior, Chicago, IL 60611, USA
* Corresponding author.
E-mail address: Christina.LewickyGaupp@nm.org
Twitter: @cgauppmd (C.L.-G.)

Gastroenterol Clin N Am 51 (2022) 177–193
https://doi.org/10.1016/j.gtc.2021.10.011
0889-8553/22/© 2021 Elsevier Inc. All rights reserved.

or vaginal scar" prolapse).[5] Although anterior vaginal wall prolapse is the most common,[6] many POP cases involve multiple anatomic compartments (**Fig. 1**).

ANATOMIC DEFINITIONS AND CONSIDERATIONS

The primary support structures for the organs within the female pelvis include the levator ani muscles (consisting of the puborectalis, iliococcygeus, and pubococcygeus) and connective tissues/fascias. These connective tissues fuse together to form the cardinal ligaments as well as the uterosacral ligaments. Defects or weaknesses in any of these support structures lead to various forms of prolapse. Anatomic levels of support (**Fig. 2; Table 1**) have been described by DeLancey[7] and are helpful in understanding what structures have been compromised in specific anatomic defects.

PREVALENCE

It is difficult to assess the true prevalence of POP, as many women do not seek medical attention for their symptoms. However, large reviews of the literature have found that symptomatic POP has a prevalence of 3% to 6%, and anatomic prolapse occurs in up to 50% of women. Prevalence for surgery for prolapse ranges from 6% to 18%. The incidence of POP surgery ranges from 1.5 to 1.8 per 1000 women years and peaks in women aged 60 to 69 years.[8]

These figures stress the importance of distinguishing whether or not POP is symptomatic as treatment of asymptomatic anatomic prolapse is rarely indicated.

In the early 2000s, Boyles and colleagues found that more than 200,000 women undergo prolapse repair procedures yearly,[9] and in a large retrospective cohort study from 1997 of more than 149,000 women, Olsen and colleagues found an 11.1% lifetime risk of undergoing a surgical procedure for prolapse or incontinence.[10] More recently, evidence derived from 2007 to 2011 US insurance claims data indicates that close to 13% of American women undergo surgery for POP by age 80 years.[11] However, it should be noted that these numbers likely under-represent true

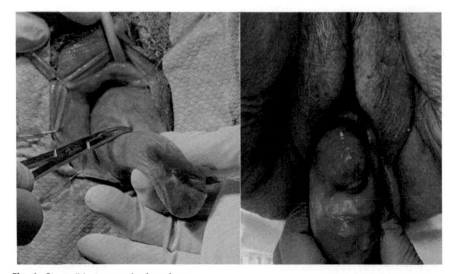

Fig. 1. Stage IV uterovaginal prolapse.

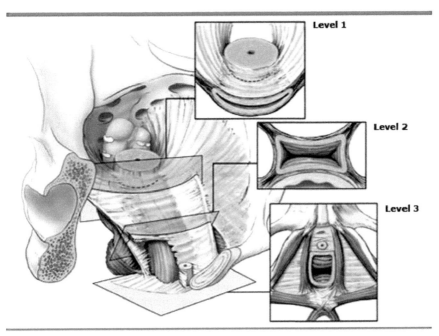

Fig. 2. DeLancey levels of vaginal support. Level I consists of the cardinal and uterosacral ligaments and suspends the vaginal apex. Level II consists of the endopelvic fascia connections to the arcus tendinous fascia pelvis, which attaches the vagina to the aponeurosis of the levator ani. Level III consists of the perineal body and includes interlacing muscle fibers of the bulbospongiosus, transverse perinei, and external anal sphincter. (*From* Walters MD, Karram MM. Urogynecology and reconstructive pelvic surgery, 3rd ed, Mosby-Elsevier, 2007. Copyright © 2007 Elsevier; with permission)

prevalence, as many women with symptomatic prolapse do not undergo surgical correction and instead manage their symptoms expectantly or with more conservative therapies.

RISK FACTORS

There are various risk factors associated with the development of POP, but the etiology of prolapse is multifactorial, which are discussed more specifically in the following:

- *Parity and Mode of Delivery*—It is well established that both parity and mode of delivery affect a woman's risk of developing prolapse. For example, in the Oxford Family Planning Association Study of more than 17,000 women, parity was more closely associated with POP than age or weight, and women with 4 or more children had an 11-fold increase in the risk of developing prolapse when compared with nulliparous women, with most of the risk occurring after 2 children.[12] Similarly, in a study of more than 4400 women, Lukacz and colleagues found that the adjusted odds of developing prolapse increased significantly with vaginal delivery compared with cesarean section; the number needed to treat analysis showed that 7 women would have to deliver by cesarean section to prevent one woman from having a pelvic floor disorder.[13]

Table 1 DeLancey levels of support		
Level of Support	Anatomic Structures	Pathology if Loss of Support
Level 1: Apical	Cardinal and uterosacral ligaments attach uterus, cervix, and upper vagina to sacrum and lateral sidewall	Prolapse of uterus or vaginal apex
Level 2: Midlevel	Paravaginal attachments along vagina to arcus tendineus fascia pelvis ("white line" of the pelvis)	Anterior compartment prolapse
Level 3: Distal	Perineal body and membrane, superficial transverse perineal muscles support distal vagina	Anterior loss: urethral hypermobility Posterior loss: posterior compartment prolapse

Numerous studies have shown operative vaginal delivery with either forceps or vacuum to be associated with the development of POP.[14,15] This is most likely explained by levator ani defects or avulsions, which are more likely to occur in operative vaginal deliveries compared with spontaneous ones. For example, Kearney and colleagues showed that in a cohort of primiparous women, major levator ani defects were detected on MRI in 42% of those delivered by forceps for a short second stage, 63% of those delivered by forceps for second stage arrest of descent, and in only 6% of women who delivered spontaneously.[16] Similarly, in a prospective cohort study of 62 primiparous women with obstetric anal sphincter injuries, women who underwent forceps-assisted vaginal deliveries were more likely to have a major avulsion on ultrasound compared with those who had a spontaneous delivery (65.6% vs 26.7%, odds ratio 5.9; 95% confidence interval 1.5–24.5, P = .014).[17] Numerous studies also have shown the association of these levator ani defects with POP. In a case-control study of more than 200 women (151 with at least stage II prolapse and 135 without prolapse), women with prolapse were 7.3-fold more likely to have a major levator ani defect than controls.[18]

- *Aging*—Aging is a known risk factor for the development of POP. In a subanalysis of the Women's Health Initiative Study, women in their sixties and seventies had significantly higher odds of apical, anterior and posterior prolapse compared with women aged 50 to 59 years.[6] In another observational study of more than 1000 women aged 18 to 83 years who were seen at an outpatient gynecology clinic, multivariate analysis revealed that the prevalence of prolapse (defined as descent to or beyond 0.5 cm above the hymen) increased by 40% with every decade of life.[19]
- *Obesity*—The data regarding obesity and the development of POP has been inconsistent. Overall, however, in a recent meta-analysis of 22 studies, Giri and colleagues concluded that although more prospective studies are needed, the current body of evidence suggests that overweight (body mass index [BMI] 25–30 kg/m^2) and obese women (BMI > 30 kg/m^2) are more likely to have POP compared with women of normal range BMI.[20] In another case-control study looking at women undergoing surgery for pelvic floor disorders, women with a BMI of greater than 26 kg/m^2 were 3-fold more likely to undergo surgery for POP than women with a lower BMI.[14] Given that obesity is a modifiable condition, encouraging women to maintain a normal BMI may be a mitigating factor in the prevention of POP as well.

- *Genetics*—There is evidence that genetics may play a role in the development of POP. In a 2011 study of high-risk familial case group participants in Utah, 6 single-nucleotide polymorphisms were found to be significantly associated with POP.[21] In a study by Jelovsek and colleagues looking at prediction models for the development of prolapse and other pelvic floor disorders, a family history of prolapse was the second strongest predictor after mode of delivery.[22] In more recent systematic reviews and metanalyses, a family history of POP significantly increased the risk for POP and POP recurrence. However, the authors did note the potential limitations of many of the studies, including recall bias and confounding.[23,24]

EVALUATION AND CLASSIFICATION OF PROLAPSE

Anatomic POP is diagnosed on physical examination, namely pelvic examination. To assess the maximum extent of prolapse, an examination can be done in standard lithotomy position with the patient performing a Valsalva maneuver, but if this does not reproduce the woman's maximum extent of prolapse by her report, a standing evaluation should be done as well. It is also important to assess which vaginal compartments are affected. Using the posterior blade of a standard bivalve gynecologic speculum, the posterior compartment of the vagina can be retracted, and the support of the anterior compartment can be assessed. The blade can then be placed to reduce the anterior vagina to allow evaluation of the posterior compartment. Assessment of apical descent can be performed digitally as the patient maximally strains if her apical prolapse is above the hymen or visually if the apex descends below the hymen. In some patients, the apex can be visualized descending with strain while a slightly open speculum is slowly withdrawn from the vagina. A rectal examination is useful in assessing anal sphincter integrity, the distal posterior vaginal wall, and the perineal body.

Since 1996, the Pelvic Organ Prolapse Quantitation system (POPQ) has become the gold standard in describing and staging prolapse in research, education, and clinical practice.[25] This system uses site-specific measurements (in centimeters) to describe anterior, apical, and posterior vaginal prolapse objectively using the hymen as a reference point at maximum Valsalva (**Fig. 3**).[26] All measurement points are taken along the vaginal epithelium, identifying the most dependent point of the prolapse in all compartments relative to the hymenal ring, which is essentially the tissue located just at the opening of the vagina (see **Fig. 3**). Points Aa and Ba refer to the anterior vaginal compartment. Point Aa is a fixed point along the midline of the anterior vaginal wall, 3 cm proximal to the urethral meatus; this point roughly represents the urethrovesical junction. The quantitative value of point Aa is anywhere from −3 (when there is no prolapse) to +3. Point Ba, on the other hand, is not a fixed point. It is merely a measurement of where the most dependent part of the anterior prolapse is located relative to the hymen; in a woman with no prolapse, the quantitative value is −3; however, if, for example, stage IV prolapse is present, this point can be as much as + total vaginal length beyond the hymen. Point C marks the location of either the cervix or vaginal cuff (if the patient is posthysterectomy) relative to the hymen, and point D marks the location of the posterior fornix, where the uterosacral ligaments meet the cervix. If the patient is posthysterectomy, point D is marked as an "X." Points Ap and Bp are similar to their anterior compartment counterparts; Ap is a fixed location 3 cm proximal to the hymenal ring along the midline posterior vaginal wall (quantitative values range from −3 to +3), and Bp marks the location of the most dependent portion of the posterior prolapse with values ranging from −3 (no prolapse) to + total vaginal length

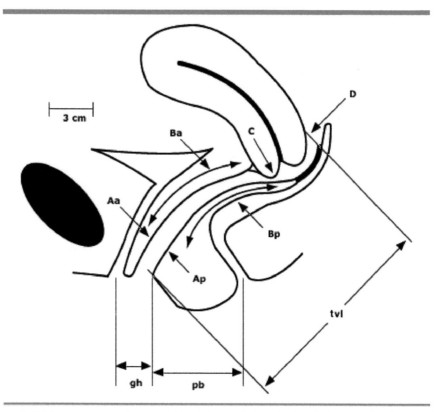

Fig. 3. Pelvic organ support quantitation. Six sites (points Aa, Ba, C, D, Bp, and Ap), genital hiatus (gh), perineal body (pb), and total vaginal length (tvl) used for pelvic organ support quantitation. (*From* Bump RC, Mattiasson A, Bø K, et al. The standardization of terminology of female pelvic organ prolapse and pelvic floor dysfunction. Am J Obstet Gynecol. 1996;175(1):10 to 17. https://doi.org/10.1016/s0002-9378(9670243-0) with permission)

(stage IV prolapse). Total vaginal length is defined by the distance (in centimeters) from the hymenal ring to the posterior fornix or cuff at rest. Genital hiatus is easily measured as the distance from the urethral meatus to the posterior midline hymenal ring, and the perineal body is the distance from the posterior hymenal ring to the mid anus. These POP-Q measurements are then used to assign a stage of prolapse, ranging from 0 to IV (**Table 2; Fig. 4**).

Once a history is obtained and a physical examination is performed, further evaluation is dependent on the individual patient. Standard in-office assessments for most patients include a urinalysis and postvoid residual volume measurement with either a catheter or ultrasonic bladder scanner. Urodynamic testing and imaging will be addressed in more detail in the following sections.

NONSURGICAL MANAGEMENT OF POP

Options for treating POP are varied and are most often dictated by patients' preference and degree of bother.

Table 2
Stages of pelvic organ prolapse

Stage of Prolapse	Definition
0	No prolapse
I	The most distal part of prolapse is >1 cm beyond the hymenal ring
II	The most distal part of the prolapse is >1 cm proximal or distal to the hymenal ring
III	The most distal part of the prolapse is >1 cm below the hymenal ring, but not further than 2 cm less than the total vaginal length
IV	The most distal part of the prolapse is at least the total vaginal length minus 2 cm below the hymen; complete eversion of the total length of the vagina

- Expectant management—Expectant management of POP is often a viable option. Many women are not bothered enough by their prolapse to pursue treatment. Women can be counseled that expectant management of prolapse is safe, and treatment can be reconsidered if symptoms become bothersome. One caveat to this occurs when the patient is exhibiting significant urinary retention, hydronephrosis (from distal ureteral kinking due to the prolapse), or significant vaginal erosions due to friction on the exposed prolapse, which can lead to bleeding, infection, and in rare cases, visceral injury.
- Pelvic floor physical therapy—Although studies consistently demonstrate the effectiveness of pelvic floor physical therapy (PFPT) for symptoms of urinary and fecal incontinence,[27] the role of PFPT in the prevention and management of POP is unclear. One study has shown that pelvic floor muscle exercises can prevent worsening anterior prolapse in older women.[28]
- Vaginal pessaries—The ancient Egyptians were the first to describe the treatment of POP with space-occupying vaginal devices, the precursors to modern pessaries.[29] Today, vaginal pessaries are the most common nonsurgical treatment method for POP. Pessaries are silicone devices and come in varying shapes and sizes (**Fig. 5**). Numerous studies support the use of pessaries as a low-risk, noninvasive, and cost-effective strategy for the management of symptomatic POP.[30,31] Studies have shown that most symptoms of prolapse (bulge, pressure) improve in 71% to 90% of women with pessary use.[32,33] Even in women who are sexually active, pessary use is feasible.[34]

Stage I   **Stage II**   **Stage III**   **Stage IV**

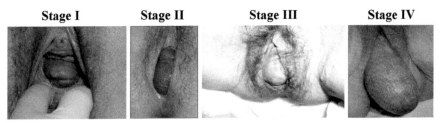

Fig. 4. Stages of prolapse. Stage I: With exposure, the cervix visible. While it has descended, it is still 2 cm above the hymenal ring. Stage II: With Valsalva, the anterior wall of the vagina is 1 cm below the level of the hymenal ring. Stage III: With Valsalva, the anterior vaginal wall comes to 3 cm below the level of the hymenal ring. Stage IV: With Valsalva, the entire vaginal vault is everted.

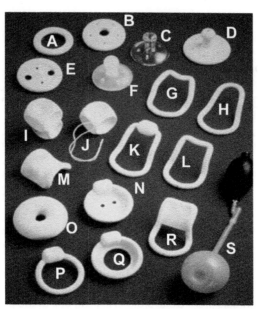

Fig. 5. Commonly used pessaries. Various types of pessaries: (*A*) Ring, (*B*) Shaatz, (*C*) Gellhorn, (*D*) Gellhorn, (*E*) Ring with support, (*F*) Gellhorn, (*G*) Risser, (*H*) Smith, (*I*) Tandem cube, (*J*) Cube, (*K*) Hodge with knob, (*L*) Hodge, (*M*) Gehrung, (*N*) Incontinence dish with support, (*O*) Donut, (*P*) Incontinence ring, (*Q*) Incontinence dish, (*R*) Hodge with support, (*S*) Inflatoball (latex) (*Photo courtesy of* Milex Products, Inc., Chicago, IL).

Pessaries are fitted in the outpatient clinical setting and can be managed by the patient herself if her manual dexterity is intact or if necessary, by the practitioner in the office setting. Patient characteristics associated with successful pessary fitting include a total vaginal length of more than 8 cm with a smaller genital hiatus (genital hiatus/TVL ratio of <0.9)[35] and lower BMI.[36] The most common complications associated with pessary use are vaginal discharge, expulsion, and erosions of the vaginal epithelium. If the vaginal epithelium is atrophic, the initiation of vaginal estrogen cream can be recommended at the time of pessary fitting. Should erosions occur despite vaginal estrogen use, the pessary can be removed for a period, often 2 weeks, during which nightly use of the estrogen is recommended. When self-managing their pessaries, women can remove and replace the devices more frequently, such as weekly, leaving the pessary out overnight to temporarily relieve pressure against the vaginal epithelium. Traditional teaching suggested that when managed in the office, pessaries should be removed and cleaned every 3 months. However, in a recently published study by Probst and colleagues, investigators found that office-based management of ring, Gellhorn, or incontinence dish pessaries every 6 months was not inferior to traditional management every 3 months; vaginal epithelial abnormalities did not differ between the groups.[37]

The more serious complications associated with pessary use are rare and generally occur in cases of neglected devices. These include pessary impaction (which may require surgical removal), vesicovaginal or rectovaginal fistula formation due to pressure necrosis, and urosepsis.[38] When offering a pessary for management of POP, it is imperative to discuss the plan of pessary maintenance and care with the patient to minimize these risks.

SURGICAL TECHNIQUES

The surgical treatment of POP in women has evolved over the decades as evidence on the safety, efficacy, and morbidity of various techniques and approaches has accumulated. Specific procedures have been categorized in several ways over the years as well. In one classification symptom, for example, procedures are grouped by functional goal, including "obliterative" procedures (which obliterate the vaginal canal), "reconstructive" procedures (designed to create a functional and anatomically normal vagina), and "compensatory" procedures, which create a functional vagina but anatomically overcorrect prolapse and elongate the vagina, as seen in sacral colpopexy.[39] Procedures can also be classified by compartment (apical, anterior, and posterior), approach (vaginal; minimally invasive or open abdominal), and suspension technique (native tissue or graft-augmented).[40,41]

In early 2020, a joint report from the American Urogynecologic Society (AUGS) and the International Urogynecological Association (IUGA) on the terminology for surgery to treat POP was published.[42] This comprehensive document was created by an international writing group including clinical and academic experts in Female Pelvic Medicine and Reconstructive Surgery (FPMRS). It was written to provide standardized terminology for POP surgeries for use by educators, learners, researchers, and clinicians. This joint report categorizes procedures as reconstructive or obliterative. Reconstructive procedures are further classified by compartment (apical, anterior, and posterior) and by whether or not graft material is used. Graft materials can be biologic or synthetic, and synthetic grafts can be either absorbable, permanent, or a combination of absorbable and permanent materials. The procedures in the document include *sacrocolpopexy* (including sacral colpoperineopexy), *sacrocervicopexy*, *uterosacral ligament suspension, sacrospinous ligament fixation, iliococcygeus fixation, hysteropexy* (including sacrohysteropexy, uterosacral hysteropexy, sacrospinous hysteropexy, anterior abdominal wall hysteropexy, and Manchester procedure), *anterior prolapse procedures* (including anterior vaginal repair, anterior vaginal repair with graft, and paravaginal repair), *posterior prolapse procedures* (including posterior vaginal repair, posterior vaginal repair with graft, levator plication, and perineal repair), and *obliterative prolapse repairs* (including colpocleisis with hysterectomy, colpocleisis without hysterectomy, and colpocleisis of the vaginal vault). Detailed descriptions of these procedures are provided in the document, but the most commonly performed surgeries will briefly be summarized here.

Prolapse repairs that use the anterior longitudinal ligament (ALL) over the sacrum as a fixation point, including *sacrocolpopexy*, *sacrocervicopexy*, and *sacrohysteropexy* (**Fig. 6**), are performed from an abdominal approach, which can involve an open laparotomy incision but which more commonly is performed through a minimally invasive (laparoscopic or robotic-assisted laparoscopic) approach to decrease risk and morbidity. These repairs include the surgical exposure of the ALL and the attachment of a lightweight, macroporous, monofilamentous polypropylene mesh to the vagina along its full length, with or without the cervix and/or uterus in situ, with suture material. The vagina is positioned anatomically, and the mesh is sutured to the ALL at S1 to secure it in place.[42]

Prolapse repairs that use the uterosacral ligaments as a fixation point for apical suspension, including *uterosacral ligament suspension* (**Fig. 7**) and *uterosacral hysteropexy*, can be performed from an abdominal or a vaginal approach. These repairs involve placement of permanent, delayed absorbable, or a combination of both types of sutures through the posteromedial aspect of the proximal uterosacral ligaments and securing these sutures to the vaginal apex or cervical tissue. Those repairs using the

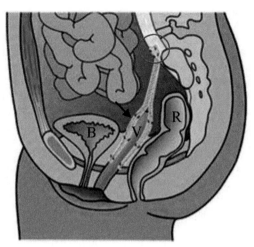

Fig. 6. Sacrocolpopexy. Arrow indicates mesh along the anterior and posterior vagina, and the red circle indicates mesh attachment to the anterior longitudinal ligament. B, bladder; R, rectum; V, vagina.

sacrospinous ligament as a suspension site, including *sacrospinous ligament fixation* (**Fig. 8**) and *sacrospinous hysteropexy*, often use the right-sided ligament alone but can use the left ligament or both ligaments. These repairs can also be performed with or without graft material.[42]

Obliterative procedures, or *colpocleisis* (**Fig. 9**), are effective for the treatment of prolapse in women who no longer desire penetrative sexual intercourse. They involve denuding the anterior and posterior surfaces of the vagina and suturing them together such that the vaginal canal is obliterated. This can be performed with the uterus in situ or after a hysterectomy, and in the former case, epithelialized tunnels usually are created to communicate with the cervix to allow drainage to exit.[42] In women who have not undergone a hysterectomy before colpocleisis, concomitant vaginal hysterectomy at the time of colpocleisis is associated with longer operating times and with an increased risk of serious medical complications compared with women who undergo colpocleisis alone.[43] This added risk should be balanced against the individual patient's risk of uterine pathology during surgical planning.

Repairs of the anterior and posterior walls, termed *anterior vaginal wall repair* and *posterior vaginal wall repair*, are performed vaginally with or without the use of graft material. They involve the opening and mobilization of the vaginal epithelium and the plication of the underlying fibromuscular tissue, either in the midline or to close specific defects identified. *Perineal repairs* similarly involve incising and mobilizing vaginal and perineal epithelium away from the underlying fibromuscular tissue, which is approximated in the midline to narrow the introitus.

Other less commonly performed repairs discussed in the joint report include *iliococcygeus fixation*, *anterior abdominal wall hysteropexy*, *Manchester procedure*, *paravaginal repair*, and *levator ani plication*. These procedures are succinctly described and well-illustrated in the joint report.[42]

There is an extensive body of literature describing comparative effectiveness research in surgery to correct POP. Although a comprehensive discussion of this broad field of study is outside the scope of this document, a summary of some of the most important findings that guide modern practice is warranted. First, hysterectomy alone in women with uterovaginal prolapse is not adequate.[44] Instead, whether

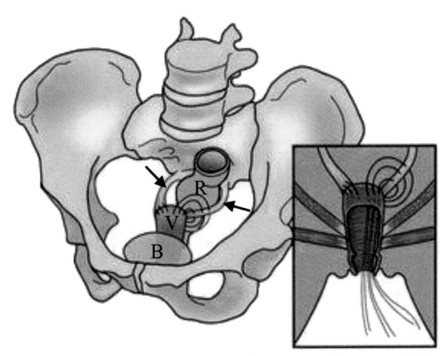

Fig. 7. Uterosacral ligament suspension. Arrows indicate uterosacral ligaments. B, bladder; R, rectum; V, vagina.

or not a hysterectomy is performed at the time of surgery for apical uterovaginal prolapse, an apical suspension is essential.[45,46] Next, many studies have shown that sacrocolpopexy is associated with a lower rate of prolapse symptoms, anatomic prolapse, repeat surgery for prolapse, and dyspareunia compared with vaginal repairs.[47] There is significant controversy about the use of *transvaginally* placed synthetic polypropylene mesh in surgery to treat female pelvic floor disorders. Because of a combination of growing medicolegal concerns in the medical community, patient fear exacerbated by sensational reports in the lay press, and corporate interests, devices marketed for the placement of transvaginal mesh (TVM) for the repair of POP are no longer available in the United States.[14] Clinical trial data have been equivocal about the efficacy and risk of these devices, and several well-designed trials were incomplete at the time of the FDA's official order. However, available outcome data show that although prolapse symptoms, anatomic prolapse, and repeat surgery for recurrent prolapse are less common after TVM-augmented procedures for prolapse, overall reoperation rates are higher after TVM procedures because of mesh complications, including mesh exposure.[48] Providers must determine for the individual patient whether offering surgeries involving TVM appropriately balances risk and benefit. Lastly, there is a growing body of evidence to support the safety and efficacy of hysteropexy in women without uterine pathology who desire uterine preservation at the time of surgery for uterovaginal prolapse.[49]

IMAGING

Historically, a thorough history and a detailed pelvic examination have been the mainstays of the evaluation of women seeking treatment, including surgery, for POP. This

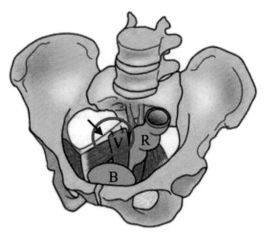

Fig. 8. Sacrospinous ligament suspension. Arrow indicates sacrospinous ligament. B, bladder; R, rectum; V, vagina.

is largely still true in modern practice. However, with the advent of more sophisticated imaging technology, additional options, including MRI and ultrasound-based studies, are available to augment physical examination findings. Both MRI and ultrasound can help identify specific viscera involved in prolapse; MRI can overstate the severity of

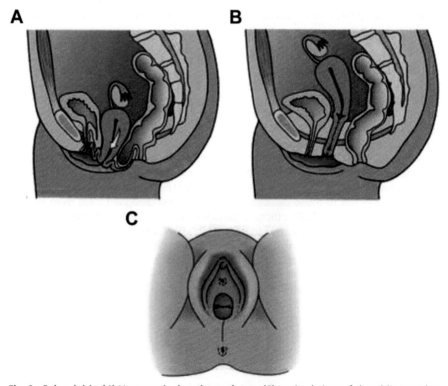

Fig. 9. Colpocleisis. (*A*) Uterovaginal prolapse shown (*B*) sagittal view of the obliterated vagina and (*C*) obliterated vagina in the dorsal lithotomy position.

anatomic prolapse compared with operative findings,[50,51] whereas ultrasound findings correlate well with POPQ measurements.[52] Although imaging is not required in the evaluation of women with POP, it can be a valuable adjunct in addressing specific anatomic or functional questions to optimize treatment planning and patient counseling.[53]

Additional Testing

Before a woman undergoes surgery for POP, a full assessment of her voiding function, including the likely impact of the planned procedure on her continence, is warranted. Particularly when surgery is planned for anterior vaginal wall and/or apical prolapse beyond the hymen, an assessment for occult stress urinary incontinence (SUI) should be performed.[44] Occult SUI refers to the unmasking of SUI, the involuntary loss of urine on effort or physical exertion, or on sneezing or coughing[1] after POP is reduced in women who previously did not have symptoms of SUI. Prolapse involving the anterior vaginal wall can anatomically kink the urethra, creating an obstruction in an otherwise weak urethra. When the obstruction is resolved with the treatment of prolapse, SUI may be observed. Occult SUI can be detected in 20% to 30% with preoperative full-bladder, prolapse-reduced testing in women who are stress continent before prolapse surgery.[54] Unfortunately, de novo SUI can occur after prolapse surgery, even in women who did not have occult SUI on preoperative testing,[55] but cough stress testing or urodynamic testing with the prolapse reduced[44] is recommended.

Because there is increasingly reassuring evidence that uterine-sparing surgery for POP is safe and effective,[49] hysterectomy at the time of surgery for uterovaginal prolapse is not universally performed. Decisions surrounding concomitant removal of the uterus, cervix, fallopian tubes, and ovaries at the time of prolapse surgery should incorporate contemporary literature as well as a thorough consideration of the individual patient's risks. This requires a review of the gynecologic history to ensure that gynecologic problems, such as episodes of postmenopausal bleeding and abnormalities in cervical cancer screening, have been satisfactorily evaluated. A concerning family history or a known genetic predisposition to gynecologic or breast malignancy or a personal history of malignant or premalignant conditions may influence decisions around removal of the uterus, cervix, fallopian tubes, and ovaries. Similarly, the evaluation of a woman planning surgery for POP is an opportunity to review colon cancer screening and gastrointestinal history with her. This may minimize unexpected colorectal findings in the pelvis at the time of surgery or prompt patients who have been delaying colonoscopy to schedule testing.

SUMMARY

Treatment planning for POP is an ideal opportunity for shared decision-making, an approach to counseling that involves a collaborative discussion between physician and patient to make an individualized, joint decision.[56] Shared decision-making is particularly beneficial for clinical scenarios in which there are no clearly superior treatment options.[57] This applies to surgeries for POP, a benign condition for which the goal of treatment is improvement in quality of life. Promising outcomes have been observed with shared decision-making instruments in women's health, especially computer-based decision analysis tools, which provide information to patients and assess their goals and values.[58] One such instrument was designed specifically for women choosing between surgeries for POP. Preliminary studies show that patients who use this instrument are more likely to choose to undergo sacrocolpopexy, which is associated with improved satisfaction with decision-making using a validated questionnaire.[59]

CLINICS CARE POINTS

- The most common presenting symptom of POP is a sensation of a "bulge" that is protruding to the opening or outside of the vagina.
- Prolapse can also present with urinary incontinence, a sensation of incomplete bladder emptying, difficulty with defecation, and needing to splint to either empty the bladder or rectum fully.
- A thorough history and physical examination are sufficient to diagnose POP.
- The Pelvic Organ Prolapse Quantitation system (POPQ) is the gold standard in describing and staging prolapse.
- The vaginal pessary is the most common form of nonsurgical treatment of prolapse and can be managed by the patient herself or up to every 6 months in the office.
- Surgical procedures to treat POP vary by surgical risk, recurrence risk, and functional outcome. Decisions regarding surgery to treat POP should be made through shared decision-making in which medical and surgical considerations are balanced with the individual patient's treatment goals and personal values.

DISCLOSURE

Dr S. Collins is an expert witness for Gynecare, Johnson & Johnson, and a content expert for MCG. Dr C. Lewicky-Gaupp is on the medical advisory board for Caldera Medical.

REFERENCES

1. Haylen BT, de Ridder D, Freeman RM, et al. An International Urogynecological Association (IUGA)/International Continence Society (ICS) joint report on the terminology for female pelvic floor dysfunction. Int Urogynecol J 2010;21(1):5–26.
2. Tan JS, Lukacz ES, Menefee SA, et al, San Diego Pelvic Floor C. Predictive value of prolapse symptoms: a large database study. Int Urogynecol J Pelvic Floor Dysfunct 2005;16(3):203–9 [discussion: 209].
3. Ellerkmann RM, Cundiff GW, Melick CF, et al. Correlation of symptoms with location and severity of pelvic organ prolapse. Am J Obstet Gynecol 2001;185(6): 1332–7, discussion: 1337-1338].
4. Jelovsek JE, Barber MD. Women seeking treatment for advanced pelvic organ prolapse have decreased body image and quality of life. Am J Obstet Gynecol 2006;194(5):1455–61.
5. Haylen BT, Maher CF, Barber MD, et al. An International Urogynecological Association (IUGA)/International Continence Society (ICS) joint report on the terminology for female pelvic organ prolapse (POP). Int Urogynecol J 2016;27(4):655–84.
6. Hendrix SL, Clark A, Nygaard I, et al. Pelvic organ prolapse in the Women's Health Initiative: gravity and gravidity. Am J Obstet Gynecol 2002;186(6):1160–6.
7. Stepp KJ, Walters MD. Anatomy of the lower urinary tract, rectum, and pelvic floor. In: Walters M, Karram M, editors. Urogynecology and reconstructive pelvic surgery. 3rd edition. Philadelphia (PA): Mosby Elsevier; 2007. p. 27.
8. Barber MD, Maher C. Epidemiology and outcome assessment of pelvic organ prolapse. Int Urogynecol J 2013;24(11):1783–90.
9. Boyles SH, Weber AM, Meyn L. Procedures for pelvic organ prolapse in the United States, 1979-1997. Am J Obstet Gynecol 2003;188(1):108–15.

10. Olsen AL, Smith VJ, Bergstrom JO, et al. Epidemiology of surgically managed pelvic organ prolapse and urinary incontinence. Obstet Gynecol 1997;89(4): 501–6.

11. Wu JM, Matthews CA, Conover MM, et al. Lifetime risk of stress urinary incontinence or pelvic organ prolapse surgery. Obstet Gynecol 2014;123(6):1201–6.

12. Mant J, Painter R, Vessey M. Epidemiology of genital prolapse: observations from the Oxford Family Planning Association Study. Br J Obstet Gynaecol 1997;104(5): 579–85.

13. Lukacz ES, Lawrence JM, Contreras R, et al. Parity, mode of delivery, and pelvic floor disorders. Obstet Gynecol 2006;107(6):1253–60.

14. Moalli PA, Jones Ivy S, Meyn LA, et al. Risk factors associated with pelvic floor disorders in women undergoing surgical repair. Obstet Gynecol 2003;101(5 Pt 1):869–74.

15. Gurel H, Gurel SA. Pelvic relaxation and associated risk factors: the results of logistic regression analysis. Acta Obstet Gynecol Scand 1999;78(4):290–3.

16. Kearney R, Fitzpatrick M, Brennan S, et al. Levator ani injury in primiparous women with forceps delivery for fetal distress, forceps for second stage arrest, and spontaneous delivery. Int J Gynaecol Obstet 2010;111(1):19–22.

17. Heliker BD, Kenton K, Leader-Cramer A, et al. Adding Insult to Injury: Levator Ani Avulsion in Women With Obstetric Anal Sphincter Injuries. Female Pelvic Med Reconstr Surg 2020. https://doi.org/10.1097/SPV.0000000000000954.

18. DeLancey JO, Morgan DM, Fenner DE, et al. Comparison of levator ani muscle defects and function in women with and without pelvic organ prolapse. Obstet Gynecol 2007;109(2 Pt 1):295–302.

19. Swift S, Woodman P, O'Boyle A, et al. Pelvic Organ Support Study (POSST): the distribution, clinical definition, and epidemiologic condition of pelvic organ support defects. Am J Obstet Gynecol 2005;192(3):795–806.

20. Giri A, Hartmann KE, Hellwege JN, et al. Obesity and pelvic organ prolapse: a systematic review and meta-analysis of observational studies. Am J Obstet Gynecol 2017;217(1):11–26.e13.

21. Allen-Brady K, Cannon-Albright L, Farnham JM, et al. Identification of six loci associated with pelvic organ prolapse using genome-wide association analysis. Obstet Gynecol 2011;118(6):1345–53.

22. Jelovsek JE, Chagin K, Gyhagen M, et al. Predicting risk of pelvic floor disorders 12 and 20 years after delivery. Am J Obstet Gynecol 2018;218(2):222.e1-e19.

23. Samimi P, Jones SH, Giri A. Family history and pelvic organ prolapse: a systematic review and meta-analysis. Int Urogynecol J 2021;32(4):759–74.

24. Lince SL, van Kempen LC, Vierhout ME, et al. A systematic review of clinical studies on hereditary factors in pelvic organ prolapse. Int Urogynecol J 2012; 23(10):1327–36.

25. Brubaker L, Norton PA. Current clinical nomenclature for description of pelvic organ prolapse. J Pelvic Surg 1996;2(5):257.

26. Bump RC, Mattiasson A, Bo K, et al. The standardization of terminology of female pelvic organ prolapse and pelvic floor dysfunction. Am J Obstet Gynecol 1996; 175(1):10–7.

27. Wilson P, Berghmans B, Hagen S, et al. Adult conservative management. Incontinence 2005;2:855–964.

28. Piya-Anant M, Therasakvichya S, Leelaphatanadit C, et al. Integrated health research program for the Thai elderly: prevalence of genital prolapse and effectiveness of pelvic floor exercise to prevent worsening of genital prolapse in elderly women. J Med Assoc Thai 2003;86(6):509–15.

29. Morice P, Josset P, Colau JC. [Gynecology and obstetrics in ancient Egypt]. J Gynecol Obstet Biol Reprod (Paris) 1994;23(2):131–6.

30. Mutone MF, Terry C, Hale DS, et al. Factors which influence the short-term success of pessary management of pelvic organ prolapse. Am J Obstet Gynecol 2005;193(1):89–94.

31. Powers K, Lazarou G, Wang A, et al. Pessary use in advanced pelvic organ prolapse. Int Urogynecol J Pelvic Floor Dysfunct 2006;17(2):160–4.

32. Clemons JL, Aguilar VC, Tillinghast TA, et al. Patient satisfaction and changes in prolapse and urinary symptoms in women who were fitted successfully with a pessary for pelvic organ prolapse. Am J Obstet Gynecol 2004;190(4):1025–9.

33. Fernando RJ, Thakar R, Sultan AH, et al. Effect of vaginal pessaries on symptoms associated with pelvic organ prolapse. Obstet Gynecol 2006;108(1):93–9.

34. Brincat C, Kenton K, Pat Fitzgerald M, et al. Sexual activity predicts continued pessary use. Am J Obstet Gynecol 2004;191(1):198–200.

35. Markle D, Skoczylas L, Goldsmith C, et al. Patient characteristics associated with a successful pessary fitting. Female Pelvic Med Reconstr Surg 2011;17(5):249–52.

36. Mao M, Ai F, Zhang Y, et al. Predictors for unsuccessful pessary fitting in women with symptomatic pelvic organ prolapse: a prospective study. BJOG 2018;125(11):1434–40.

37. Propst K, Mellen C, O'Sullivan DM, et al. Timing of Office-Based Pessary Care: A Randomized Controlled Trial. Obstet Gynecol 2020;135(1):100–5.

38. Trowbridge ER, Fenner DE. Practicalities and pitfalls of pessaries in older women. Clin Obstet Gynecol 2007;50(3):709–19.

39. Bent AE, Swift SE, Cundiff GW, editors. Ostergard's urogynecology and pelvic floor dysfunction. 6th edition. Philadelphia (PA): Lippincott, Williams & Wilkins; 2008.

40. Walters MD, Karram M, editors. Urogynecology and reconstructive pelvic surgery. 4th edition. Philadelphia (PA): Saunders, an imprint of Elsevier Inc.; 2015.

41. Handa VL, Van Le L, editors. Te linde's operative gynecology. 12th edition. Philadelphia (PA): Wolters Kluwer; 2020.

42. Joint Report on Terminology for Surgical Procedures to Treat Pelvic Organ Prolapse. Female Pelvic Med Reconstr Surg 2020;26(3):173–201.

43. Bochenska K, Leader-Cramer A, Mueller M, et al. Perioperative complications following colpocleisis with and without concomitant vaginal hysterectomy. Int Urogynecol J 2017;28(11):1671–5.

44. Pelvic Organ Prolapse: ACOG Practice Bulletin, Number 214. Obstet Gynecol 2019;134(5):e126–42.

45. Eilber KS, Alperin M, Khan A, et al. Outcomes of vaginal prolapse surgery among female Medicare beneficiaries: the role of apical support. Obstet Gynecol 2013;122(5):981–7.

46. Cruikshank SH, Kovac SR. Randomized comparison of three surgical methods used at the time of vaginal hysterectomy to prevent posterior enterocele. Am J Obstet Gynecol 1999;180(4):859–65.

47. Maher C, Feiner B, Baessler K, et al. Surgery for women with apical vaginal prolapse. Cochrane Database Syst Rev 2016;10:CD012376.

48. Maher C, Feiner B, Baessler K, et al. Transvaginal mesh or grafts compared with native tissue repair for vaginal prolapse. Cochrane Database Syst Rev 2016;2:CD012079.

49. Meriwether KV, Antosh DD, Olivera CK, et al. Uterine preservation vs hysterectomy in pelvic organ prolapse surgery: a systematic review with meta-analysis and clinical practice guidelines. Am J Obstet Gynecol 2018;219(2):129–46.e2.

50. Broekhuis SR, Kluivers KB, Hendriks JC, et al. POP-Q, dynamic MR imaging, and perineal ultrasonography: do they agree in the quantification of female pelvic organ prolapse? Int Urogynecol J Pelvic Floor Dysfunct 2009;20(5):541–9.

51. Fauconnier A, Zareski E, Abichedid J, et al. Dynamic magnetic resonance imaging for grading pelvic organ prolapse according to the International Continence Society classification: which line should be used? Neurourol Urodyn 2008; 27(3):191–7.

52. Dietz HP. Pelvic Floor Ultrasound: A Review. Clin Obstet Gynecol 2017;60(1): 58–81.

53. International Urogynecological Consultation (IUC): Clinical definition of Pelvic Organ Prolapse (POP) (2021). Int Urogynecol J In Press

54. Visco AG, Brubaker L, Nygaard I, et al, Pelvic Floor Disorders N. The role of preoperative urodynamic testing in stress-continent women undergoing sacrocolpopexy: the Colpopexy and Urinary Reduction Efforts (CARE) randomized surgical trial. Int Urogynecol J Pelvic Floor Dysfunct 2008;19(5):607–14.

55. Alas AN, Chinthakanan O, Espaillat L, et al. De novo stress urinary incontinence after pelvic organ prolapse surgery in women without occult incontinence. Int Urogynecol J 2017;28(4):583–90.

56. Charles C, Gafni A, Whelan T. Decision-making in the physician-patient encounter: revisiting the shared treatment decision-making model. Soc Sci Med 1999;49(5):651–61.

57. Tucker Edmonds B. Shared decision-making and decision support: their role in obstetrics and gynecology. Curr Opin Obstet Gynecol 2014;26(6):523–30.

58. Dugas M, Shorten A, Dube E, et al. Decision aid tools to support women's decision making in pregnancy and birth: a systematic review and meta-analysis. Soc Sci Med 2012;74(12):1968–78.

59. Collins SA, Mueller MG, Geynisman-Tan J, et al. Impact of a Web-Based Decisional Aid on Satisfaction in Women Undergoing Prolapse Surgery. Female Pelvic Med Reconstr Surg 2021;27(2):e309–14.

Endometriosis and Pelvic Pain for the Gastroenterologist

Sukhbir S. Singh, MD, FRCSC[a], Stacey A. Missmer, ScD[b,c], Frank F. Tu, MD, MPH[d,*]

KEYWORDS

- Endometriosis • Hormonal therapy • Laparoscopy • Dyschezia

KEY POINTS

- Endometriosis is an estrogen-driven disorder with pain symptoms resulting from cyclical activation of ectopic endometrial-like cells, generally invading into the peritoneal lining.
- Endometriosis should be considered whenever a patient has severe dysmenorrhea unresponsive to conventional hormonal therapy.
- Dyschezia, especially worsening during the menstrual cycle, should prompt a pelvic examination with the consideration of additional pelvic imaging (MRI or ultrasound by specialty-trained radiologist) to ensure deep infiltrative disease with endometriosis is not missed.
- Hormonal therapy to suppress period pain and peritoneal inflammation is a first-line treatment of endometriosis.
- Excisional therapy for patients failing to respond to conventional endometriosis therapy may provide relief in up to 2/3 of women; bowel involvement, although rare, may require specialized treatment including lesion shaving, disc excision, or segmental resection.

Coming together is a beginning. Keeping together is progress. Working together is success.

—Henry Ford

[a] Department of Obstetrics and Gynecology, The Ottawa Hospital, University of Ottawa, Women's Health Center, 7th Floor, Riverside Campus, 1967 Riverside Drive, Ottawa, Ontario K1H 7W9, Canada; [b] Department of Obstetrics, Gynecology, and Reproductive Biology, College of Human Medicine, Michigan State University, 15 Michigan Street Northeast, Grand Rapids, MI 49503, USA; [c] Department of Epidemiology, Harvard T.H. Chan School of Public Health, Boston, MA, USA; [d] Department of Obstetrics and Gynecology, NorthShore University HealthSystem, Pritzker School of Medicine at the University of Chicago, Walgreen's 1507, 2650 Ridge Avenue, Evanston, IL 60201, USA
* Corresponding author.
E-mail address: tfsheng@gmail.com

Gastroenterol Clin N Am 51 (2022) 195–211
https://doi.org/10.1016/j.gtc.2021.10.012
0889-8553/22/© 2021 Elsevier Inc. All rights reserved.
gastro.theclinics.com

INTRODUCTION

When patients present with pelvic pain, the approach and differential diagnosis may differ depending on the clinician they meet. A gynecologist is trained to focus the evaluation on reproductive organs and related pathology, while a gastroenterologist is typically tasked to consider functional or structural gastrointestinal (GI) causes. Sharing knowledge and working together with other health care providers will ultimately ensure patients get the right treatment, of the right condition(s), in the right time frame. This article aims to help guide the gastroenterologist (or GI surgeon) through endometriosis and its correlated pelvic conditions that may present to their practices. It is important to note that the discussion in This paper applies to those assigned female sex at birth. However, transgender patients, including non-binary and gender nonconforming, should also be included when approaching complex chronic pelvic pain.

ENDOMETRIOSIS – THE BASICS

Endometriosis is a chronic inflammatory condition defined as the implantation of endometrial-like tissue outside the uterus, often presenting with severe pain and infertility.[1] In March 2021 the World Health Organization released an Endometriosis Fact Sheet, stating that, "The World Health Organization (WHO) recognizes the importance of endometriosis and its impact on people's sexual and reproductive health, quality of life, and overall well-being."(https://www.who.int/news-room/fact-sheets/detail/endometriosis) Up to 70% of women with chronic pelvic pain (CPP), 75% of adolescents with pain unresponsive to oral contraceptives or nonsteroidal antiinflammatory treatments, and approximately 5-10% of all individuals with female reproductive organs are diagnosed with endometriosis.[2]

Endometriosis may present as lesions, plaques, cysts, or nodules that may be located along intraabdominal peritoneal surfaces including the ovaries, uterus, fallopian tubes, and beyond.[1] The disease may be found throughout the abdomen from the diaphragm to distal bowel, including the appendix and rectum. Extraabdominal disease may be found in the thoracic cavity and prior surgical skin incisions.

Endometriosis has 3 main visualized phenotypic disease subtypes including superficial peritoneal surface involvement, deep endometriosis, and ovarian endometriomas (**Fig. 1**).[3] Deep endometriosis, defined by the presence of endometriotic nodules with >5 mm depth of penetration, is often the most complex subtype to treat, as it frequently presents with tissue obliterating fibrosis and may involve the bowel, bladder, ureter, nerves, or diaphragm.

The heritability of endometriosis (the proportion of disease risk in the population attributable to genetic factors) is ~50%,[4] with 14 loci robustly replicated across 10

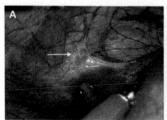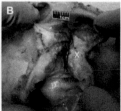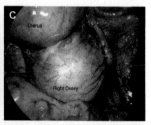

Fig. 1. Subtypes of endometriosis (*A*-peritoneal, *B*- deep [intestinal], *C*- ovarian endometrioma). (*Courtesy of* Dr. Sukhbir S. Singh, MD, Ontario, Canada.)

genome-wide association studies to date.[5] Associated risk factors emerging across the life-course include Müllerian anomalies, low birth weight, earlier age at menarche, shorter menstrual cycle length, lean body size, exposure to endocrine-disrupting chemicals, and higher consumption of transfats and red meat.[2]

Delays in diagnosis and access to treatment have been a major issue for those with endometriosis and CPP. A four-to-eleven year delay in diagnosis has been reported in developed countries and is in large part due to the lack of recognition of this disease, lack of high-quality imaging, and lack of education among clinicians and the public.[6] Further complicating the diagnosis is the overall stigma of discussing menstrual health and related issues such as dysmenorrhea or heavy menstrual bleeding. Normalizing discussion of reproductive health is an essential strategy to improve timely care. Unfortunately, potential early interventions (such as using oral contraceptives for dysmenorrhea) have not been shown to prevent the emergence of endometriosis; however, extensive studies in the general pain literature suggest the benefit of promptly alleviating acute pain to reduce the emergence of chronic pain.[7,8]

SYMPTOMS

Patients affected by endometriosis may present with classic symptoms of dysmenorrhea (80%), dyspareunia (30%), dysuria, and dyschezia (the 4-D's).[3] A key feature of these symptoms is their association with menses or cyclic variation (among those with at least one functional ovary) (**Table 1**). Endometriosis should be considered in any female patient with a cyclic pattern to their abdominal, pelvic, nerve, or thoracic symptoms.[9]

Pain and infertility can have a substantially negative impact on the physical, mental, sexual, and social well-being of women. In an analysis of the US Health Interview Survey, 50% of women reporting endometriosis had stayed in bed all day because of their condition at some time during the past year, with an average number of 17.8 bed days per year.[10] A recent multicenter study, in tertiary care settings, found that women affected by endometriosis report losing an average of 10.8 hours of work weekly because of the disease, a substantial loss of work productivity.[11]

Some individuals with endometriosis are asymptomatic; however, many may ignore symptoms they may have dismissed as "normal." GI and bowel symptoms are commonly associated among those diagnosed with endometriosis or suspected to have this condition.[12] Abdominal bloating, rectal or abdominal pain, rectal bleeding, constipation, diarrhea, and changes in bowel frequency or consistency have all been reported among these patients. Comorbid chronic overlapping pain conditions (ie, irritable bowel syndrome [IBS]) may explain many of these symptoms as well. Studies have documented that as many as two-thirds of adults with endometriosis met the criteria for IBS and were more likely to have an IBS diagnosis compared with adults without endometriosis.[13–15] A recent study of more than 300 adolescents revealed five times greater odds of IBS among those with endometriosis compared with those without.[12] Luminal obstruction can occur among those with deep endometriosis affecting the bowel, with the cecum and recto-sigmoid colon most commonly affected.

CHRONIC PAIN AND ENDOMETRIOSIS

While cyclic (catamenial) symptoms of pain prompt us to consider endometriosis, nonmenstrual pelvic pain (NMPP) should also be evaluated. Life-impacting moderate to severe dysmenorrhea is reported by one-third of premenopausal girls and women,[16]

Table 1
Overview of key symptoms, examination, imaging, GI investigations, and therapy options for endometriosis

Clinical History	Symptoms
	• Dysmenorrhea
	• Dyspareunia
	• Dyschezia
	• Dysuria
	• Catamenial or cyclical symptoms:
	   ○ Constipation
	   ○ Rectal bleeding
	   ○ Diarrhea
	   ○ Constipation
	   ○ Abdominal bloating ± pain

Examination	Abdominal examination • Masses (e.g., endometrioma, uterine leiomyoma, or other concomitant pathology) • Pain examination to include evaluation for allodynia, hyperalgesia, and focal pain (e.g., Carnett's sign) Pelvic examination • Nodularity and/or pain in the posterior fornix (under the cervix) • Rectal or recto-vaginal mass (larger or more painful at menses)
Imaging	Transvaginal ultrasound – primary imaging modality • Rectal/bowel assessment limited to those with expertise MRI – established endometriosis protocols • Assess vagina, cervix, uterus relationship to rectum/sigmoid colon • Assess urinary tract system if bowel mass detected due to correlation with ureteric and bladder involvement • Allows for expanded bowel evaluation (beyond pelvis) for disease that may involve cecum or small bowel
GI investigations	Colonoscopy • Rule out other concomitant conditions (e.g., malignancy, inflammatory bowel disease) • May not visualize endometriosis lesions if not invading through mucosa or if not done at the time of menses • Consider if external mass or acute angulation CT colonography or other testing as needed • For example, colonic transit study if concomitant bowel functional disorders
Treatment options	Watchful waiting • In asymptomatic patients without obvious intestinal obstruction or ureteric involvement Medical Therapies • Manage symptoms with hormonal suppression (e.g., oral contraceptives, progestins, GnRH agonists or antagonists) • Manage pain and bowel symptoms as required Surgery • Performed by experienced surgeons with possible collaboration with colorectal or general surgery • Excision of endometriosis, release of fibrotic adhesions to restore anatomy • Lesion shaving, disc excision, or segmental bowel resection for deep bowel involvement (See text) Postoperative follow-up • Post-operative medical therapy will assist with reducing symptom recurrence • Important to follow-up long term due to the risk of recurrence

while CPP (noncyclical pelvic pain lasting for more than 6 months) is a disorder affecting up to 27% of the female population.[17] Dysmenorrhea itself can be debilitatingly painful and present with nausea, bowel dysfunction, fatigue, and other symptoms that diminish the quality of life *cyclically*. CPP—in part due to its unpredictable onset and frequency throughout the menstrual cycle—is a well-established cause for *constant* diminished quality of life, increased levels of depression and anxiety, decreased work productivity, and high health care expense.[18,19] A British study of 1671 reproductive-aged women found that of the 24% of women with CPP, 19.3% also reported dysmenorrhea, 9.7% reported dyspareunia, with 8% reporting all 3 conditions.[17]

On recall, many patients with endometriosis endorse a classic history of pain that began as cyclic in nature in adolescence and later developed into daily pelvic or abdominal pain. Pelvic pain may be inflammatory as well as neuropathic in nature, characterized by the potential sensitization of the central nervous system that can result in persistent pain even after endometriotic lesions have been excised.[20] This finding of pain without visible disease may represent a shift from nociceptive pain (pain due to inflammation and local tissue damage) to centralized pain. Bidirectional cross-sensitization of the pelvic visceral nerves may further account for the substantial overlap of CPP disorders.[21]

EXTRAPELVIC MANIFESTATIONS OF ENDOMETRIOSIS

Among those with deep endometriosis, the disease may commonly involve the urinary tract. Cyclic hematuria may represent bladder invasion and severe ureteric obstruction may result in silent kidney death.[9] A rectovaginal endometriosis nodule greater than 3 cm increases the chance of ureteric involvement and should be considered in perioperative planning.[22] Thoracic endometriosis may present with cyclic hemothorax or pneumothorax. Diaphragmatic endometriosis presents with right shoulder pain and/ or cyclical upper abdominal or chest pain. Nerve involvement may occur with deep disease including sciatic endometriosis (cyclic sciatica) or pudendal nerve entrapment (with radiating pain into perineum, superficial dyspareunia, and difficulty sitting).[23]

EXAMINATION FOR ENDOMETRIOSIS

A patient with suspected endometriosis can truly benefit from an intentional, symptom-directed examination. Among those who present with pain, a detailed abdominal/pelvic examination is essential. Initial evaluation should consider signs of central sensitization along the abdomen and vulva including examining for allodynia or hyperalgesia. Abdominal/pelvic masses may be detected on palpation, bimanual pelvic, or rectal exam (see **Table 1**). Vaginal and/or rectal examination may reveal tenderness, a palpable mass, or direct invasion through the vagina (**Fig. 2**) or rectal mucosa (often, but not limited to lesions blue/black in color on inspection or sigmoidoscopy).

Identification of myofascial involvement (hypertonicity) along the abdominal and pelvic floor is essential to allow for the direction of therapy for either primary levator ani myofascial dysfunction or secondary pelvic floor guarding in response to the chronic pain experience. Pelvic floor spasm is more common among women with deep endometriosis, and as a result, may explain some of the symptoms related to pain and pelvic floor dysfunction.[24]

Finally, accurate and repetitive documentation of pain and tenderness locations, and the intensity of pain (score) during ambulatory visits can be crucial for identifying the relevant sources of pain and following response to treatment.

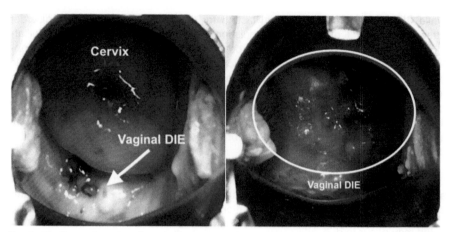

Fig. 2. Findings of Vagina deep infiltrating endometriosis (DIE) on examination. (*Courtesy of* Dr. Sukhbir S. Singh, MD, Ontario, Canada.)

IMAGING

The goal of imaging is to help rule out other pathology that may be contributing to the patient's symptoms while helping to "diagnose" endometriosis in specific circumstances.

Pelvic ultrasound, with a transvaginal (TVUS) probe when possible, is the first-line imaging modality recommended for those with pelvic pain. It can readily exclude issues with uterine leiomyoma or nonendometriotic ovarian masses. However, the quality of imaging is highly variable, and aside from excellent results for assessing ovarian involvement, experience with identifying sonographic markers for endometriosis or deep endometrial lesions is lacking.

TVUS helps confirm endometriosis if there is an obvious endometrioma (ovarian endometriosis cyst) due to its classic appearance. Beyond this finding, expert-guided imaging to detect pelvic endometrial nodules or masses along the vagina/rectum is required. Expert imaging guidelines have been developed and can aid in diagnosis and planning for subsequent procedural treatment.[25] Urinary tract and bowel examinations are essential in cases of deep endometriosis. For GI tract disease beyond 25 cm from the anal verge, an assessment for bowel involvement often requires additional testing such as magnetic resonance imaging (MRI). Peritoneal endometriosis is often beyond the spatial resolution of conventional imaging.

ALTERNATIVE IMAGING FOR ENDOMETRIOSIS

MRI is widely used when evaluating for deep endometriosis and eliminates user variability seen with ultrasound. It has high sensitivity and specificity for bowel involvement (88% and 98%, respectively).[26] Importantly, the radiologist reviewing the images should ideally be experienced in diagnosing and describing endometriosis, with an independent review ideally performed by the gynecologic surgeon involved in the patient's care. MRI is more accurate than TVUS in cases of extrapelvic disease (eg, bowel disease above the level of the recto-sigmoid colon).[27] Other imaging modalities may be indicated if there is multi-system involvement (CT scan, urogram, etc.).

THE ROLE OF A GASTROENTEROLOGIST – A GYNECOLOGIST'S PERSPECTIVE

Referral to GI specialists is essential for the care of those affected with endometriosis and CPP. In general, gynecologists will seek out consultation for the following:

- Identification and management of functional or inflammatory bowel disorders that may be overlapping with the current presentation
- Colonoscopy among those with suspected deep involvement, hematochezia, or rectal bleeding to help rule out other conditions, including malignancy, and to allow preoperative biopsy for diagnosis (**Fig. 3**)
- Assistance in planning for surgical intervention when indicated (e.g., tattoo of bowel lesions, describe the extent of involvement, and location)

A key point among those who manage endometriosis is that a colonoscopy alone is of little utility to rule out endometriosis that may have bowel involvement. The disease may not be easily biopsied or identified. Extrinsic compression of the rectum/sigmoid colon may occur to due enlarged pelvic organs or an impression from peritoneal surface disease. Complete erosion/invasion through the mucosa is a relatively rare manifestation and most likely to coincide with menses (or time of menses among those without a uterus). In some cases of deep endometriosis, as seen laparoscopically (**Fig. 4**), the bowel may densely adhere to the pelvic peritoneum, limiting the success of a colonoscopic evaluation.

OVERVIEW OF TREATMENT

Treatment of endometriosis is usually symptom-based unless imaging is suspicious for concomitant malignancy or there are associated issues with infertility. Most studies have focused largely on menstrual pain and NMPP as outcomes, and largely ignored the impact of bowel disorders like IBS, which may be present in at least a third of patients presenting with endometriosis-associated pelvic pain (EAPP). It is important to note that patients with significant symptoms related to overlapping pelvic conditions may need to have all relevant issues addressed to meaningfully reduce overall symptom burden. In rare instances of acute ureter or bowel obstruction, surgical treatment clearly should be prioritized. Otherwise, shared decision making regarding initial medical or surgical options can be undertaken. For patients with milder symptoms, it is

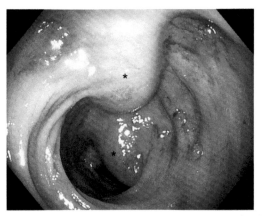

Fig. 3. Endometriosis of the rectum at colonoscopy and Ultrasound (*submucosal endometriosis nodules). (*Courtesy of* Dr. Sukhbir S. Singh, MD, Ontario, Canada.)

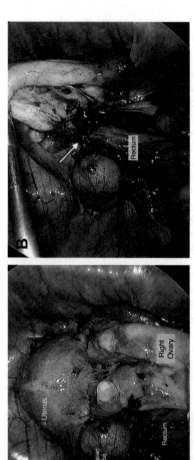

Fig. 4. (*A, B*) Example of obliterated cul-de-sac with rectum adhered to back of uterus, ovaries. (*Courtesy of* Dr. Sukhbir S. Singh, MD, Ontario, Canada.)

reasonable to support exercise, dietary optimization, body movement education with yoga, or cognitive behavioral therapy (particularly if there is a stress-related component exacerbating symptoms) as initial interventions. While they may only offer modest benefits, these general care approaches promote general wellness and use can complement more advanced therapies as well. **Fig. 5** summarizes the recursive nature of management of this often chronic disease.

PHARMACOLOGIC APPROACHES

Treatment of pelvic pain symptoms is essential to help improve the patient's quality of life and function. Furthermore, early management of pain in some women may prevent a shift from purely nociceptive, peripheral pain to a state of central sensitization that maintains chronic pain over time. Most often among those with endometriosis, the predominant symptom requiring management is dysmenorrhea, which may be addressed with nonsteroidal antiinflammatory drugs (NSAIDs) or with hormonal suppression of painful menstrual withdrawal bleeding.

Combined oral contraceptives, progestins, and gonadotropin-releasing hormone (GnRH) agonists/antagonists all have data supporting their use for reducing pain related to endometriosis (**Table 2**).[28] The mechanism is thought to be secondary to a reduction in estrogen-related stimulation of implant growth and/or peripheral afferent activation associated with bleeding-related inflammation—particularly if using doses sufficient to induce amenorrhea. Of note, GnRH targeting agents, although FDA approved, are typically only used for a period of 6 to 24 months due to concerns about bone loss and may be less well tolerated by individuals with significant mood disorders or comorbid chronic overlapping pain conditions.[29,30] They are frequently

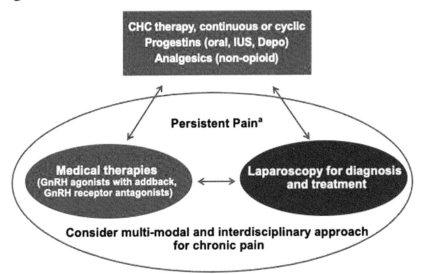

Target - Endometriosis-Associated Pain

Fig. 5. Management of endometriosis-associated pain. [a] pain may persist due to incomplete response or intolerance to first-line therapy. CHC, combined hormonal contraceptive; GnRH, gonadotrophin-releasing hormone; IUS, intrauterine system. (*Courtesy of* Dr. Sukhbir S. Singh, MD, Ontario, Canada.)

Table 2
Selected treatments for endometriosis-associated pelvic pain

Class	Examples	Side Effects to Consider
Oral contraceptives and progestins	ethinylestradiol combined with a progestin (e.g., norethindrone, levonorgestrel, norgestimate, drospirenone) OR progestins (norethindrone, norethindrone acetate, medroxyprogesterone acetate, drospirenone, micronized progesterone, dienogest)	Nausea, vomiting, worsened mood, venous thromboembolism (potential lower risk with progestin-only regimen)
GnRH agonist/antagonists[a]	leuprolide acetate, elagolix May be used with hormonal "add-back therapy" to prevent side effect profile or and reduce the risk of bone loss	Symptoms of hypoestrogenism (hot flashes, vaginal dryness), mood changes or exacerbation of underlying conditions, rare dramatic weight gain
Aromatase inhibitor	anastrozole, letrozole	Hypoestrogenism, worsened mood, formation of functional ovarian cysts (at initiation)
Nonsteroidal antiinflammatory	ibuprofen, naproxen, celecoxib, ketorolac, etodolac	Gastritis, nephropathy among those at risk with chronic use
Muscle relaxants	cyclobenzaprine, tizanidine, methocarbamol, baclofen	Sedation, impaired cognition
Tricyclic antidepressants	nortriptyline, desipramine, amitriptyline, imipramine	dizziness, somnolence, dry mouth, blurry vision, constipation, weight gain, arrhythmia in older individuals
Selective serotonin/ norepinephrine reuptake inhibitors	duloxetine, venlafaxine	somnolence, dizziness, dry mouth, some reports difficult to wean off
Gabapentinoids	gabapentin, pregabalin	Somnolence, dizziness, impaired cognition

[a] FDA approved for endometriosis indication.

coadministered with "add-back" hormonal therapy (estrogen/progestin combinations or norethindrone acetate alone) to limit their hypoestrogenic side effects. This may allow for prolonged off-label use if bone health continues to be monitored.[31] For episodic relief of pelvic pain, NSAIDs and muscle relaxants (ie, intermittent cyclobenzaprine, tizanidine, or methocarbamol) are reasonable options, especially if treating intermittent uterine cramping. Patients should be informed about key side effects (see **Table 2**).

SURGICAL INTERVENTIONS

Surgery for endometriosis requires an understanding of the heterogeneity of the disease, patient presentation, patient goals, impact on future fertility, and long-term outcomes. Ultimately the decision to pursue surgery is not simple and ideally should encompass a thoughtful and personalized approach embracing shared decision making with the patient.

Key principles related to the role of surgery are as outlined later in discussion:[32]

- There is a limited role for purely "diagnostic laparoscopy": With proper history, examination, and imaging, diagnostic laparoscopy in high-volume endometriosis centers has been replaced with thoughtful and well-planned "one-stop" excisional surgeries for management of identified or suspected endometriosis. In cases of a "surprise" finding of endometriosis at the surgery with less experienced surgeons, it may be best to document the extent of involvement (clinical photos) and refer to a gynecologist with experience in managing this disorder.
- Surgery for those with pelvic pain and endometriosis is indicated in the following circumstances:
  - Patients who decline, do not respond to, do not tolerate, or have contraindications to hormonal medical therapy
  - Presentation with acute surgical or new severe pain event
  - Deep endometriosis involving the urinary tract, GI tract or causing other significant organ obstruction or dysfunction
  - Concomitant management of coexisting disease: for example, managing colorectal cancer in a patient with severe disease obliterating the pelvic cul-de-sac
  - Females with pelvic pain planning immediate efforts at conception, as hormonal medical therapies prevent pregnancy
  - Large ovarian endometriomas with pain or with a suspicion of malignancy based on radiologic risk scores

How do we advise patients when it's appropriate to consider laparoscopic excisional therapy for lesions? If clinical findings and imaging suggest purely peritoneal disease, if symptoms are predominantly cyclical, we embrace a shared decision-making approach, favoring simple hormonal suppression for a 3-month trial. However, individual circumstances (such as pregnancy planning, as listed above) are also considered, and we may offer laparoscopic treatment directly; ultimately, the plan is based on the entire assessment and patient goals.

Although the literature is relatively scant, predictors of persistent postsurgical pain following conservative laparoscopic excisional therapy include the following: coexistence of multiple overlapping pain conditions; coexisting mood disorders; catastrophizing; history of significant emotional trauma; or younger operative age.

For conservative excision of endometriosis, we encourage the removal of all visible peritoneal disease, while sparing vital structures unless significantly contributing to symptoms. Laparoscopic excision using three to four 5 mm abdominal access incisions can be conducted using radiofrequency/ultrasonic/or laser-based energy sources. Excision allows for pathologic evaluation and provides symptom relief. An experienced endometriosis surgeon will mitigate the risk of damage to adjacent organs with the proper technique by gentle site-specific dissection whereby vital structures can be freed from implants. Of note, disease around the uterosacral ligaments and posterior cul-de-sac, in particular, seems to be crucial to address nonspecific pain. This is due in part to the convergence of many sensory afferents within the hypogastric nerves.[33] Studies suggest selective surgery for peritoneal-only disease can provide 60% of women with meaningful relief, and that the duration of relief may last between 2 to 5 years.[34] Complication rates from laparoscopic surgery are low: there is an approximate 2% to 5% overall risk of a surgical site infection, or bleeding requiring transfusion, and approximately a 1/1000 risk of iatrogenic bowel, bladder or ureteral injury or deep venous thrombosis.

When bowel ($\sim$5–15% cases) or urogenital involvement ($\sim$1%) is suspected by history and examination and supported by preoperative imaging, a general (colorectal) surgeon or urologist, respectively, may be consulted preoperatively as international consensus promotes a "team-based" approach for optimal outcomes. Bowel surgery may be required in cases of deep endometriosis, most often involving the rectum and sigmoid colon. Durable symptom relief rates have been reported by high volume centers of expertise (closer to 80%),[35,36] but these outcomes are not generalizable to most clinical settings, and prospective trials are necessary to quantify short and long term outcomes.[37] A basic overview of bowel-related surgical procedures is summarized in **Box 1**. When bowel surgery is required for endometriosis, major complication rates (in expert centers) range from 10% to 25%. Complications that may be encountered include anastomotic bleeding, leaks, stenosis, and rectovaginal fistulas.

Hysterectomy (with excision of endometriosis also if needed) is also considered in cases with strong uterine pain components, and when child-bearing is no longer being contemplated. Approximately 70+% of women will achieve long-term pain relief posthysterectomy, but this percentage approaches 90+% if bilateral oophorectomy is performed concurrently.[38] Based on computer models of mortality following oophorectomy, we encourage most women under the age of 50 to keep their ovaries to maintain hormonal protection of the heart and bones.[39] Patients who opt for ovarian removal despite the increased mortality risk often do so because of persistent severe obliterative disease involving the adnexa or failure of multiple prior surgeries for pain.

Role of Medical Therapy After Surgical Intervention

A recent meta-analysis of postoperative hormonal therapy concluded that such approaches prolong the surgery-free interval following conservative excisional therapy.[40] One convenient option for women not seeking immediate conception is the insertion of a levonorgestrel intrauterine device. Persistent postoperative use of oral contraceptives and progestins for ovarian endometriomas also significantly reduces the recurrence of these lesions.[31] Among those individuals not seeking immediate pregnancy, long-term medical management is seen as an important adjunct to surgical therapy.

Box 1
Bowel endometriosis surgical approaches

Shaving – conservative removal from wall, without full-thickness exposure, followed by suture repair, best for less than 1 cm lesion, higher recurrence risk

Disc Excision – removal of isolated 1 to 3 cm lesions followed by primary closure (stapler or suture)

Segmental resection – best for larger lesions, multifocal disease, proximal lesions

CONSIDERATIONS WHEN THERE IS A CLEAR CONTRIBUTION FROM COMORBID PELVIC CONDITIONS

Although a complete approach to managing overlapping chronic overlapping pain conditions of the pelvis (IBS, bladder pain syndrome, vulvar pain syndrome) when presenting alongside EAPP is not entirely possible within this review, a couple of key considerations should guide the practitioner. Almost one-half of EAPP cases will involve overlapping pain syndromes.[41] In these instances, pain complaints derived from disorders of viscera–brain interaction like irritable bowel or bladder pain syndromes can be treated with neuromodulators (see **Table 2**).[42] Other treatment modalities may also be integrated (**Fig. 6**, courtesy of SS). In patients with pain clearly emanating from bladder dysfunction, the American Urologic Association (AUA) has published standard treatment guidelines (**Box 2**).[43] Importantly, physical therapy has been used extensively, and is one of the few treatments shown to reduce related bladder pain and dysfunction.[44]

Less is known about the role of integrative approaches in treating EAPP. Vitamin E, calcium supplementation, melatonin, and acupuncture all have shown some benefits in prior studies.[45–47] Other strategies including antiinflammatory diets, exercise, mindfulness practice, and pain neurophysiology educational strategies may work by altering neuro-immuno-endocrine system dysregulation underlying EAPP. Further studies are warranted.

In summary, endometriosis is a common condition in reproductive-age women and a key contributor to dysmenorrhea and CPP states. Diagnosis requires laparoscopic tissue biopsy, but careful pelvic examination, and/or specialized imaging with either ultrasound or MRI, may identify patients who should receive empiric first-line therapy, which can include both hormonal suppressive approaches as well as standard approaches for chronic pain disorders. The presence of dyschezia, especially if worsened cyclically, should raise suspicion for bowel or rectovaginal septum involvement, which may be more likely to require some degree of surgical intervention for optimal relief. Although medical and complementary therapy can be quite effective, earlier surgical intervention may be critical for patients with deep infiltrating disease, or those failing to respond to an initial 3 to 6 months of suppressive therapy.

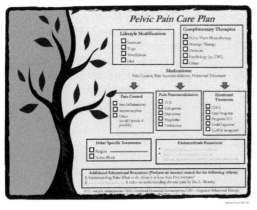

Fig. 6. Clinical guide for managing endometriosis. (*Courtesy of* Dr. Sukhbir S. Singh, MD, Ontario, Canada.)

Box 2
American Urologic Association (AUA) guideline for the treatment of bladder pain syndrome, highlights

First line - conservative management including behavioral changes, diet alteration, heat/cold packs, home pelvic floor exercises, stress reduction

Second line – pelvic floor physical therapy; oral medications (tricyclic antidepressants, antihistamines, pentosan polysulfate sodium [need to periodically screen for maculopathy]), or bladder instillations

Third line – bladder cystoscopic hydrodistention, fulguration of Hunner's lesions.

Fourth line – botulinum toxin, denervation of bladder, or sacral nerve stimulator

CLINICS CARE POINTS

- Concurrent dyschezia and dysmenorrhea should prompt consideration for endometriosis in reproductive-age women.
- Expert guided ultrasound for endometriosis can help detect deep disease; however, routine pelvic ultrasound is often only able to identify ovarian endometriomas and may miss other lesions.
- Pelvic MRI has high sensitivity and specificity for bowel endometriosis when reviewed by an individual with disease-specific expertise.
- Hormonal therapy, neuromodulators, and pelvic floor physical therapy are all viable nonsurgical treatment options for some endometriosis cases.
- Bowel surgery for endometriosis can be highly effective for the relief of pain and obstructive symptoms; however, outcomes and complications are highly dependent on surgical experience and techniques used.

DISCLOSURE

Dr S.S. Singh has served on Advisory Boards for AbbVie, Myovant, and Bayer; has received speaker fees from Abbvie and Bayer for CME events and has been an investigator in trials sponsored by Abbvie and Bayer through his local institution. Dr S.A. Missmer has served on Advisory Boards for AbbVie and Roche, as a Statistical Editor for Human Reproduction, and as the Field Chief Editor for Frontiers in Reproductive Health; she currently has research grant awards from the U.S. National Institutes of Health (NIH), the U.S. Department of Defense (DoD), the J. Willard and Alice S. Marriott Foundation, and AbbVie. Dr F.F. Tu has done consulting for AbbVie, Myovant, and UroShape. He has been on speaker's bureau for AbbVie and receives royalties from Wolters Kluwer. He has research grant awards from the U.S. National Institutes of Health (NIH), Eximis, and Dot Laboratories.

REFERENCES

1. Zondervan KT, Becker CM, Missmer SA. Endometriosis. N Engl J Med 2020; 382(13):1244–56.
2. Shafrir AL, Farland LV, Shah DK, et al. Risk for and consequences of endometriosis: A critical epidemiologic review. Best Pract Res Clin Obstet Gynaecol 2018; 51:1–15.

3. Vercellini P, Viganò P, Somigliana E, et al. Endometriosis: pathogenesis and treatment. Nat Rev Endocrinol 2014;10(5):261–75.

4. Saha R, Pettersson HJ, Svedberg P, et al. Heritability of endometriosis. Fertil Steril 2015;104(4):947–52.

5. Sapkota Y, Steinthorsdottir V, Morris AP, et al. Meta-analysis identifies five novel loci associated with endometriosis highlighting key genes involved in hormone metabolism. Nat Commun 2017;8:15539.

6. Agarwal SK, Chapron C, Giudice LC, et al. Clinical diagnosis of endometriosis: a call to action. Am J Obstet Gynecol 2019;220(4):354.e1-12.

7. Tu FF, Du H, Goldstein GP, et al. The influence of prior oral contraceptive use on risk of endometriosis is conditional on parity. Fertil Steril 2014;101(6):1697–704.

8. Schliep KC, Mumford SL, Peterson CM, et al. Pain typology and incident endometriosis. Hum Reprod 2015;30(10):2427–38.

9. Vilasagar S, Bougie O, Singh SS. A Practical Guide to the Clinical Evaluation of Endometriosis-Associated Pelvic Pain. J Minim Invasive Gynecol 2020;27(2): 270–9.

10. Kjerulff KH, Erickson BA, Langenberg PW. Chronic gynecological conditions reported by US women: findings from the National Health Interview Survey, 1984 to 1992. Am J Public Health 1996;86(2):195–9.

11. Nnoaham KE, Hummelshoj L, Webster P, et al. Impact of endometriosis on quality of life and work productivity: a multicenter study across ten countries. Fertil Steril 2011;96(2):366–73.e8.

12. DiVasta AD, Vitonis AF, Laufer MR, et al. Spectrum of symptoms in women diagnosed with endometriosis during adolescence vs adulthood. Am J Obstet Gynecol 2018;218(3):324.e1-11.

13. Ballard KD, Seaman HE, de Vries CS, et al. Can symptomatology help in the diagnosis of endometriosis? Findings from a national case-control study–Part 1. BJOG 2008;115(11):1382–91.

14. Seaman HE, Ballard KD, Wright JT, et al. Endometriosis and its coexistence with irritable bowel syndrome and pelvic inflammatory disease: findings from a national case-control study–Part 2. BJOG 2008;115(11):1392–6.

15. Wu C-Y, Chang W-P, Chang Y-H, et al. The risk of irritable bowel syndrome in patients with endometriosis during a 5-year follow-up: a nationwide population-based cohort study. Int J Colorectal Dis 2015;30(7):907–12.

16. Bettendorf B, Shay S, Tu F. Dysmenorrhea: contemporary perspectives. Obstet Gynecol Surv 2008;63(9):597–603.

17. Zondervan KT, Yudkin PL, Vessey MP, et al. The community prevalence of chronic pelvic pain in women and associated illness behaviour. Br J Gen Pract 2001; 51(468):541–7.

18. Brawn J, Morotti M, Zondervan KT, et al. Central changes associated with chronic pelvic pain and endometriosis. Hum Reprod Update 2014;20(5):737–47.

19. Souza CA, Oliveira LM, Scheffel C, et al. Quality of life associated to chronic pelvic pain is independent of endometriosis diagnosis–a cross-sectional survey. Health Qual Life Outcomes 2011;9:41.

20. He W, Liu X, Zhang Y, et al. Generalized hyperalgesia in women with endometriosis and its resolution following a successful surgery. Reprod Sci 2010;17(12): 1099–111.

21. Pezzone MA, Liang R, Fraser MO. A model of neural cross-talk and irritation in the pelvis: implications for the overlap of chronic pelvic pain disorders. Gastroenterology 2005;128(7):1953–64.

22. Knabben L, Imboden S, Fellmann B, et al. Urinary tract endometriosis in patients with deep infiltrating endometriosis: prevalence, symptoms, management, and proposal for a new clinical classification. Fertil Steril 2015;103(1):147–52.

23. Lemos N, D'Amico N, Marques R, et al. Recognition and treatment of endometriosis involving the sacral nerve roots. Int Urogynecol J 2016;27(1):147–50.

24. Dos Bispo APS, Ploger C, Loureiro AF, et al. Assessment of pelvic floor muscles in women with deep endometriosis. Arch Gynecol Obstet 2016;294(3):519–23.

25. Guerriero S, Condous G, van den Bosch T, et al. Systematic approach to sonographic evaluation of the pelvis in women with suspected endometriosis, including terms, definitions and measurements: a consensus opinion from the International Deep Endometriosis Analysis (IDEA) group. Ultrasound Obstet Gynecol 2016;48(3):318–32.

26. Bazot M, Darai E, Hourani R, et al. Deep pelvic endometriosis: MR imaging for diagnosis and prediction of extension of disease. Radiology 2004;232(2):379–89.

27. Guerriero S, Saba L, Pascual MA, et al. Transvaginal ultrasound vs magnetic resonance imaging for diagnosing deep infiltrating endometriosis: systematic review and meta-analysis. Ultrasound Obstet Gynecol 2018;51(5):586–95.

28. Guzick DS, Huang LS, Broadman BA, et al. Randomized trial of leuprolide versus continuous oral contraceptives in the treatment of endometriosis-associated pelvic pain. Fertil Steril 2011;95(5):1568–73.

29. Ling FW. Randomized controlled trial of depot leuprolide in patients with chronic pelvic pain and clinically suspected endometriosis. Pelvic Pain Study Group. Obstet Gynecol 1999;93(1):51–8.

30. Taylor HS, Giudice LC, Lessey BA, et al. Treatment of Endometriosis-Associated Pain with Elagolix, an Oral GnRH Antagonist. N Engl J Med 2017;377(1):28–40.

31. Hornstein MD, Surrey ES, Weisberg GW, et al. Leuprolide acetate depot and hormonal add-back in endometriosis: a 12-month study. Lupron Add-Back Study Group. Obstet Gynecol 1998;91(1):16–24.

32. Singh SS, Suen MWH. Surgery for endometriosis: beyond medical therapies. Fertil Steril 2017;107(3):549–54.

33. Kelm Junior AR, Lancellotti CLP, Donadio N, et al. Nerve fibers in uterosacral ligaments of women with deep infiltrating endometriosis. J Reprod Immunol 2008; 79(1):93–9.

34. Abbott JA, Hawe J, Clayton RD, et al. The effects and effectiveness of laparoscopic excision of endometriosis: a prospective study with 2-5 year follow-up. Hum Reprod 2003;18(9):1922–7.

35. Donnez J, Squifflet J. Complications, pregnancy and recurrence in a prospective series of 500 patients operated on by the shaving technique for deep rectovaginal endometriotic nodules. Hum Reprod 2010;25(8):1949–58.

36. Roman H, Tuech J-J, Huet E, et al. Excision versus colorectal resection in deep endometriosis infiltrating the rectum: 5-year follow-up of patients enrolled in a randomized controlled trial. Hum Reprod 2019;34(12):2362–71.

37. Jago CA, Nguyen DB, Flaxman TE, et al. Bowel surgery for endometriosis: A practical look at short- and long-term complications. Best Pract Res Clin Obstet Gynaecol 2021;71:144–60.

38. Shakiba K, Bena JF, McGill KM, et al. Surgical treatment of endometriosis: a 7-year follow-up on the requirement for further surgery. Obstet Gynecol 2008; 111(6):1285–92.

39. Evans EC, Matteson KA, Orejuela FJ, et al. Salpingo-oophorectomy at the Time of Benign Hysterectomy: A Systematic Review. Obstet Gynecol 2016;128(3): 476–85.

40. Zakhari A, Delpero E, McKeown S, et al. Endometriosis recurrence following post-operative hormonal suppression: a systematic review and meta-analysis. Hum Reprod Update 2021;27(1):96–107.
41. Stratton P, Khachikyan I, Sinaii N, et al. Association of chronic pelvic pain and endometriosis with signs of sensitization and myofascial pain. Obstet Gynecol 2015;125(3):719–28.
42. Horne AW, Vincent K, Hewitt CA, et al. Gabapentin for chronic pelvic pain in women (GaPP2): a multicentre, randomised, double-blind, placebo-controlled trial. Lancet 2020;396(10255):909–17.
43. Hanno PM, Burks DA, Clemens JQ, et al. AUA guideline for the diagnosis and treatment of interstitial cystitis/bladder pain syndrome. J Urol 2011;185(6): 2162–70.
44. Fitzgerald MP, Payne CK, Lukacz ES, et al. Randomized multicenter clinical trial of myofascial physical therapy in women with interstitial cystitis/painful bladder syndrome and pelvic floor tenderness. J Urol 2012;187(6):2113–8.
45. Darling AM, Chavarro JE, Malspeis S, et al. A prospective cohort study of Vitamins B, C, E, and multivitamin intake and endometriosis. J Endometr 2013;5(1): 17–26.
46. Schwertner A, Conceição Dos Santos CC, Costa GD, et al. Efficacy of melatonin in the treatment of endometriosis: a phase II, randomized, double-blind, placebo-controlled trial. Pain 2013;154(6):874–81.
47. Xu Y, Zhao W, Li T, et al. Effects of acupuncture for the treatment of endometriosis-related pain: A systematic review and meta-analysis. PLoS One 2017;12(10):e0186616.

Printed and bound by CPI Group (UK) Ltd, Croydon, CR0 4YY

03/10/2024

01040408-0003